Discrete Distributions

WILEY SERIES IN PROBABILITY AND STATISTICS

Established by WALTER A. SHEWHART and SAMUEL S. WILKS

A complete list of the titles in this series appears at the end of this volume.

Discrete Distributions

Applications in the Health Sciences

Daniel Zelterman

*Division of Biostatistics,
Epidemiology and Public Health,
Yale University, USA*

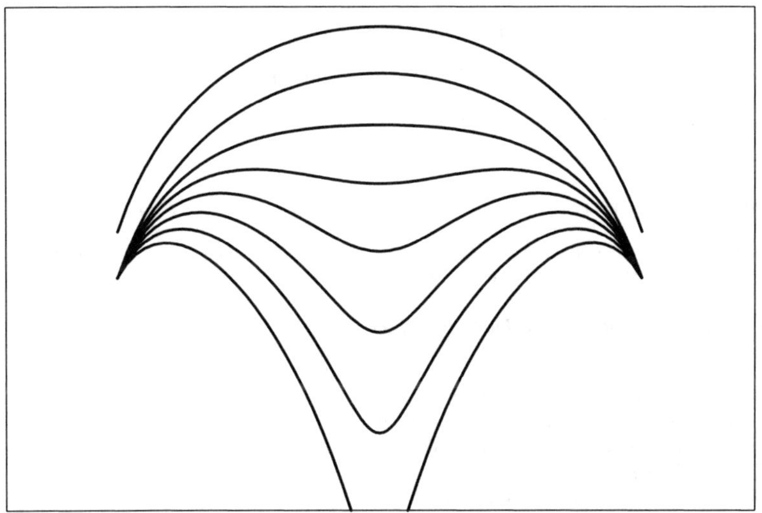

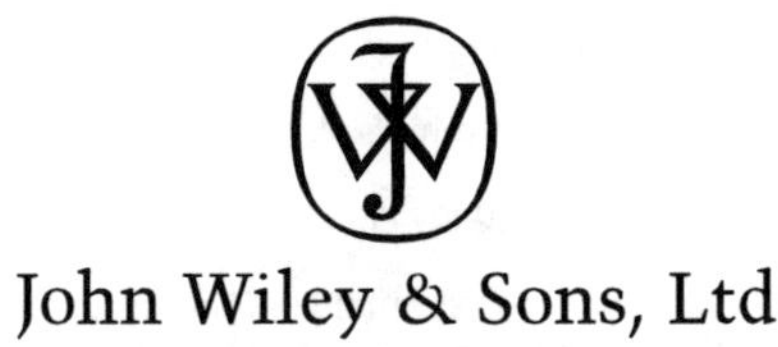

John Wiley & Sons, Ltd

Telephone (+44) 1243 779777

Email (for orders and customer service enquiries): cs-books@wiley.co.uk
Visit our Home Page on www.wileyeurope.com or www.wiley.com

Reprinted April 2005

Other Wiley Editorial Offices

John Wiley & Sons Inc., 111 River Street, Hoboken, NJ 07030, USA

Jossey-Bass, 989 Market Street, San Francisco, CA 94103-1741, USA

Wiley-VCH Verlag GmbH, Boschstr. 12, D-69469 Weinheim, Germany

John Wiley & Sons Australia Ltd, 33 Park Road, Milton, Queensland 4064, Australia

John Wiley & Sons (Asia) Pte Ltd, 2 Clementi Loop #02-01, Jin Xing Distripark, Singapore 129809

John Wiley & Sons Canada Ltd, 22 Worcester Road, Etobicoke, Ontario, Canada M9W 1L1

Wiley also publishes its books in a variety of electronic formats. Some content that appears in print may not be available in electronic books.

Library of Congress Cataloging-in-Publication Data

Zelterman, Daniel.
Discrete distributions : applications in the health sciences / Daniel Zelterman.
p. cm.—(Wiley series in probability and statistics)
Includes bibliographical references and index.
ISBN 0-470-86888-0 (alk. paper)
1. Medical sciences—Mathematics. 2. Medical sciences—Mathematical models. 3. Medicine—Mathematics. 4. Distribution (Probability theory) 5. Probabilities. I. Title. II. Series.

RA853.M3Z456 2004
610′.1′5118—dc22 2004041199

British Library Cataloguing in Publication Data

A catalogue record for this book is available from the British Library

ISBN 10: 0-470-86888-0 ISBN 13: 978-0-470-86888-1

Typeset in 10/12pt Times by Laserwords Private Limited, Chennai, India
Printed and bound in Great Britain by TJ International, Padstow, Cornwall
This book is printed on acid-free paper responsibly manufactured from sustainable forestry in which at least two trees are planted for each one used for paper production.

To the memory of my father, M.Z.

D.Z.

Contents

Preface

This book describes a number of new discrete distributions that arise in the statistical examination of real examples. These examples are drawn from my interactions with researchers studying cancer, epidemiology, demography, and other health-related disciplines. In every case, an understanding of the issues surrounding the data provides the chief motivation for the subsequent development of the mathematical models. Without the data and the helpful discussions with others in these different disciplines, this book would not have been possible.

The work here represents several years' experience of looking at several examples of real data. In each of these examples, there was an important question to be answered through the use of statistical modeling. The principal examples that gave rise to these models are as follows:

- A design of a medical screening protocol for a genetic marker (Chapters 2 and 3)
- A measure of the association in lifespans of twins (Chapters 4 and 5)
- Multiple cases of a disease occurring in the same family or animal litter (Chapters 6 through 9).

The distributions that came about in the examination of these three examples have analogies to sampling two different colored balls from an urn. Sampling balls from an urn is a useful teaching tool but, unfortunately, tends to lack practical importance. Similarly, the urn models will be briefly mentioned when they are applicable but will not be emphasized. The distributions developed here describe sampling procedures from the urn

- until c of each color are observed (Chapter 3),
- two balls at a time until the urn is emptied (Chapter 4),
- a handful of balls at a time until the urn is emptied (Chapter 6),

respectively, corresponding to the three motivating situations. Table 1 is an outline of the distributions discussed in this book and their specific references to the text that follows.

The original source material for all of these examples and distributions has been published by myself and with coauthors, in some cases. The published material has appeared in various journals and book chapters. My first aim is to unify these results in one place.

A second aim is to provide additional detail for the various models. One drawback to journal publication is the terse nature required of the authors of such articles. I anticipate a more leisurely style that includes more discussion of the motivation of the methods, rather than the headlong rush to obtain mathematical results.

Software will allow the reader to repeat the data analyses presented here and extend these to other data sets as well. S-Plus or R© provide a higher-level platform, allowing the user to omit many of the tedious bookkeeping chores that FORTRAN or C++ ask of the programmer. There are several settings here where extensive iterations are needed and these programs are written in FORTRAN. These situations appear in Chapters 5 and 6, where exact significance levels are obtained only after completely enumerating huge numbers of all possible outcomes. There are also settings in Chapters 4 and 8 where the data takes a tabular form and the regression diagnostics in SAS make that language the ideal tool for the data analysis. I expect that the software that is included in this text will be posted on a web site.

The audience I am aiming at are those doing an advanced graduate level course and those doing research in the field. There are a number of useful techniques identified here that reappear in several places. These methods will prove useful to others doing work in the study of discrete distributions.

The work of Johnson, Kotz, and Kemp (*Univariate Discrete Distributions*, 1992, Wiley) is a popular book, now in its second edition. I would expect that individuals who bought that book would be interested in this book as well. The Johnson text is an outstanding reference encyclopedia of methods and references. The companion volume covering multivariate distributions is that by Johnson, Kotz, and Balakrishnan (1997).

The recent book by Balakrishnan and Koutras (2002) also describes a large number of discrete distributions. Two out-of-print books, *Urn Models* (1977) by Johnson and Kotz and *Random Allocations*, the translation of *Случайные размещения* by Kolchin, Sevast'yanov and Chistyakov (1978), are specific to the mathematical development of urn models and do not put any special emphasis on applications. In contrast, I want to cover less material, include new material, and motivate these ideas by several intriguing numerical examples.

Brief overview of contents

A brief overview of the models described in this volume is given in Table 1. These distributions can be divided into the two categories as to sampling from either an infinite or from a finite sized population. Finite-sized populations are assumed to be sampled without replacement. In a finite population, the probability of future events

Table 1 Comparison of related sampling distributions

Sampling scheme	Infinite population or with replacement	Finite population without replacement
Predetermined number of items	Binomial distribution (1.6)	Hypergeometric distribution (1.17)
Until c successes	Negative binomial distribution (1.13)	Negative hypergeometric distribution (1.21)
Until either c successes or c failures	Riff shuffle or the minimum negative binomial distribution (2.1)	Minimum negative hypergeometric distribution (3.5)
Until at least c successes and c failures	Maximum negative binomial distribution (2.4)	Maximum negative hypergeometric distribution (3.6), (3.7)
Two items at a time		The twins distribution (4.2)
A handful of items at a time		The family frequency distribution (6.3)

depends on the composition of individuals already sampled. In infinite populations, the distribution of future events is independent of those of the past.

The binomial distribution describes the number of successes when a predetermined number of items are independently sampled from an infinitely large Bernoulli population. The hypergeometric distribution is the corresponding model when the population has a finite size. The negative binomial and negative hypergeometric distributions describe the number of trials necessary in order to obtain a specified number of 'successes.'

The minimum and maximum distributions of Table 1 refer to the number of trials necessary in order to observe at least a specified number of successes and/or failures. The maximum negative binomial is the distribution of the number of trials needed in order to obtain at least c successes and c failures. One example of this is the problem facing Noah when stocking the ark. How many wild animals need to be captured in order to obtain one (or seven) of both sexes? The original motivation for the development of these distributions arose in connection with a genetic screening clinical trial among colon-cancer patients. The maximum negative hypergeometric distribution is the finite population analogy to this model. These distributions are described in Chapters 2 and 3.

The twins distribution describes the behavior of samples from a finite population (or 'urn') taken two at a time. This distribution is described in Chapter 4. Generalizations of this distribution that examine dependent observations are given

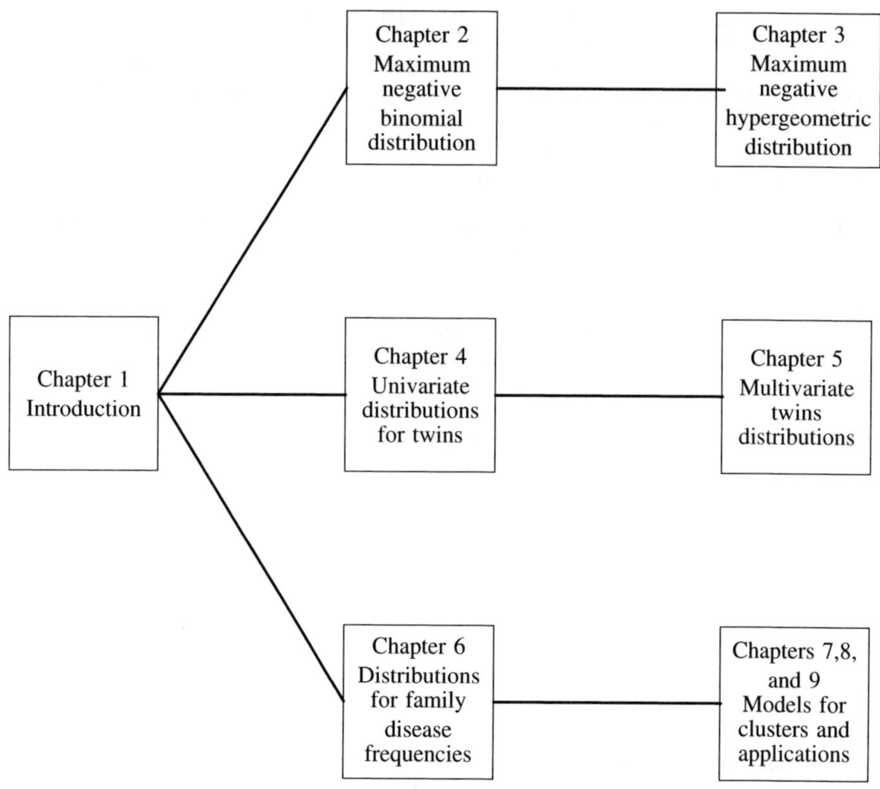

Figure 1 Logical ordering of subject matter in chapters

in Chapter 5. The motivating question behind this distribution was the search for a gene for human longevity. What evidence do we have for it, and if it exists, what possible benefit in lifespan does it confer upon those who are born with it? A dataset summarizing the joint lifespans of twin pairs is examined to provide some answers to these questions.

Twins represent families all of size two, and the corresponding generalizations to families of arbitrary sizes are given in Chapter 6. These family frequency distributions correspond to sampling a finite population taken "a handful" at a time. These observed samples are of different sizes and correspond to the number of children in various families. Chapter 6 provides the distribution when there is no dependence among various family members. The motivating examples in this chapter include clusters of childhood cancers, incidence of infections in family units, among others.

Chapters 7 and 8 list a variety of methods that measure the degree of dependence among family members. These methods are applied to teratology experiments in Chapter 9. These experiments are based on litters of small laboratory animals exposed to toxic substances.

The logical ordering of the subject matter in the chapters is described in Fig.1. The introductory material in Chapter 1 can be followed by Chapters 2 and 3 on the maximum negative distributions. Similarly, Chapters 4 and 5 describe distributions of twins but do not depend on the material in Chapters 2 and 3. Finally, Chapter 6 introduces data and methods for family-level data. Models for disease clustering appear in Chapters 7 and 8. These are applied to additional examples in Chapter 9. Finally, there is a section of Complements that provides a list of open-ended problems that the reader might wish to pursue. The author would be grateful to hear about any published results that relate to items on this list.

And special thanks to . . .

I want to thank Chang Yu, a colleague and friend, for many useful conversations, hikes in the woods and for reminding me to keep life on the lighter side, and Elizabeth Johnston who continues to advocate my work behind the scenes. I also wish to thank Barbara Burtness, Michael Boehnke, Lee Schacter, James Vaupel, Tom Louis, Lance Waller, Dean Follmann, Priya Wickramarantne, Ellen Matloff, Segun George, N. Balakrishnan, Ramesh Gupta, Heping Zhang, Joel Dubin, Hani Doss, and Emile Salloum for helpful discussions. I am grateful to Yan Li for a careful reading of an early version of the manuscript and to John Zhang who taught me many things. Anonymous reviewers provided innumerable useful comments along the way. And most of all, I want to thank my wife Linda for her constant support and encouragement.

Daniel Zelterman
Hamden, CT
February 19, 2004

Acknowledgements

The following material has been reprinted with permission.

The translation of Genesis 7:2–3 appearing in *Etz Hayim* is used with permission from the Rabbinical Assembly, New York, N.Y.

Material in Chapter 2 is reprinted from Z. Zhang, B.A. Burtness, and D. Zelterman 2000, 'The maximum negative binomial distribution', *Journal of Statistical Planning and Inference*, **87**, 1–19, with permission from Elsevier.

Material in Chapter 7 is reprinted from *Statistics & Probability Letters*, **57**, pages 363–73, 2002, C. Yu and D. Zelterman, 'Sums of dependent Bernoulli random variables and disease clustering', with permission from Elsevier.

Material in Table 1.4 is reprinted from Innes *et al.* (1969). Oxford University Press, copyright holder of *Journal of the National Cancer Institute* indicated that this material is in the public domain.

Financial, salary, and other support is acknowledged from the following institutions and grants:

American Cancer Society TURSGO1-174-01

Susan G. Komen Foundation: BCTR 0100202

National Institutes of Health:

NIMH: P30 MH62294-01A1 Center for Interdisciplinary Research on AIDS

NICHD: P50 HD25802-11 The Center for the Study of Learning and Attention Disorders

NCI: P30 CA16359-28 Yale Cancer Center Core Grant; R21 CA093002; R21 CA98144

NHLBI: R01 HL047193

National Science Foundation: DMS 0241160

About the Author

Daniel Zelterman, PhD, is Professor of Epidemiology and Public Health, Division of Biostatistics, at Yale University. His application areas include work in AIDS and cancer. Before moving to Yale in 1995, he was on the faculty of the University of Minnesota and of the State University of New York at Albany. He is an elected Fellow of the American Statistical Association and is an Associate Editor of *Biometrics* and several other statistical journals. In his spare time, he plays the bassoon in several amateur chamber and orchestral groups in the New Haven area.

Other books by the author:
Models for Discrete Data, Oxford University Press, Oxford, 1999.
Advanced Log-Linear Models Using SAS, SAS Publishing, Cary, N.C., 2002.

About the Author

1

Introduction

These are the fundamental properties, definitions, and general building blocks for everything that follows. Section 1.1 describes discrete distributions in general. The following sections of this chapter provide specific examples of useful and popular models. The reader is referred to (Johnson, Kotz, and Kemp (1992)) as a more comprehensive and definitive resource to this material for univariate distributions. Johnson, Kotz, and Balakrishnan (1997) is the corresponding reference for multivariate discrete distributions.

1.1 Discrete Distributions in General

We will describe properties of a discrete valued random variable Y whose support is taken to be $0, 1, \ldots$ or a finite subset of these nonnegative integers. In general, random variables are denoted by capital letters and their observed values by lower case letters.

The simplest example of a random variable is the *Bernoulli random variable* for which

$$\Pr[\,Y = 1\,] = p \quad \text{and} \quad \Pr[\,Y = 0\,] = 1 - p \tag{1.1}$$

for probability parameter p satisfying $0 \leq p \leq 1$. The values of $Y = 1$ and $Y = 0$ are often referred to as successes and failures, respectively.

More generally, for $y = 0, 1, \ldots$ let

$$\Pr[\,Y = y\,] = p_y$$

for $p_y \geq 0$ with $\sum p_y = 1$.

The function

$$f(y) = p_y$$

Discrete Distributions Daniel Zelterman
 ISBN: 0-470-86888-0 (PPC)

for $y = 0, 1, \ldots$ and zero elsewhere is called the *probability mass function* or the *mass function*.

The function

$$F(y) = \sum_{j=0}^{y} p_j = \Pr[\, Y \le y\,]$$

is called the *cumulative distribution function* or the *distribution function*.

The value $\tilde{y}$ for which $p_{\tilde{y}}$ is a maximum is called the *mode* of the distribution. The mode may not be unique. There may be local modes as well. These ideas are illustrated in the distribution plotted in Fig. 2.3 and discussed in Section 2.2.3.

The *expected value of a function* $g(Y)$ of the random variable Y is

$$\mathrm{E}[\, g(Y)\,] = \sum_y g(y) \Pr[\, Y = y\,] = \sum_y g(y) f(y)$$

provided this sum converges.

Expectation is a linear operation so

$$\mathrm{E}[\, g(Y) + h(Y)\,] = \mathrm{E}[\, g(Y)\,] + \mathrm{E}[\, h(Y)\,].$$

The specific example in which $g(Y)$ is a power of Y is called a *moment*. The expectation

$$\mathrm{E}[\, Y^j\,] = \sum_y y^j \Pr[\, Y = y\,]$$

for $j = 1, 2 \ldots$ is called the *jth moment* of Y or sometimes the *jth moment about zero*.

The first moment $\mathrm{E}[Y]$ is called the *mean* or the *expected value*. Let us denote the mean of Y by μ. Moments of Y about its mean are called *central moments* so that

$$\mathrm{E}[\, (Y - \mu)^j\,]$$

is called the *jth central moment*.

The first central moment is zero and the second central moment is called the *variance* of Y. This is denoted by

$$\mathrm{Var}[\, Y\,] = \mathrm{E}[\, (Y - \mu)^2\,]$$

Expanding the square here shows

$$\mathrm{Var}[\, Y\,] = \mathrm{E}[\, Y^2\,] - \mu^2.$$

The square root of the variance is the *standard deviation*.

Higher central moments are usually standardized by the standard deviation. The third central standardized moment

$$\mathrm{E}[\, (Y - \mu)^3\,]/\{\mathrm{Var}[\, Y\,]\}^{3/2}$$

is called the *skewness*.

The *moment generating function* of Y

$$M_Y(t) = \mathrm{E}[\,\mathrm{e}^{tY}\,] = \sum_y \mathrm{e}^{ty}\,\Pr[\,Y = y\,]$$

is the expected value of e^{tY} and may only be defined for values of t in a neighborhood of zero.

The moment generating function is so called because successive derivatives at zero are equal to the moments for many distributions. Specifically, for all of the distributions we will discuss

$$(\mathrm{d}/\mathrm{d}t)^j M_Y(t)\Big|_{t=0} = \mathrm{E}[\,Y^j\,]$$

for every $j = 1, 2, \ldots$. In all generality, not all the moments exist for all the distributions and the moment generating function may fail to generate the moments even when these exist.

The *characteristic function* of Y

$$\phi_Y(t) = \mathrm{E}[\,\mathrm{e}^{itY}\,] = \sum_y \mathrm{e}^{ity}\,\Pr[\,Y = y\,]$$

is the expected value of e^{itY}, where $i^2 = -1$. Unlike the moment generating function, the characteristic function always exists.

The *probability generating function* is

$$G(t) = \mathrm{E}[\,t^Y\,] = \sum_y t^y\,\Pr[\,Y = y\,]. \tag{1.2}$$

The probability generating function has the property that successive derivatives at $t = 0$ are equal to the individual probabilities of Y in the sense that

$$(\mathrm{d}/\mathrm{d}t)^j G(t)\Big|_{t=0} = j!\,\Pr[\,Y = y\,]$$

for $j = 0, 1, \ldots$.

The relation between the probability generating function and the characteristic function is

$$\phi_Y(t) = G_Y(\mathrm{e}^{it}).$$

For many discrete distributions, the factorial moments are available in a convenient functional form. For $k = 1, 2, \ldots,$ define the *factorial polynomial*

$$z^{(k)} = z(z-1)\cdots(z-k+1) \tag{1.3}$$

and $z^{(0)} = 1$.

The *factorial moments* of Y are then

$$\mathrm{E}[\,Y^{(k)}\,] = \mathrm{E}[\,Y(Y-1)\cdots(Y-k+1)\,].$$

These are also referred to as the *descending factorial moments* by some authors.

Similarly, we have

$$\mathrm{E}[\,Y\,] = \mathrm{E}[\,Y^{(1)}\,]$$

and

$$\mathrm{Var}[\,Y\,] = \mathrm{E}[\,Y^{(2)}\,] + \mathrm{E}[\,Y\,] - \{\mathrm{E}[\,Y\,]\}^2.$$

The *factorial moment generating function* is

$$G(t+1) = \mathrm{E}[\,(t+1)^Y\,],$$

where G is the probability generating function given in (1.2).

The factorial moment generating function has the property

$$(\mathrm{d}/\mathrm{d}t)^j\, G(1+t)\Big|_{t=0} = \mathrm{E}[\,Y^{(j)}\,]$$

for many distributions.

There are, of course, many other useful generating functions available with important relationships between them. Those listed here are limited to those specifically referred to in the volume. The reader is referred to (Johnson, Kotz, and Kemp (1992, Section 1.B)) for a more thorough treatment of the subject.

1.2 Multivariate Discrete Distributions

The joint mass function of the random variables $\{X_1, \ldots, X_k\}$ is the function

$$f(x_1, \ldots, x_k) = \Pr[\,X_1 = x_1, \ldots, X_k = x_k\,].$$

The mass function is never negative over the range of $\{X_1, \ldots, X_k\}$ and sums to one:

$$\sum_{x_1} \cdots \sum_{x_k} f(x_1, \ldots, x_k) = 1.$$

Marginal distributions are obtained by summing over individual random variables in their joint mass function. So for $1 \le j < k$,

$$\begin{aligned} f(x_1, \ldots, x_j) &= \Pr[\,X_1 = x_1, \ldots, X_j = x_j\,] \\ &= \sum_{x_{j+1}} \cdots \sum_{x_k} f(x_1, \ldots, x_k). \end{aligned}$$

The summations are over the range of the random variables being summed.

Conditional probability mass functions are obtained using the laws of probability so that for $1 \le j < k$ we write

$$\begin{aligned} &f(x_1, \ldots, x_j \mid x_{j+1}, \ldots, x_k) \\ &\quad = \Pr[\,X_1 = x_1, \ldots, X_j = x_j \mid X_{j+1} = x_{j+1}, \ldots, X_k = x_k\,] \\ &\quad = \Pr[\,X_1 = x_1, \ldots, X_k = x_k\,] / \Pr[\,X_{j+1} = x_{j+1}, \ldots, X_k = x_k\,] \\ &\quad = f(x_1, \ldots, x_k)/f(x_{j+1}, \ldots, x_k). \end{aligned}$$

Multivariate moments are taken with respect to the joint mass function. Specifically, the expectation of the function $g(X_1, \ldots, X_k)$ is

$$\mathrm{E}[\, g(X_1, \ldots, X_k)\,] = \sum_{x_1} \cdots \sum_{x_k} g(x_1, \ldots, x_k)\, f(x_1, \ldots, x_k),$$

provided this summation converges.

Multivariate moments can also be defined. The *covariance* between random variables X_1 and X_2 is

$$\begin{aligned}\mathrm{Cov}[\, X_1, X_2\,] &= \mathrm{E}[\,(X_1 - \mathrm{E}[X_1])\,(X_2 - \mathrm{E}[X_2])\,] \\ &= \mathrm{E}[\, X_1 X_2\,] - \mathrm{E}[\, X_1\,]\mathrm{E}[\, X_2\,]\end{aligned}$$

and their *correlation* is

$$\mathrm{Corr}[\, X_1, X_2\,] = \mathrm{Cov}[\, X_1, X_2\,]/\{\mathrm{Var}[\, X_1\,]\,\mathrm{Var}[\, X_2\,]\}^{1/2}.$$

The correlation is always between -1 and 1. The correlation is a measure of the strength of the linear relationship between two random variables. If the random variables are independent then their correlation is zero, but zero correlation does not imply independence. There are also higher-order analogies to the correlation coefficient that extend to more than two random variables at a time. These are introduced and used in Section 7.3.

Another example of multivariate moments are the *joint factorial moments*. Specifically, for nonnegative integers $r_1, \ldots, r_k$ the joint factorial moments of $X_1, \ldots, X_k$ are

$$\mathrm{E}[\, X_1^{(r_1)} \cdots X_k^{(r_k)}\,] = \sum_{x_1} \cdots \sum_{x_k} \left[\prod_i x_i^{(r_i)} \right] f(x_1, \ldots, x_k).$$

Conditional moments are taken with respect to the conditional distribution. In particular, we have the *iterated expectation*

$$\mathrm{E}[\, X_1\,] = \mathrm{E}\{\mathrm{E}[\, X_1 \mid X_2\,]\}, \tag{1.4}$$

where the outer expectation is taken with respect to X_2.

Similarly,

$$\mathrm{Var}[\, X_1\,] = \mathrm{Var}\,\{\mathrm{E}[\, X_1 \mid X_2\,]\} + \mathrm{E}\{\,\mathrm{Var}[\, X_1 \mid X_2\,]\}. \tag{1.5}$$

The sections that follow illustrate these definitions with reference to specific discrete distributions.

1.3 Binomial Distribution

The binomial distribution is the sum of n independent, identically distributed Bernoulli p random variables. The valid parameter values are $0 \le p \le 1$ and

$n = 1, 2, \ldots$. The parameter n is often referred to as the *index* or the *sample size* of the binomial distribution.

The probability that the sum of n independent and identically distributed Bernoulli random variables is equal to y is

$$\Pr[\,Y = y\,] = \binom{n}{y} p^y (1-p)^{n-y}, \tag{1.6}$$

defined for $y = 0, 1, \ldots, n$ and zero otherwise. Bernoulli random variables are defined in (1.1).

We can reverse the roles of success and failure. Specifically if Y behaves as binomial with parameters n and p, then $n - Y$ behaves as binomial with parameters n and $1 - p$.

Figure 1.1 illustrates the binomial distribution for $n = 10$ and parameter $p = 0.2$, 0.5, and 0.8. For $p = 0.5$, the binomial distribution is symmetric. The distribution has a longer left or right tail, depending on whether $p > 0.5$ or $p < 0.5$, respectively.

The proof that the probabilities in (1.6) sum to one is provided by the expansion of the binomial polynomial

$$[p + (1-p)]^n \; = \; 1.$$

The terms in this expansion are the individual binomial probabilities in (1.6). This relationship has led to the name of the binomial distribution.

The mean of Y in the binomial distribution (1.6) is $\mathrm{E}[Y] = np$ and the variance is $\mathrm{Var}[Y] = np(1-p)$. The variance is smaller than the mean.

The third central moment

$$\mathrm{E}[\,(Y - np)^3\,] = np(1-p)(1-2p)$$

is positive for $0 < p < 1/2$, negative for $1/2 < p < 1$, and zero when $p = 1/2$. This symmetry and asymmetry can be seen in Fig. 1.1.

The moment generating function of the binomial distribution is

$$M(t) = \mathrm{E}[\,\mathrm{e}^{tY}\,] = (1 - p + p\mathrm{e}^t)^n.$$

The factorial moment generating function is

$$G(t) = \mathrm{E}[\,(1+t)^Y\,] \; = (1 + pt)^n.$$

For $r = 1, 2, \ldots$ the factorial moments of the binomial distribution are

$$\mathrm{E}[\,Y^{(r)}\,] = n^{(r)} p^r.$$

The sum of two independent binomial random variables with respective parameters $(n_1,\ p_1)$ and $(n_2,\ p_2)$ behaves as binomial $(n_1 + n_2,\ p_1)$ when $p_1 = p_2$. If the parameters p_1 and p_2 are not equal, then the sum of the two independent binomial random variables does not behave as binomial.

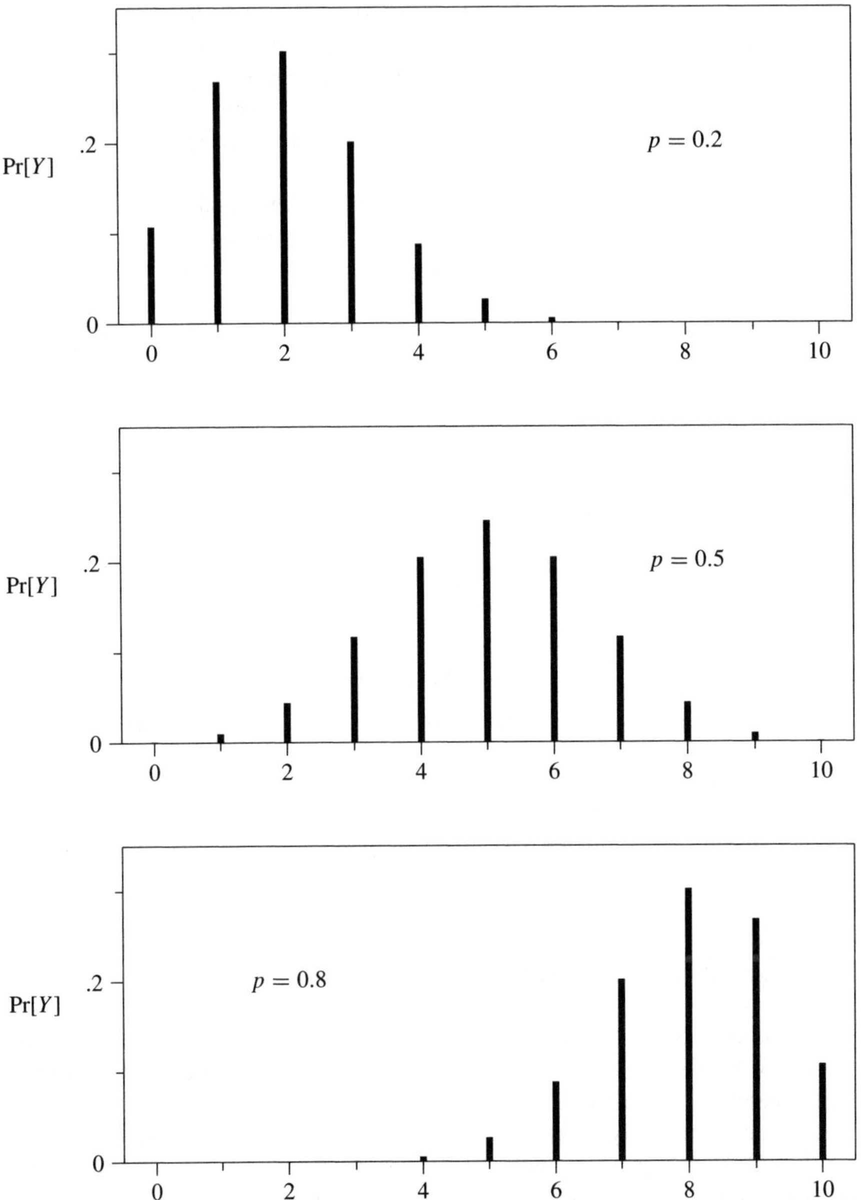

Figure 1.1 The binomial distribution probability mass function is illustrated for $n = 10$ with parameters $p = 0.2$, 0.5, and 0.8.

If n is large and p is not close to either 0 or 1 so that the variance is also large, then the binomial can be approximated by the normal distribution. If n is large and p is very close to zero, then the binomial can be approximated by the Poisson distribution. Similarly, if p is very close to 1 then $n - Y$ will behave approximately as Poisson. The Poisson distribution and these approximations are discussed in Section 1.5.

Chapter 7 describes several generalizations of the binomial distribution when we drop the assumption of independence among the individual Bernoulli indicators.

In another generalization, if the binomial p parameter varies according to the beta distribution, then the marginal distribution of Y is beta-binomial. Specifically, suppose that Y conditional on p behaves as binomial (n, p) and that p behaves as a beta random variable with density function

$$f_{\alpha\beta}(p) = \frac{\Gamma(\alpha+\beta)}{\Gamma(\alpha)\,\Gamma(\beta)}\, p^{\alpha-1}\,(1-p)^{\beta-1}$$

for $0 \leq p \leq 1$ and parameters $\alpha > 0$ and $\beta > 0$.

The marginal mass function of Y is then

$$\begin{aligned}\Pr[\,Y = y\,] &= \int_0^1 \binom{n}{y} p^y\,(1-p)^{n-y}\, f_{\alpha\beta}(p)\,\mathrm{d}p \\ &= \frac{n!\,\Gamma(\alpha+\beta)\,\Gamma(\alpha+y)\,\Gamma(\beta+n-y)}{y!\,(n-y)!\,\Gamma(\alpha)\,\Gamma(\beta)\,\Gamma(\alpha+\beta+n)}. \qquad (1.7)\end{aligned}$$

This is the mass function of the beta-binomial distribution and is derived in another fashion in Section 7.2.4. More details about this distribution are available in Johnson, Kotz, and Kemp (1992, pp 239–42).

The gamma function $\Gamma(\cdot)$ is a generalization of the definition of the factorial function extended to nonintegers. The gamma function and its approximations are described in Section 1.8.

1.4 The Multinomial Distribution

The multinomial distribution is the generalization of the binomial to more than two mutually exclusive categories. This multivariate distribution is used to describe the joint frequencies of several possible outcomes.

Consider n mutually independent experiments, each of which results in one of k $(k = 2, 3, \ldots)$ possible mutually exclusive and exhaustive outcomes. The probability of each of these outcomes is $p_1, \ldots, p_k$, where $p_i \geq 0$ and $\sum p_i = 1$. After n independent replications of this experiment, let $\{N_1, \ldots, N_k\}$ denote the set of joint frequencies of each of the k outcomes. Each of these frequencies can take on the values $0, 1, \ldots, n$ and satisfy

$$\sum_i^n N_i = n. \qquad (1.8)$$

The k frequencies $\{N_1, \ldots, N_k\}$ represent a $k - 1$ dimensional random variable as a result of this constraint.

The joint probability mass function of $\{N_1, \ldots, N_k\}$ is

$$\Pr[\, N_1 = n_1, \ldots, N_k = n_k \,] = \frac{n!}{n_1! \cdots n_k!} \prod_{i}^{k} p_i^{n_i} \tag{1.9}$$

for nonnegative integers $\{n_i\}$ that satisfy $\sum n_i = n$.

All of the probabilities in (1.9) represent the complete expansion of the polynomial

$$(p_1 + p_2 + \cdots + p_k)^n .$$

This polynomial is equal to 1 because $\sum p_i = 1$, demonstrating that (1.9) is a valid mass function and sums to unity.

The marginal distribution of each N_i is binomial with parameters n and p_i. The conditional distribution of N_1, given $N_2 = n_2$ is binomial with parameters $n - n_2$ and $p_1/(1 - p_2)$. The joint marginal distribution of $\{N_1,\, N_2,\, n - N_1 - N_2\}$ is multinomial $(k = 3)$, with parameters n and $\{p_1,\, p_2,\, 1 - p_1 - p_2\}$.

The joint factorial moments of $\{N_1, \ldots, N_k\}$ are

$$\mathrm{E}\left[\prod_i N_i^{(r_i)} \right] = n^{(r_+)} \prod_i p_i^{r_i}$$

for $r_i = 0, 1, \ldots$ and $r_+ = \sum r_i$.

In particular, the covariance of N_1 and N_2 is

$$\mathrm{Cov}\,[\, N_1,\, N_2 \,] = \mathrm{E}[\, (N_1 - np_1)(N_2 - np_2) \,] = -np_1 p_2 .$$

This covariance is negative, reflecting the constraint (1.8) that the sum of the N_i is fixed.

The correlation between a pair of frequencies

$$\mathrm{Corr}\,[\, N_1,\, N_2 \,] = -\left[\frac{p_1}{1 - p_1} \frac{p_2}{1 - p_2} \right]^{1/2}$$

is related to the product of the two odds for the frequencies.

There are two approximations to the multinomial distribution when the sample size n is large. Suppose n is large and (p_1, p_2) become small at a rate such that the limits $\lambda_1 = np_1$ and $\lambda_2 = np_2$ are bounded above and away from zero. Then (N_1, N_2) will jointly behave approximately as independent Poisson random variables with parameters (λ_1, λ_2).

A second approximation occurs when n is large and the variances of (N_1, N_2) are both large. Then the joint behavior of (N_1, N_2) is approximately bivariate normal.

1.5 Poisson Distribution

The Poisson distribution is often described as an approximation to the binomial distribution. It is useful in settings where the binomial n parameter is large and p is small. These parameters approach limits in such a way that the mean, denoted by $\lambda = np$, remains moderate and bounded away from zero. Under these conditions, the binomial distribution can be approximated by the Poisson distribution.

This approximation is based on the sum of a large number of independent and identically distributed Bernoulli random variables. The Poisson distribution is also the approximate behavior of a large number of independent Bernoulli indicators that are not identically distributed but all of whose p parameters are uniformly small.

The probability mass function for the Poisson distribution with mean parameter $\lambda > 0$ is

$$\Pr[\,Y = y\,] = \mathrm{e}^{-\lambda}\lambda^{y}/y! \tag{1.10}$$

defined for $y = 0, 1, \ldots$ and zero otherwise.

The mean and variance of the Poisson distribution are both equal to λ. The third central moment of the Poisson distribution

$$\mathrm{E}[\,(Y-\lambda)^3\,] = \lambda$$

is also equal to λ.

Higher Poisson central moments do not continue this pattern. For example, the fourth central moment is

$$\mathrm{E}[\,(Y-\lambda)^4\,] = 3\lambda^2 + \lambda.$$

For $r = 1, 2, \ldots,$ the factorial moments of the Poisson distribution are

$$\mathrm{E}[\,Y^{(r)}\,] = \lambda^r \tag{1.11}$$

and the factorial moment generating function is

$$\mathrm{E}[\,(t+1)^Y\,] = \mathrm{e}^{t\lambda}.$$

The moment generating function is

$$M_Y(t) = \mathrm{E}[\,\mathrm{e}^{tY}\,] = \exp[\lambda(\mathrm{e}^t - 1)].$$

When the mean parameter λ is large, then the Poisson distribution can be approximated by the normal distribution. This normal approximate distribution becomes more apparent in Fig. 1.2 as λ grows larger.

The sum of two independent Poisson random variables will also behave as Poisson. Specifically, if Y_1 and Y_2 are independently distributed as Poisson with parameters λ_1 and λ_2, respectively, then $Y_1 + Y_2$ will follow the Poisson distribution with parameter $\lambda_1 + \lambda_2$.

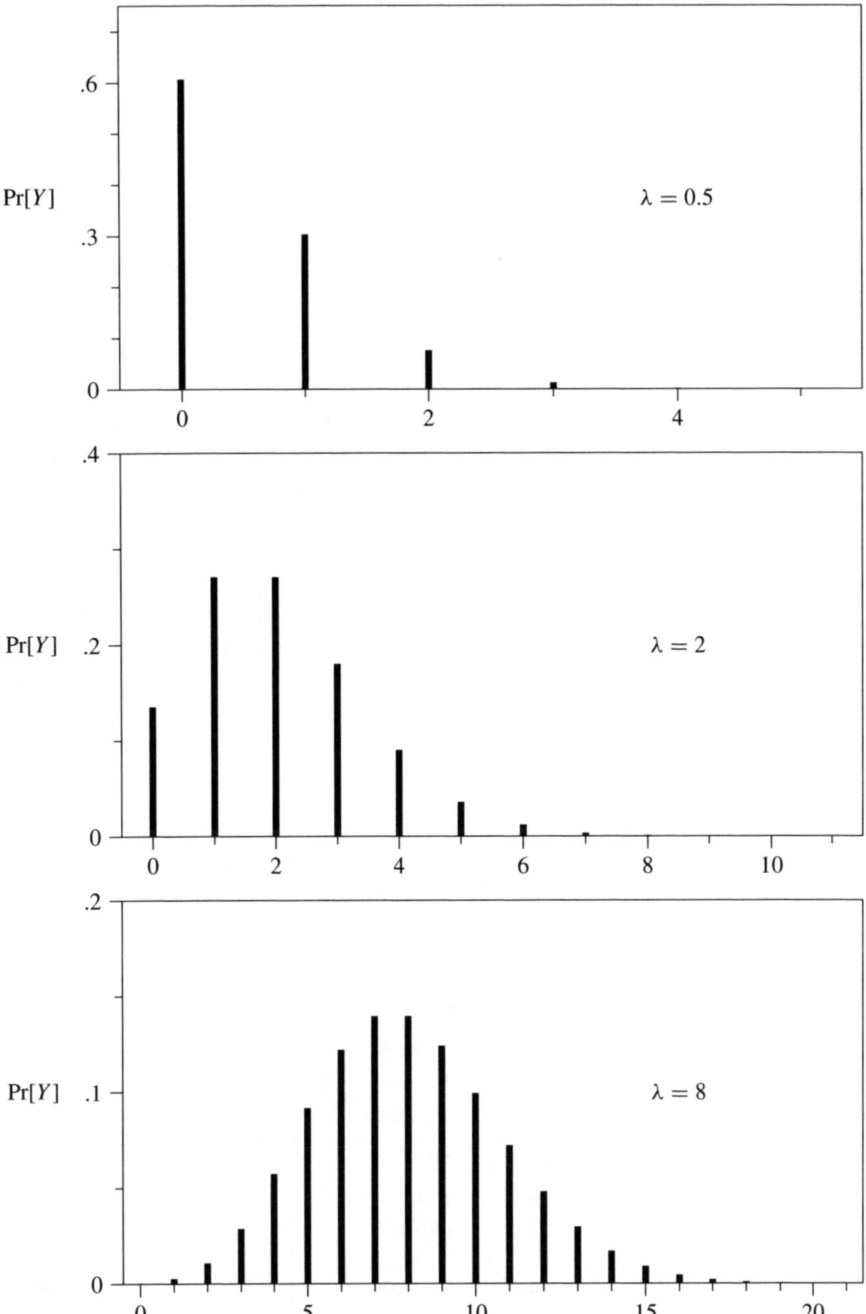

Figure 1.2 The Poisson distribution illustrated for $\lambda = 0.5$, 2, and 8.

Similarly, the distribution of Y_1 conditional on the value of $Y_1 + Y_2$ is binomial with parameters

$$n = Y_1 + Y_2$$

and

$$p = \lambda_1/(\lambda_1 + \lambda_2).$$

Finally, there is a close relationship between the Poisson and the negative binomial distribution that is described in the following section.

As a numerical example of the Poisson distribution, consider the data in Table 1.1 reported by Student (1907) on the distribution of yeast cells using a hemocytometer. WS Gosset was employed by the Guinness brewery and published under the *nom de plume* Student. The hemocytometer is a glass slide with a tiny 20×20 grid etched into its surface. It was commonly used to count dilute samples of blood cells, or in this example, yeast cells under the microscope.

The distribution of a sample of 272 yeast cells across the 400 compartments on the glass slide is given in the second column of Table 1.1. Specifically, in 213 of the 400 compartments there were no yeast cells, in 128 compartments there was exactly one yeast cell, and so on. The expected counts and the corresponding χ^2 values are also given.

The argument we use to justify the Poisson distribution is based on its approximation to the binomial model. In terms of the binomial model there are a large number of $n = 400$ compartments but there are not so many yeast cells relative to this number. We expect approximately

$$272/400 = 0.680$$

yeast cells per compartment. There is a very small probability that any one compartment is occupied by a given yeast cell. In particular, more than half of the 400 compartments are unoccupied. Kolchin *et al.* (1978, Ch. 2) contains a large

Table 1.1 Observed yeast cell frequencies and fitted Poisson distribution.

Count	Observed frequency	Fitted Poisson frequency	Components of χ^2
0	213	202.342	.561
1	128	137.897	.710
2	37	46.989	2.123
3	18	10.674	} 6.667
4+	4	2.098	
Totals	400	400	10.061

Source: Student (1907)

number of limiting distributions of occupancy problems such as described by this example.

The maximum likelihood estimate $\widehat{\lambda} = 0.6815$ is obtained by numerically maximizing the likelihood function

$$\begin{aligned}\Lambda(\lambda) &= 213 \log \Pr[\,Y = 0 \mid \lambda\,] + 128 \log \Pr[\,Y = 1 \mid \lambda\,] \\ &\quad + 37 \log \Pr[\,Y = 2 \mid \lambda\,] + 18 \log \Pr[\,Y = 3 \mid \lambda\,] \\ &\quad + 4 \log \Pr[\,Y \geq 4 \mid \lambda\,] \qquad (1.12)\end{aligned}$$

This estimate of 0.6815 is slightly larger than 272/400=0.680 because of how we treat the category listed as containing four or more yeast cells.

The expected counts using the fitted value of $\widehat{\lambda} = 0.6815$ are given in Table 1.1. The last two categories of three and four or more yeast cells are combined in order to increase the small expected counts in these compartments when calculating the χ^2 statistic. The $\chi^2 = 10.06$ with 2 df has a significance level of .007 indicating a poor fit of the Poisson model.

The large values of the components of the χ^2 statistic show that the lack of fit is due to those compartments with large numbers of yeast cells. This is probably because the yeast cells cling together resulting in compartments with unusually large numbers of cells. The Bernoulli events of cells occupying compartments on the slide are then not independent, so a binomial distribution might be in question. Similarly, the Poisson approximation to this binomial distribution might not be appropriate either. This example is examined again in Section 1.6.

1.6 Negative Binomial Distribution

Suppose we continue to sample Bernoulli distributed events with probability parameter p until we obtain c successes or 1's. The value of $c = 1, 2, \ldots$ is determined before the sampling begins. The sampling process ends with the observation of the $c-$th success. The negative binomial distribution describes the number of failures (0's) observed before the cth success has been achieved.

The number of failures Y until the cth success follows the negative binomial distribution with mass function

$$\Pr[\,Y = y\,] = \binom{c + y - 1}{c - 1} p^c (1 - p)^y. \qquad (1.13)$$

for $y = 0, 1, \ldots$.

The name 'negative binomial' and the proof that the mass function (1.13) sums to one comes from the following expansion. For P near zero, we have

$$(Q - P)^{-c} = Q^{-c} + \frac{c}{1!} P Q^{-c-1} + \frac{c(c+1)}{2!} P^2 Q^{-c-2} + \cdots.$$

Then set $Q = P + 1$ and write

$$Q^{-c} = [(Q - P)/Q]^c = (1 - P/Q)^c$$

to show

$$(Q - P)^{-c} = (1 - P/Q)^c + \frac{c}{1!}(P/Q)(1 - P/Q)^c + \frac{c(c+1)}{2!}(P/Q)^2(1 - P/Q)^c + \cdots .$$

These terms are the same as those in (1.13), where

$$P = (1 - p)/p.$$

The expected value of the negative binomial random variable with mass function in (1.13) is

$$\mathrm{E}[\,Y\,] = \mu = c(1 - p)/p \tag{1.14}$$

and the variance is

$$\mathrm{Var}[\,Y\,] = c(1 - p)/p^2.$$

The variance of the negative binomial distribution is always larger than its mean.

The probability generating function is

$$G(t) = \mathrm{E}[\,t^Y\,] = [(1 - p)/(1 - pt)]^c.$$

The factorial moment generating function is

$$G(1 + t) = \mathrm{E}[\,(1 + t)^Y\,] = [\,1 - (1 - p)t/p\,]^{-c}$$

and the factorial moments of the negative binomial distribution are

$$\mathrm{E}[\,Y^{(k)}\,] = (c + k - 1)^{(k)}[\,(1 - p)/p\,]^k$$

for $k = 0, 1, \ldots$.

If the c parameter is large and p approaches one in such a manner that the mean $c(1 - p)/p$ approaches a finite, nonzero limit λ, then the negative binomial distribution can be approximated by the Poisson with mean λ.

The negative binomial distribution is plotted in Fig. 1.3 for various values of parameters c and p. From top to bottom, this figure displays the negative binomial and Poisson mass functions with means 0.5, 2, and 8. The mass points of these discrete distributions are connected with lines in order to compare the different distributions. This will be the convention in the remainder of the book.

In Fig. 1.3, the values of the c parameters are set to 1, 2, 4, and 8. Values of the p parameters vary in order to achieve a constant value of the expected value μ. Specifically, from (1.14) we have

$$p = c/(c + \mu) \tag{1.15}$$

for mean $\mu > 0$ and parameter c.

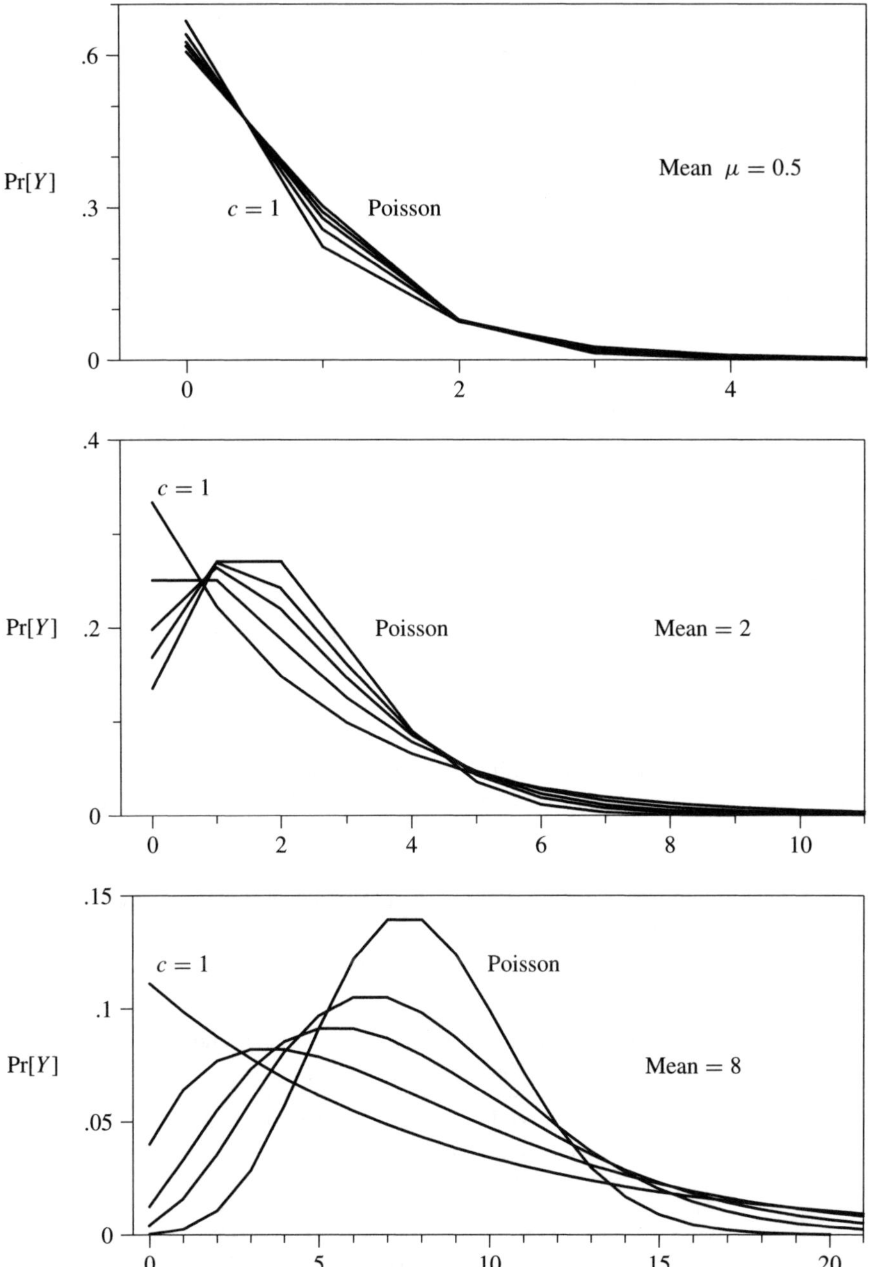

Figure 1.3 Negative binomial and Poisson mass functions with means $\mu = 0.5$, 2, and 8. The negative binomial c parameters in every figure are 1, 2, 4, and 8. The Poisson distribution is the limit for large values of c.

As the c parameter gets larger, in every case in Fig. 1.3, the negative binomial distribution looks more like the Poisson distribution with the same mean. When the mean and c are both large, then the negative binomial distribution can be approximated by the normal distribution, as seen in the bottom of this figure. The normal approximation for the negative binomial distribution is also described in Section 2.3.1.

More generally, the c parameter need not be an integer. The following derivation of the negative binomial mass function demonstrates its description as a mixture of Poisson distributions. Let Y, given λ, behave as Poisson with parameter λ and suppose λ behaves as a gamma random variable with density function

$$f_\Gamma = (c/\mu)^c \lambda^{c-1} \exp(-\lambda c/\mu)/\Gamma(c)$$

for $\lambda > 0$. This gamma distribution has mean parameter $\mu > 0$ and variance μ^2/c for shape parameter $c > 0$.

The marginal distribution of Y has mass function

$$\begin{aligned}\Pr[Y = y] &= \int_0^\infty e^{-\lambda}\lambda^y/y!\; f_\Gamma(\lambda)\, d\lambda \\ &= \frac{\Gamma(c+y)}{y!\,\Gamma(c)} \left(\frac{c}{\mu + c}\right)^c \left(\frac{\mu}{\mu + c}\right)^y, \qquad (1.16)\end{aligned}$$

which is a form of the mass function of the negative binomial distribution.

Expressions (1.13) and (1.16) coincide when c is an integer and $p = c/(\mu + c)$. The derivation of the negative binomial distribution in (1.16) helps explain why it has longer tails than the corresponding Poisson distribution with the same mean, as seen in Fig. 1.3.

Let us use this derivation of the negative binomial distribution to motivate another examination of Student's yeast example given in Table 1.1. The negative binomial distribution is fitted to this data in Table 1.2. The maximum likelihood estimates are obtained by numerically maximizing a likelihood similar to the

Table 1.2 Observed yeast cell frequencies and fitted negative binomial distribution.

Count	Observed frequency	Fitted frequency	Components of χ^2
0	213	214.330	.008
1	128	122.476	.249
2	37	45.004	1.423
3	18	13.477	1.518
4+	4	4.714	.108
Totals	400	400	3.306

function given at (1.12), namely

$$\Lambda(c, \mu) = 213 \log \Pr[\,Y = 0 \mid c, \mu\,] + 128 \log \Pr[\,Y = 1 \mid c, \mu\,]$$
$$+ 37 \log \Pr[\,Y = 2 \mid c, \mu\,] + 18 \log \Pr[\,Y = 3 \mid c, \mu\,]$$
$$+ 4 \log \Pr[\,Y \geq 4 \mid c, \mu\,]$$

with probability model $\Pr[\cdot]$ given in (1.16).

These maximum likelihood estimates are $\widehat{c} = 3.496$ and $\widehat{\mu} = .6831$. Notice that the estimate of the mean parameter $\widehat{\mu}$ is very close in value to the estimate $\widehat{\lambda} = .6815$ for the Poisson parameter that maximizes (1.12). Using the parameterization given in (1.13), we also have

$$\widehat{p} = [\,\widehat{c}/(\widehat{c} + \widehat{\mu})\,] = .8365.$$

The fitted expected counts and the components of the χ^2 statistic are given in Table 1.2. The $\chi^2 = 3.306$ value with 2 df has significance level .19, indicating a very good fit to the data. The negative binomial model has longer tails than the Poisson, so this model is better able to model the large number of compartments on the glass slide containing several yeast cells clinging together. Not all cells exhibit this phenomenon but apparently some do. Similarly, the negative binomial as a mixture of Poisson distributions is able to model some of the dependence among the yeast cells.

The negative binomial distribution is generalized in Chapter 2, in which we describe the number of trials necessary in order to obtain both c successes and c failures. The resulting distribution is the larger of two negative binomial distributions: the number of trials necessary until c successes and the number of trials needed until c failures are observed.

1.7 Hypergeometric Distribution

The binomial, Poisson, and negative binomial distributions all assume that we are sampling from an infinitely large parent population. The hypergeometric distribution is the analogy for sampling from a finite population.

Consider an urn containing N balls. Of these, suppose m are of the 'successful' color and the remaining $N - m$ are of the 'unsuccessful' type. We reach into the urn and draw out a sample of size n balls. The hypergeometric distribution describes the number of successful colored balls in our sample of size n. This sample can also be illustrated as a 2×2 table of counts as given in Table 1.3.

The probability mass function of the hypergeometric distribution is

$$\Pr[\,Y = y\,] = \binom{m}{y}\binom{N-m}{n-y} \Big/ \binom{N}{n}. \qquad (1.17)$$

Intuitively, y out of the m successful types are sampled and $n - y$ out of the $N - m$ unsuccessful types are sampled. The denominator considers all possible ways in which samples of size n can be drawn out of the total N.

Table 1.3 The hypergeometric distribution of Y, given in (1.17) displayed as a 2×2 table.

	Types of Items		
	Successful	Unsuccessful	Totals
Items drawn	Y	$X = n - Y$	n
Items not drawn	$m - Y$	$N - n - m + Y$	$N - n$
Totals	m	$N - m$	N

The support or range of the hypergeometric distribution in (1.17) is

$$\max(0, m + n - N) \le y \le \min(n, m).$$

This range assures that all counts in Table 1.3 are nonnegative.

The derivation of this distribution can be obtained as a conditional distribution of a binomial. Specifically, let X and Y denote independent binomial random variables with index parameters $N - m$ and m respectively with the same value of their p parameter.

We want the conditional distribution of Y, given $X + Y = n$. Begin by writing

$$\begin{aligned} &\Pr[\,Y = y \mid X + Y = n\,] \\ &\qquad = \Pr[\,Y = y \text{ and } X + Y = n\,]/\Pr[\,X + Y = n\,] \\ &\qquad = \Pr[\,Y = y;\; X = n - y\,]/\Pr[\,X + Y = n\,]. \end{aligned}$$

The distribution of $X + Y$ in the denominator behaves as binomial with parameters N and p. We also use the independence of X and Y to show

$$\begin{aligned} &\Pr[\,Y = y \mid X + Y = n\,] \\ &\qquad = \Pr[\,Y = y\,]\ \Pr[\,X = n - y\,]\ /\ \Pr[\,X + Y = n\,] \\ &\qquad = \binom{m}{y} p^{y}(1-p)^{m-y} \binom{N-m}{n-y} p^{n-y}(1-p)^{N-n-m+y} \\ &\qquad\qquad \Big/ \binom{N}{n} p^{n}(1-p)^{N-n}\,. \end{aligned} \tag{1.18}$$

All of the terms involving p and $1 - p$ cancel in the numerator and the denominator. The binomial coefficients that remain after this cancellation yield the mass function given in (1.17).

The expected value of this distribution is

$$\mathrm{E}[\,Y\,] = mn/N.$$

This is also the estimate used for the expected counts when we calculate the χ^2 statistic.

The variance of the hypergeometric distribution is

$$\begin{aligned}\mathrm{Var}[\,Y\,] &= mn(N-m)(N-n)/N^2(N-1)\\ &= \mathrm{E}[\,Y\,](N-m)(N-n)/N(N-1).\end{aligned}$$

The variance is always smaller than the mean.

The more general factorial moments of this distribution are

$$\mathrm{E}[\,Y^{(r)}\,] = m^{(r)}n^{(r)}/N^{(r)}$$

for $r = 1, 2, \ldots, \min(m, n)$ and zero for larger values of r.

The same method used to prove that the hypergeometric probabilities sum to one is used several times in this book. The easiest way to prove that the probabilities in (1.17) sum to one is to begin by writing the polynomial identity

$$(1+z)^N = (1+z)^m(1+z)^{N-m}. \tag{1.19}$$

This equality is true for all values of z. The coefficients of each power of z must agree on both sides of this identity. If we identify the coefficient of z^n on both sides of this identity, then we have

$$\binom{N}{n} = \sum_y \binom{m}{y}\binom{N-m}{n-y}. \tag{1.20}$$

This is the same equality we need to show that the probabilities in (1.17) sum to one. This equality is known as *Vandermonde's theorem.* The polynomial identity in (1.19) is referred to as the *generating polynomial* of the hypergeometric distribution.

1.7.1 Negative hypergeometric distribution

This distribution is the finite sample analogy to the negative binomial distribution described in Section 1.6. The *negative hypergeometric distribution* (Johnson *et al.* 1992, pp. 239–42) is the distribution of the number of unsuccessful draws, one at a time, from an urn with two different colored balls until a specified number of successful draws have been obtained. If m out of N balls are of the successful type, then the number of unsuccessful draws Y observed before c of the successful types are obtained is

$$\Pr[\,Y = y\,] = \binom{c+y-1}{c-1}\binom{N-c-y}{m-c}\bigg/\binom{N}{m}, \tag{1.21}$$

with parameters satisfying $1 \le c \le m < N$ and range $y = 0, 1, \ldots, N - m$. The expected value of Y in (1.21) is $mc/(N - m - 1)$.

This distribution is used by Kaigh and Lachenbruch (1982) in applications of resampling for nonparametric quantile estimation. This distribution is a special case of the beta-binomial when all of its parameters are positive integers. The beta-binomial distribution is described in Section 7.2.4.

1.7.2 Extended hypergeometric distribution

This distribution is the extension of (1.18) when the binomial p parameters are not the same for X and Y. Let X and Y denote independent binomial random variables with parameters $(N - m,\ p_1)$ and $(m,\ p_2)$ respectively. We want to describe the conditional distribution of Y given $X + Y = n$. This distribution is discussed in detail by Johnson, Kotz, and Kemp (1992, pp. 279–82).

Following the derivation in (1.18), write

$$\Pr[\,Y = y \mid X + Y = n\,] = \Pr[\,Y = y\,]\ \Pr[\,X = n - y\,]/\Pr[\,X + Y = n\,].$$

This denominator does not have a simple expression because $X + Y$ does not have a binomial distribution for $p_1 \neq p_2$. The denominator $\Pr[\,X + Y = n\,]$ does not depend on y.

We then have

$$\begin{aligned}
&\Pr[\,Y = y \mid X + Y = n\,] \\
&\qquad \propto \binom{m}{y} p_2^{y}\,(1 - p_2)^{m-y} \binom{N - m}{n - y} p_1^{n-y}\,(1 - p_1)^{N-n-m+y} \\
&\qquad \propto \binom{m}{y}\binom{N - m}{n - y} \exp(\lambda y),
\end{aligned} \tag{1.22}$$

where λ is the log-odds ratio

$$\lambda = \log[p_2(1 - p_1)/p_1(1 - p_2)].$$

The normalizing constant of proportionality in (1.22) depends on N, n, m, and λ but not y. Similarly, the moments and generating functions of this distribution do not have simple closed form expressions, in general. The special case of (1.22) is the hypergeometric mass function given in (1.17), when $\lambda = 0$ or equivalently when $p_1 = p_2$.

An example of the extended hypergeometric mass function is plotted in Fig. 1.4 for $m = 12$; $n = 10$ and $N = 25$. Values of λ vary from -3 to 3 in this figure, shifting the mass from the lower to the upper range of the distribution.

The most common application of this distribution is as a model for the alternative hypothesis in the analysis of 2×2 tables. The hypergeometric distribution with mass function given in (1.17) is derived by assuming $p_1 = p_2$ or independence of population and sampling parameter. This is the basis of the Fisher exact

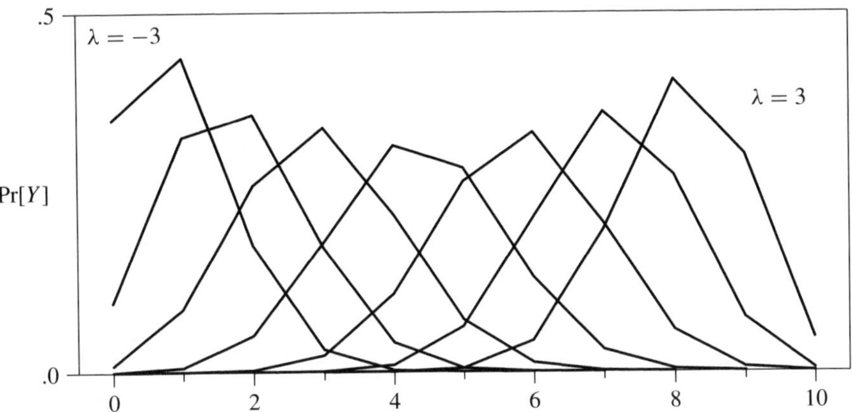

Figure 1.4 Extended hypergeometric mass function for $m = 12$, $n = 10$, and $N = 25$. Values of λ are from -3 to 3 by 1.

test of significance when examining 2×2 tables. As an alternative to the independence hypothesis, the extended hypergeometric distribution is a natural choice and provides a single parameter λ that allows expression of an alternative hypothesis.

As an example of the hypergeometric distribution in use, let us consider the data from Innes *et al.* (1969) summarized in Table 1.4. In this experiment, 16 mice were exposed to the fungicide Avadex and an additional 79 mice were kept separately under unexposed conditions. After 85 weeks, all of the 95 mice were sacrificed and their lungs were examined for tumors by pathologists. The frequencies of tumors in the exposed and unexposed mice is summarized in Table 1.4.

The χ^2 statistic for this table is 5.41 with 1 df and significance level 0.02, indicating that there is some evidence of association between exposure and the tumor outcome. The assumption made using this statistic is that the counts in the table can be approximated using the normal distribution, and the significance level of the χ^2 statistic is approximated using the corresponding asymptotic distribution.

Exact methods for analyzing data of this type require a complete enumeration of all possible outcomes consistent with the margins of the table. The observed

Table 1.4 Incidence of tumors in mice exposed to the fungicide Avadex (Innes *et al.*, 1969).

	Exposed	Control	Totals
Mice with tumors	4	5	9
No tumors	12	74	86
Totals	16	79	95

Public domain: *Journal of the National Cancer Institute*, Oxford University Press

count of $Y = 4$ exposed mice with tumors could also have taken on any of the possible values $0, 1, \ldots, 9$ for these sets of marginal totals.

These marginal totals are all considered to be fixed in the *frequentist* statistical analysis of the interaction between exposure and cancer development. The number of mice exposed or not was determined by the experimenters and has no random component. The number of mice developing tumors is an outcome that could be different if the same experiment were repeated today. Nevertheless, we also treat both sets of marginal totals as fixed in the examination of the interaction between exposure and tumor development.

The frequentist approach to the analysis of this data posits that the marginal totals contain no information about the interaction of the row and column categories. The Bayesian approach, on the other hand, might argue that the investigators knew that 16 exposed mice would be sufficient to detect a difference and hence also knew something about the interaction *a priori.*

The hypergeometric distribution in (1.17) is the model of independence of exposure status and the eventual tumor development. Four exposed mice developed tumors. Under this model of independence we expect

$$9 \times 16/95 = 1.516$$

exposed mice to develop tumors.

The observed number (=4) is larger than this expected value. The probability of four exposed mice with tumors is not the significance level. Instead, we need to examine the probability of this outcome plus all of those outcomes that are more extreme than the one observed. The exact probability of observing four or more exposed mice with tumors is

$$\Pr[\, X \geq 4 \mid N = 95,\ m = 16,\ n = 9\,] = .0411, \tag{1.23}$$

using distribution (1.17), modeling the null hypothesis of independence of fungicide exposure and tumor development.

This *exact significance level* does not rely on making any approximations or using any asymptotic assumptions. While exact methods do have many virtues, it is well recognized that they usually suffer from diminished power over other methods. In Section 6.1, there is additional discussion of the settings where exact methods are useful.

One method of increasing the power of the exact test of significance is to apply a *continuity correction*. In calculating $\Pr[Y \geq 4]$ in the current example, the value of this expression is dominated by the first term, namely $\Pr[Y = 4]$. To improve the power, we sometimes apply a correction that diminishes the effect of this first term and calculate

$$\frac{1}{2}\Pr[\, Y = 4\,] + \Pr[\, Y > 4\,] = .0236 \tag{1.24}$$

and report this value as the exact significance level. This continuity corrected significance level is very close to the corresponding value obtained by the χ^2 statistic for this data.

The examination of Table 1.4 using both exact and asymptotic χ^2 methods provides evidence that tumor incidence is increased with exposure to the fungicide in terms of their statistical significance levels that are rather small. We can also measure the effect using the extended hypergeometric distribution given in (1.22).

The empirical log-odds ratio for this table is

$$\log[\,(4 \times 74)/(5 \times 12)\,] = 1.596.$$

The maximum likelihood estimate $\widehat{\lambda}$ of λ is 1.572, which is close to the empirical ratio. The maximum likelihood estimate is the value of λ that maximizes the probability

$$\Pr[\,X = 4 \mid \lambda,\ N = 95,\ m = 16,\ n = 9\,]$$

of the observed data using the extended hypergeometric distribution (1.22).

An exact 95% confidence interval for λ is obtained by solving the equations

$$\Pr[\,X \geq 4 \mid \lambda_1,\ N = 95,\ m = 16,\ n = 9\,] = .025$$

and

$$\Pr[\,X \leq 4 \mid \lambda_2, N = 95,\ m = 16,\ n = 9\,] = .025$$

for (λ_1, λ_2) using distribution (1.22). The resulting 95% confidence interval for λ is the solution of these two equations, namely $(-.1814,\ 3.264)$.

This exact 95% confidence interval for λ contains zero, corresponding to the null hypothesis of independence of exposure and tumor development. This confidence interval is two sided. The exact significance level of λ given in (1.23) and (1.24) is less than 0.05 but these also represent one-sided tests. In contrast, we note that the χ^2 test is two-sided because it squares the difference between the observed and expected counts in its numerator.

1.8 Stirling's Approximation

This section contains a number of mathematical results that will be used in subsequent chapters.

The *gamma function* is defined by

$$\Gamma(x) = \int_0^\infty t^{x-1} \mathrm{e}^{-t}\, \mathrm{d}t$$

for $x > 0$.

The gamma function satisfies the recurrence relation

$$\Gamma(x + 1) = x\,\Gamma(x).$$

When the argument x is a positive integer, then the gamma function is equal to the factorial

$$\Gamma(x + 1) = x!.$$

Stirling's approximation to the gamma function for large values of the argument is given by

$$\Gamma(x) = \mathrm{e}^{-x}\, x^{x-1/2}\, (2\pi)^{1/2} \left[1 + 1/12x + 1/288x^2 + \cdots\right]. \tag{1.25}$$

Other useful forms of Stirling's formula include

$$x! = (2\pi)^{1/2}\, x^{x+1/2} \exp\left[-x + \theta/12x\right] \tag{1.26}$$

for $0 < \theta(x) < 1$ and

$$\log \Gamma(x) = -x + (x - 1/2)\log(x) + 1/2 \log(2\pi) + 1/12x - 1/360x^3 + \cdots . \tag{1.27}$$

These relations and many other useful approximations and properties of the gamma function are given in (Abramowitz and Stegun (1972, Ch. 6)).

2

Maximum Negative Binomial Distribution

Of every pure animal you shall take seven pairs, males and their mates,
and of every animal that is not pure, two, a male and its mate;
Of birds of the sky also, seven pairs, male and female,
to keep seed alive upon the earth.[1]

Genesis 7:2–3.

This quotation was part of the charge given to Noah in stocking the ark before the impending flood. How many wild animals and birds of each species did Noah have to plan on capturing before being reasonably sure of obtaining either 1 or 7 of each sex?

The negative binomial distribution describes the number of failures observed until c Bernoulli successes are obtained. The negative binomial distribution is described in Section 1.6. In a generalization of this sampling scheme, how many observations should we expect to sample in order to obtain both c successes and c failures? That is, how long should it take before we observe c of each?

The maximum negative binomial distribution is the distribution of the smallest number of independent Bernoulli in p trials needed in order to observe at least c successes and c failures. For Noah, we presume that there is an even balance of the two sexes, so the Bernoulli parameter p is 1/2. His sampling parameter c is either 1 or 7, depending on the species involved. In this chapter, we assume that the species has a huge number of individuals so that the population can be treated as infinitely large. In the following chapter, we consider the problem when the population is finite and sampled without replacement. Noah also faced the problem of collecting male and female representatives of endangered species.

[1]Reprinted from *Etz Hayim: Torah and Commentary* pages 44, © 2001, The Rabbinical Assembly. (2001) used with permission of the Rabbinical Assembly. Scholars suggest that the reference to an animal's purity describes its suitability for sacrifice, not its suitability for human consumption.

Discrete Distributions Daniel Zelterman
© 2004 John Wiley & Sons, Ltd ISBN: 0-470-86888-0 (PPC)

The distribution discussed in this chapter is also motivated by a different problem with applications in genetics. In this second application, the Bernoulli parameter p can be very different from 1/2. In the (infinite) population, let p denote the frequency of the presence (or absence) of a certain genetic marker. If p is very close to one, then almost everybody has the marker and there is little to be learned by testing for it. Similarly, if p is extremely close to zero then routine testing for it also has limited value. To avoid either of these situations, we need an efficient plan for testing whether p is moderate (not too far from 1/2), or else p is extreme (close to either zero or one).

The proposed method to test these hypotheses in the genetics problem is to sequentially examine members of the population at random until we have observed at least c of each genotype. If we observe at least c of each of the two genotypes for a single genetic marker in a small sample, then we can conclude that p is moderate and not too far from 1/2. If a large sample is required in order to observe c of each, then this provides good statistical evidence that p is extreme. We can also terminate the sampling experiment early if a large number of observations has not yet provided c of both genotypes.

In this second example, we see that the same distribution is involved at a greater degree of generality than how it is used to describe the problem facing Noah in the first example. We want to sample independent Bernoulli (p) observations until we observe c successes and c failures. For Noah, the p parameter is 1/2 but, more generally, it can be any valid probability.

We describe the moments and modes for this sampling distribution in Sections 2.2.2 and 2.2.3. When c is large, there are normal and half-normal approximate distributions. These approximations are given in Sections 2.3.1 and 2.3.2. If the Bernoulli p parameter is extremely close to either zero or one, then a gamma approximate distribution is demonstrated in Section 2.3.3. Estimation of the Bernoulli parameter is a difficult problem for this distribution because we do not know if we are estimating p or $1 - p$. A number of estimation procedures are described in Section 2.4 using the EM algorithm and a Bayesian prior distribution.

2.1 Introduction

If we want to draw inference from the Bernoulli p parameter, the most common approach is to sample n observations $X_1, \ldots, X_n$ and count the number of successes $X_+ = \sum X_i$. If the sample size n is specified in advance, then X_+ behaves as a binomial distributed random variable. The binomial distribution should be familiar to the reader, and important properties of this popular distribution are given in Section 1.3.

Other sampling distributions appear in response to specific statistical problems or perhaps as a cost-saving effort. If we wanted to test the hypothesis of $p > 1/2$, for example, we might sample until we observed two successes. If we obtain two successes quickly, then this provides us good evidence that p is indeed greater than

1/2. If, however, we do not obtain two successes after a large number of Bernoulli observations, then we can stop the experiment prematurely and be confident that p is less than 1/2.

The reader will recognize that the number of trials necessary to obtain two, or more generally, c successes follows the negative binomial distribution. The negative binomial distribution is described more fully in Section 1.6. The maximum negative binomial distribution described in this chapter is the distribution of the number of trials necessary to obtain at least c successes *and* c failures.

The maximum negative binomial distribution described in this chapter is related to two other discrete distributions. Uppuluri and Blot (1970) and Lingappiah (1987) studied the riff-shuffle or minimum negative binomial distribution. The riff-shuffle distribution is the smallest number of Bernoulli trials needed in order to observe either c successes or c failures. The probability mass function of the riff-shuffle distribution is

$$\binom{c+y-1}{y}\left(p^c q^y + p^y q^c\right) \tag{2.1}$$

for $y = 0, 1, \ldots, c-1$.

The number of trials required to obtain either the earlier or later of c successes and/or c failures is also referred to as the 'sooner' and 'later times' in the work of Ebneshahrashoob and Sobel (1990) and Balasubramanian, Viveros, and Balakrishnan (1993). Such problems are also called 'frequency quotas', in which we want to know how many trials are needed until a specified number of c successes and d failures. There is also a literature on 'runs quotas', which model the number of trials necessary to obtain a run of specified length of successes and a specified run of failures. A run of successes, for example, is a series of successes uninterrupted by a single failure. The maximum negative binomial distribution is also related to a generalization of the coupon collector's distribution (Knuth (1981), pp. 62–63), in which a game is won after the contestant collects c of each of two different coupons that occur with frequency p and $1-p$. The usual coupon collector's distribution is that of the number of trials needed in order to collect one each of several equally likely coupons.

The development of the distribution described in this chapter and the following arises in a design for a medical study in which we want to draw inference from the parameter p in a Bernoulli distribution. The frequency, p, of an abnormal Ki-*ras* gene in the screen of colon cancer patients may prove, in future research, to be a useful predictor of subsequent disease progression. If p is extremely close to either zero or one, then knowledge of the status of this genetic defect will not have any useful prognostic value except for those few rare cases. Simply put, if we know that virtually everybody (or nobody) exhibits that genotype, then there is little to be gained by testing for it. The present statistical problem, then, is to design an efficient study to test the null hypothesis that p is 'moderate' (close to 1/2) against the alternative hypothesis that p is 'extreme' or close to either zero or one.

Our plan to study the problem is as follows. For a pre-specified value of the positive integer–valued parameter c, we will sequentially screen patients for the presence of a mutated Ki-*ras* gene until we have observed at least c normal (wild type) and c abnormal blood tests. If we need to sample a large number of patients, then this provides evidence that p is close to either zero or one. Similarly, if we observe c normal and c abnormal genotypes relatively quickly, then we are led to believe that p is moderate. The critical value of this distribution depends on the values of the parameters p and c. This chapter and the following describe properties of the sampling distribution arising from this design.

Let $X_1, X_2, \ldots$ denote a sequence of independent, identically distributed Bernoulli trials with parameter p $(0 < p < 1)$, and let c denote a positive integer. Define the random variable Y to be the smallest nonnegative integer for which there are at least c zeros and c ones in $\{X_1, \ldots, X_{Y+2c}\}$.

In other words, the random variable Y is defined as

$$Y = \arg\min_n \left\{ \sum_{i=1}^{n} X_i \geq c, \text{ and } \sum_{i=1}^{n} (1 - X_i) \geq c \right\} - 2c. \tag{2.2}$$

The valid values of Y are $0, 1, \ldots$.

The random variable $Y + 2c$ denotes the smallest number of trials needed to obtain at least c successes and c failures. The random variable Y counts the 'excess' number of trials needed beyond the minimum of $2c$. This chapter describes properties of the random variable Y.

Let $N_p = N_p(X_1, X_2, \ldots)$ denote the number of zeros in $\{X_1, X_2, \ldots\}$ before the cth one is recorded. Then N_p is a random variable with the negative binomial distribution and its mass function is denoted by

$$a_k(p) = \Pr[N_p = k] = \binom{c+k-1}{c-1} p^c q^k \tag{2.3}$$

defined for $k = 0, 1, \ldots$.

The random variable $Y + c$ is equal to the larger of $N_p(X_1, X_2, \ldots)$ and $N_q = N_q(1 - X_1, 1 - X_2, \ldots)$, where $q = 1 - p$. From this property, we refer to Y as having the *maximum negative binomial distribution*. The random variables N_p and N_q are not independent because they are defined on the same sequence of Bernoulli trials $X_1, X_2, \ldots$. The riff-shuffle distribution given in (2.1) is the smaller of N_p and N_q.

The distribution of Y can be determined from the value of X_{Y+2c} that ends the sequence in (2.2). If $X_{Y+2c} = 1$, then the probability of Y is $a_{Y+c}(p)$, where $a(\cdot)$ is given in (2.3). When $X_{Y+2c} = 0$, the probability of Y is $a_{Y+c}(q)$. These two events are mutually exclusive so the probability of $Y = k$ is the sum of $a_{k+c}(p)$ and $a_{k+c}(q)$.

In other words, waiting for the cth success, the probability of $Y + c$ failures is

$$\binom{Y+2c-1}{c-1} p^c q^{Y+c}$$

and waiting for the cth failure, the probability of $Y + c$ successes is

$$\binom{Y+2c-1}{c-1} p^{Y+c} q^{c}$$

The sum of these two probabilities shows that the maximum negative binomial probability mass function is

$$\Pr(Y = k) = \binom{2c+k-1}{c-1} (p^k + q^k)\,(p\,q)^c \tag{2.4}$$

defined for $k = 0, 1, \ldots$.

To confirm that (2.4) is a valid probability distribution and sums to one, we need to show

$$\Pr(N_p \geq c) + \Pr(N_q \geq c) = 1$$

for every value of the positive integer c parameter.

The events $\{N_p \geq c\}$ and $\{N_q \geq c\}$ are the same as the events $\{N_p > N_q\}$ and $\{N_p < N_q\}$, respectively. Since N_p and N_q cannot be equal, equation (2.4) defines a valid probability distribution.

The terms in the probability in (2.4) can be intuitively explained as follows. There are c successes (1's) and c failures (0's) whose probability is $(pq)^c$. The k remaining 'excess' trials must be either all 1's or all 0's; hence the $(p^k + q^k)$ term. The binomial coefficient describes all possible permutations of the $2c + k$ Bernoulli trials. The last of these trials must be either the cth 0 or 1 that ends the sequence.

We also note that p and $q = 1 - p$ are not identifiable in (2.4). The same maximum negative binomial distribution results if the roles of p and q are reversed. This problem of identifiability is raised in Section 2.4 in which we discuss parameter estimation. At that point we run into a special challenge because it is not clear whether we are estimating p or $1 - p$.

2.1.1 Outfitting the ark

The special case of the maximum negative binomial distribution with parameter $p = 1/2$ is illustrated here. Specifically, we want to know how many animals of each species must be captured in order to be reasonably assured that c of each sex are obtained. We assume that males and females are equally likely to be captured and an equal effort is spent pursuing each sex. The problem facing Noah was to obtain either $c = 1$ or $c = 7$, depending on the species involved.

In this application, we assume that there is a large number of animals available and this justifies the assumption of sampling with replacement, or from an infinite population. In other words, a small sample does not markedly change the composition of the population. We also assume that a captured animal is equally likely to be either male or female.

Stirzaker (2003) identifies this problem for an endangered species. Sampling from a finite population is described in the following chapter. This problem also appears in Andel (2001, pp. 136–9) in which pairs of wyverns are needed. A wyvern (also spelled wivern) is a mythical dragon.

Figure 2.1 displays the cumulative maximum negative binomial distribution (2.4) for each value of $c = 1, \ldots, 12$. Only the upper tail is presented to emphasize a high probability of successfully capturing c specimens of both sexes. Keep in mind that the sampling distribution depicted here describes the number of excess samples required, in addition to the minimum of $2c$.

The horizontal axis in Fig. 2.1 is the range of samples needed in excess of the minimum $2c$. As an example, for $c = 1$ of each sex, a minimum sample of size two will be required corresponding to $y = 0$ extra captures. With probability .9375, a total of five observations will be needed or $y = 3$ excess samples. This final sample of size five will contain four animals of one sex and one of the other, or $y = 3$ extra animals.

The expected number of animals necessary to capture is approximately 3. That is, the maximum negative binomial distribution in (2.4) has an expected value of about 1 for parameters $c = 1$ and $p = 1/2$. This suggests that, on average, one extra animal will be needed in order to capture one of each sex.

Similarly, for $c = 7$, a minimum of 14 animals will be needed. If $y = 8$ extra, or 22 total animals, are captured, then there is probability .9475, that the sample will contain at least seven of both sexes. The expected value for the maximum negative binomial distribution in (2.4) is 2.93 for $c = 7$ and $p = 1/2$.

Noah then needed to plan on capturing

$$2c + 2.93 = 16.93$$

animals in order to obtain $c = 7$ of each sex.

2.1.2 Medical screening application

Our medical application of the maximum negative binomial distribution (2.4) calls for continued sampling of Bernoulli-valued colon cancer patients $X_1, X_2, \ldots$ until we observe $c = 2$ normal (wild type) and 2 abnormal Ki-*ras* genotypes. The critical value for this experiment depends on the desired significance level, as well as the value for p considered under the null hypothesis.

As a numerical example, suppose the null hypothesis is that the Bernoulli parameter (Ki-*ras* mutation frequency) p is between 0.1 and 0.9. If we have not observed at least $c = 2$ of each of the two genotypes after the first 46 patients tested, then we will stop and declare that p is extreme. Under the null hypothesis that p is moderate and between 0.1 and 0.9 this procedure has significance level 0.05. Under the alternative hypothesis, if p is either smaller than 0.015 or greater than 0.985, then this procedure has power 0.85. If p is 0.1 (or 0.9), then this procedure is expected to terminate after 20 patients. That is, if $p = 0.1$

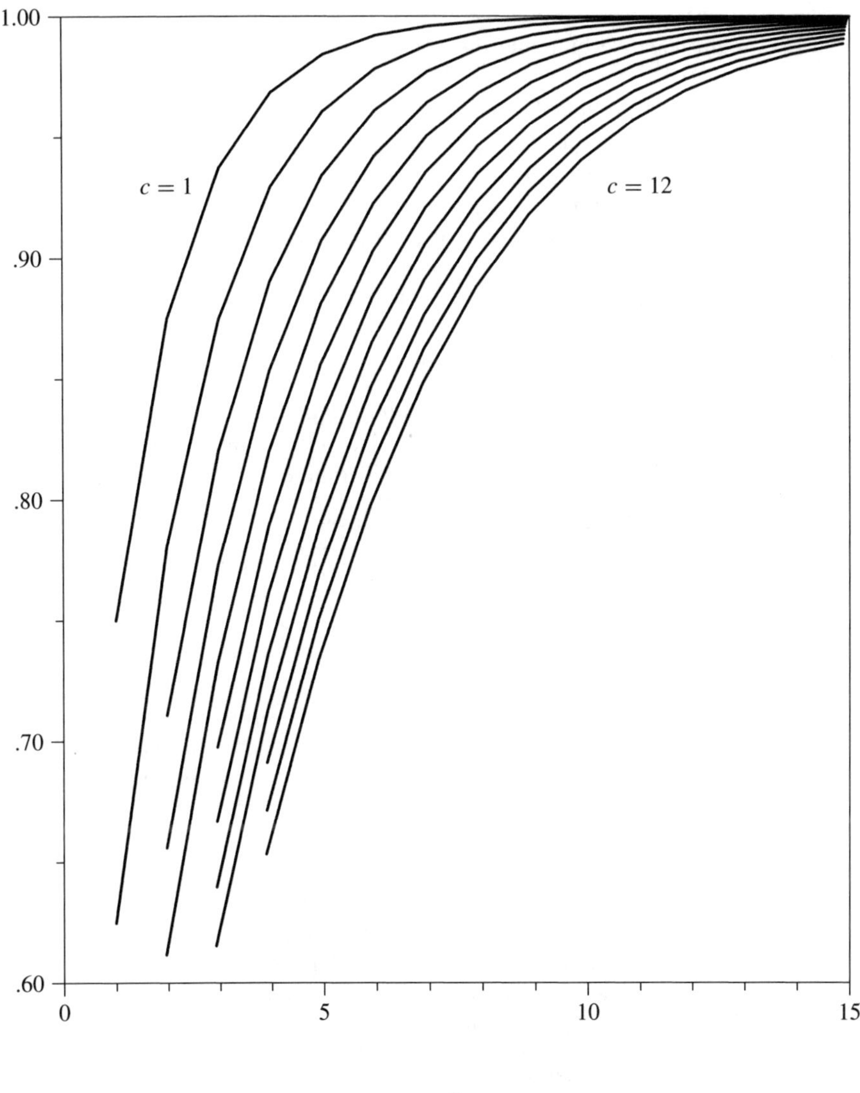

Figure 2.1 The maximum negative binomial cumulative distribution for $c = 1, \ldots, 12$ and $p = 1/2$. Noah needs to capture a total of $y + 2c$ animals in order to have this probability of having at least c of each sex.

then the expected value of the maximum negative binomial distribution (2.4) is equal to $20 - 2c = 16$. If p is 0.25 (or 0.75), then this procedure is expected to terminate after 8.29 patients.

The critical value of 46 for this test consists of the $2c = 4$ minimum required in order to observe 2 of each plus 42 excess trials. The upper 0.05 critical value of the maximum negative binomial distribution is $Y = 42$ for parameters $c = 2$ and $p = 0.1$ or 0.9.

Tables 2.1 and 2.2 provide details and examples of other settings related to this example of genetic testing. Table 2.1 provides the critical values for testing the null hypothesis of $0.1 \le p \le 0.9$ for different values of c and different significance levels. In the previous example, at significance level 0.01, if we need 64 or more observations to observe at least $c = 2$ of both genotypes, then we reject the null hypothesis that the p parameter is between 0.1 and 0.9. This sample of size 64 consists of the 0.01 significance critical value of $Y = 60$ in Table 2.1 plus the $2c = 4$ minimum additional.

Table 2.1 Critical values to test the null hypothesis of $0.1 \le p \le 0.9$ for different significance levels α. The total number of samples necessary is $2c$ more than the values given here.

	Critical values for significance level			
c	$\alpha = 0.1$	$\alpha = 0.05$	$\alpha = 0.01$	$\mathrm{E}[\,Y \mid c, p = 0.1\,]$
1	20	26	42	8.11
2	33	42	60	16.04
3	46	55	75	24.02
4	57	67	89	32.01
5	68	79	102	40.00
10	119	134	163	80.00

Table 2.2 Hypotheses concerning p and $1 - p$ that can be tested at significance level 0.05 and power 0.8 with 50 observations, including the $2c$ minimum.

c	Null hypothesis	Alternative
1	0.0582	0.0044
2	0.0914	0.0166
3	0.1206	0.0309
4	0.1478	0.0463
5	0.1738	0.0624

The critical values in Table 2.1 increase with c and with more extreme significance levels as we would anticipate. Lemma 2.3.1 shows that the expected value for this distribution is approximately $8c$ for $p = 0.1$ or $p = 0.9$.

Table 2.2 lists the hypotheses that can reasonably be tested with a budget that limits us to a total sample of size 50. This sample of size 50 includes the minimum of $2c$ needed. All of the hypotheses listed in this table are being tested with power 0.8 and significance level 0.05. The hypotheses listed in Table 2.2 are for either parameter p or $1 - p$. In this table, we see that larger values of c with a fixed sample size and power prevent us from detecting more extreme alternative hypotheses. Investigators may be reluctant to base their decision to accept or reject the null hypothesis on the basis of only $c = 1$ or two possibly aberrant observations. In Section 2.4, we see that larger values of c are more appropriate in drawing inference when p is closer to 1/2.

2.2 Elementary Properties

Let us describe some of the elementary properties of this distribution and outline the remainder of this chapter. The maximum negative binomial distribution (2.4) has a wide variety of shapes depending on the values of c and p. These are demonstrated in Figs. 2.2 through 2.6. In Section 2.2.2, we derive expressions for the mean and

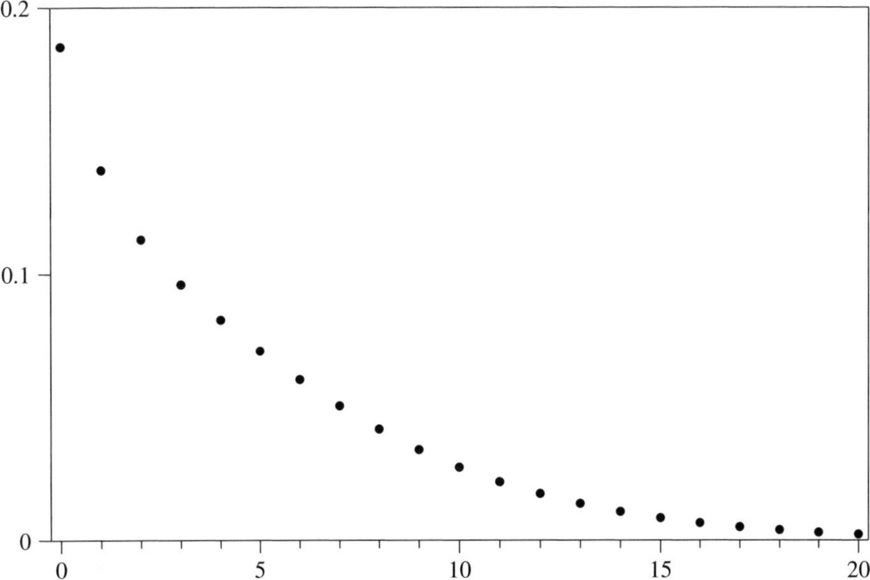

Figure 2.2 The maximum negative binomial distribution at (2.4) for $c = 3$ and $p = 0.3$ has a j-shape similar to that of the geometric distribution.

variance of Y. This distribution may have one or two local modes and these are discussed in Section 2.2.3. Section 2.3 describes asymptotic moments and approximations to the distribution of Y when c is large or when p is extremely close to 0 or 1. Section 2.4 discusses estimation of the parameter p when c is known.

2.2.1 Shapes of the distribution

There are five different shapes of the maximum negative binomial mass function (2.4) depending on the values of the parameters c and p, and these are illustrated in Figs. 2.2 through 2.6. The wide variety of these shapes is largely explained by the derivation of (2.4) as the sum of two separate negative binomial distributions. These two component distributions have mass functions that can be very dissimilar in shape.

When $c = 3$ and $p = 0.3$, Fig. 2.2 shows that the maximum negative binomial distribution has a j-shape much like the geometric distribution. Figure. 2.3 shows that the maximum negative binomial distribution is bimodal for $c = 7$ and $p = 0.3$. In Section 2.2.3, we describe the conditions under which a bimodal shaped distribution occurs.

Figure 2.4 demonstrates that for $c = 25$ and $p = 0.3$, this distribution approaches the shape of a normal distribution. The normal approximation for large values of c is discussed in Section 2.3.1.

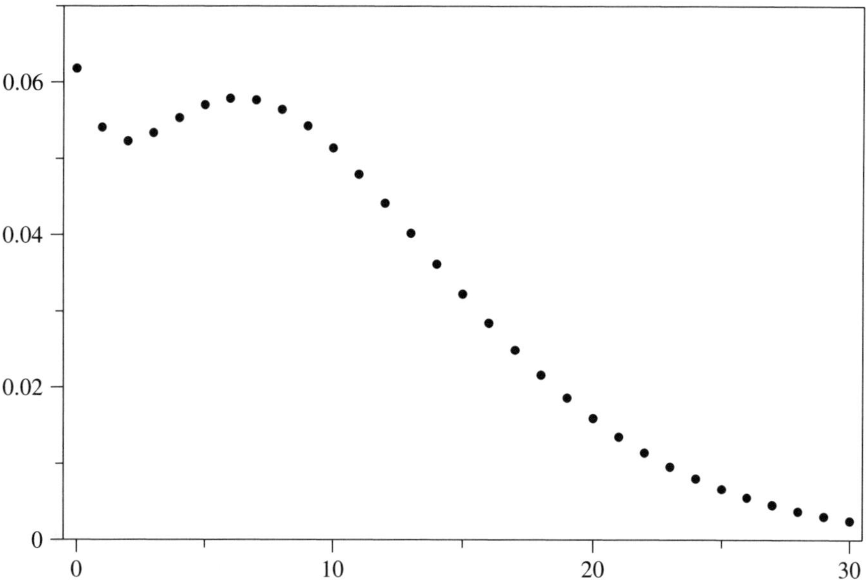

Figure 2.3 The maximum negative binomial distribution is bimodal for $c = 7$ and $p = 0.3$. Table 2.3 gives the conditions under which the distribution is unimodal.

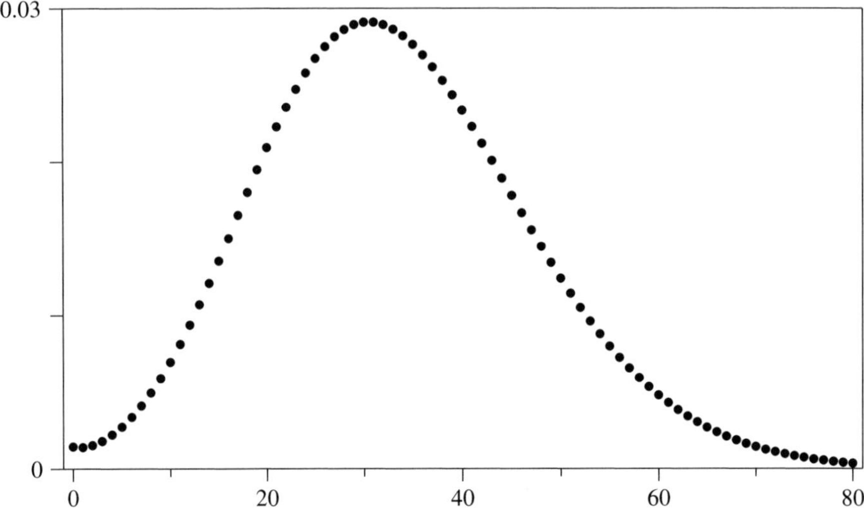

Figure 2.4 The maximum negative binomial distribution has an approximately normal shape for $c = 25$ and $p = 0.3$. An asymptotic normal limiting distribution for large values of c is proved in Lemma 2.3.1.

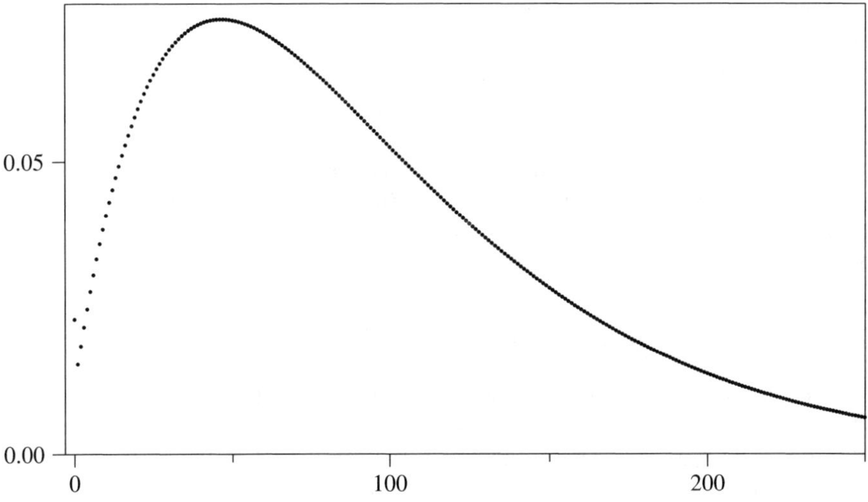

Figure 2.5 The maximum negative binomial distribution for $c = 2$ and $p = 0.02$. An approximate gamma distribution for extreme values of p is described in Lemma 2.3.3. The small local mode at zero is described in Section 2.2.1.

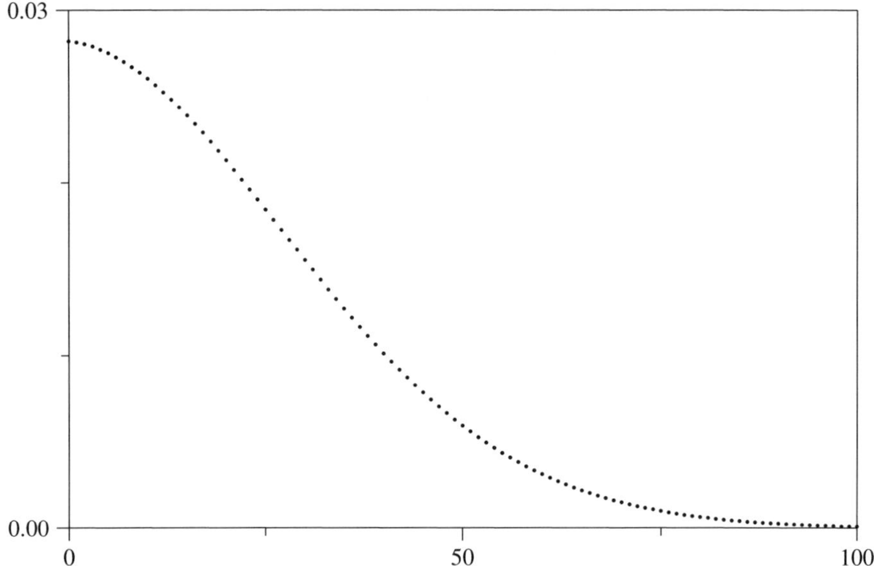

Figure 2.6 The maximum negative binomial distribution for $c = 400$ and $p = 1/2$. A folded or half-normal approximate distribution for large values of c and $p = 1/2$ is given in Lemma 2.3.2.

Figure 2.5 demonstrates another shape for $c = 2$ and $p = 0.02$. A gamma approximation is described in Section 2.3.3 for extreme values of p. The unusual left tail appearing in Fig. 2.5 exhibits a small local mode at zero because one of the two component distributions of the maximum negative binomial has almost all of its mass at zero.

A folded or half-normal distribution is observed in Fig. 2.6 when $p = 1/2$ and c is large. This half-normal approximate distribution is described in Section 2.3.2. In this section, we give expressions for the mean and variance of the maximum negative binomial random variate along with its moment generating function.

2.2.2 Moments of the distribution

The moments of Y can be expressed in terms of negative binomial tail areas. Denote $S_p = \Pr(N_p \geq c)$ where N_p is the negative binomial distributed number of zeros in $\{X_1, X_2, \ldots\}$ before the c–th one is recorded. Similarly, let $S_q = \Pr(N_q \geq c) = 1 - S_p$. There are no simple expressions for S_p (or S_q), but these functions are related to the incomplete beta function as shown below.

Let B_c denote a beta (c, c) random variable with density function

$$f_c(x) = \Gamma(2c)(\Gamma(c))^{-2}x^{c-1}(1 - x)^{c-1} \tag{2.5}$$

for $0 < x < 1$. The mean of B_c is $1/2$ and the variance of B_c is $\{4(2c + 1)\}^{-1}$.

For all p satisfying $0 < p < 1$, Morris (1963) shows

$$S_p = \Pr[B_c \leq p] = \int_0^p f_c(x)\,dx.$$

This result allows us to derive a useful expression for the moment generating function $M_Y(t)$ of the maximum negative binomial variate Y.

Lemma 2.2.1 *For values of t in a neighborhood of zero for which* $pe^t < 1$ *and* $qe^t < 1$, *the moment generating function* $M_Y(t) = \mathrm{E}[\exp(tY)]$ *is expressible as*

$$M_Y(t) = \left(\frac{p\exp(-t)}{1 - q\exp(t)}\right)^c \Pr[B_c \leq q\exp(t)] + \left(\frac{q\exp(-t)}{1 - p\exp(t)}\right)^c \Pr[B_c \leq p\exp(t)]. \tag{2.6}$$

Proof. The moment generating function of Y is expressible as

$$M_Y(t) = \mathrm{E}[\exp(Yt)] = \sum_{k=0}^{\infty} \exp(tk)\binom{2c+k-1}{c-1}(p^k + q^k)(pq)^c$$

$$= \sum_{k=0}^{\infty} \binom{2c+k-1}{c-1}[(p\exp(t))^k + (q\exp(t))^k](pq)^c$$

$$= \sum_{k=c}^{\infty} \binom{c+k-1}{c-1}[(p\exp(t))^k q^c + (q\exp(t))^k p^c]\exp(-ct).$$

Restrict values of t to a neighborhood of zero so that $pe^t < 1$. According to equation (5.30) of Johnson, Kotz, and Kemp (1992, p. 210),

$$\sum_{k=c}^{\infty} \binom{c+k-1}{c-1}[p\exp(t)]^k[1 - p\exp(t)]^c = \int_0^{p\exp(t)} f_c(x)dx = \Pr[B_c \leq p\exp(t)].$$

An analogous formula exists substituting q for p and for values of t for which $qe^t < 1$. Together these complete the proof of (2.6). ■

The expected value of Y is obtained from Lemma 2.2.1 or by conditioning on the value of the Bernoulli variate X_{Y+2c}:

$$\mathrm{E}[Y] = \mathrm{E}[Y \mid N_p \geq c]\Pr[N_p \geq c] + \mathrm{E}[Y \mid N_q \geq c]\Pr[N_q \geq c]$$

$$= S_q(cq/p) + S_p(cp/q) - c + c\binom{2c-1}{c-1}(pq)^{c-1}.$$

A similar conditioning argument or the use of (2.6) shows that the variance of Y is

$$\operatorname{Var}[Y] = cp(cp+1)q^{-2}S_p + cq(cq+1)p^{-2}S_q$$
$$+c\binom{2c-1}{c-1}\left[(c+1)(pq)^{c-2} - (2c+3)(pq)^{c-1}\right] - (\mathrm{E}[Y])^2.$$

The mean and variance of Y are minimized when $p = 1/2$ for any fixed value of c. Similarly, the mean and variance increase with c. The expected value and standard deviation of this distribution are plotted in Figs. 2.7 and 2.8 respectively for $c = 1, \ldots, 5$ and $0 < p < 1$.

In Section 2.3.1, we show that the mean and variance of the maximum negative binomial distribution both grow in proportion to c when c is large. More generally, the moment generating function (2.6) is expanded in Section 2.3 for large values of c and for extreme values of p.

2.2.3 Modes of the distribution

We next examine the modes of the maximum negative binomial distribution. The ratio of the first two masses of (2.4) satisfies

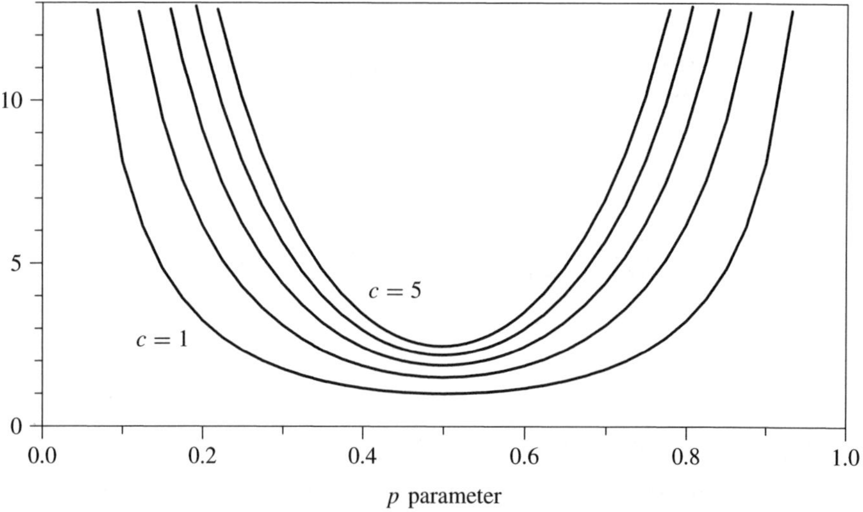

Figure 2.7 Expected value of the maximum negative binomial distribution for $c = 1, \ldots, 5$. When p is close to zero or one, then the mean is approximately c/p or $c/(1-p)$ respectively. The behavior of the distribution with extreme values of p is discussed in Section 2.3.3.

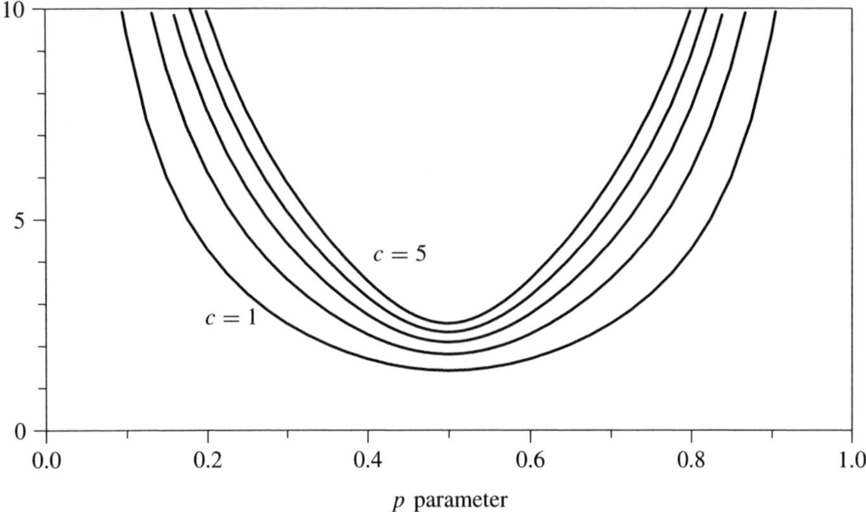

Figure 2.8 Standard deviation of the maximum negative binomial distribution for $c = 1, \ldots, 5$.

$$\frac{\Pr(Y = 0)}{\Pr(Y = 1)} = \frac{c + 1}{c} > 1,$$

showing that this distribution always has at least a local mode at $Y = 0$.

The local mode for Y at zero is clearly visible in Figs. 2.2, 2.3, 2.5, and 2.6. The local mode at zero is also present although it is very small in Fig. 2.4. There may also exist a second mode away from zero for this distribution, as seen in Figs. 2.3, 2.4, and 2.5.

Table 2.3 describes the ranges of the p parameter that give rise to distributions with a single mode at zero. If $c = 1$, then the maximum negative binomial distribution is always unimodal. For other values of c, the maximum negative binomial distribution has a single mode at zero when the parameter p is in a sufficiently small neighborhood centered around $p = 1/2$.

Roughly speaking, bimodal distributions occur when p is relatively close to either zero or one. The range of values for p that exhibit unimodal distributions becomes narrower with larger values of c. The limiting behavior of this distribution with large values of c when $p = 1/2$ is a folded normal distribution that is described in Section 2.3.2 and illustrated in Fig. 2.6.

2.3 Asymptotic Approximations

There are three useful approximations to the maximum negative binomial distribution of Y with mass function given in (2.4). For large values of c, we obtain

Table 2.3 Range of values of the p parameter with unimodal maximum negative binomial distributions.

c parameter	Range of p	
1	Always unimodal	
2	0.15	0.85
3	0.22	0.78
4	0.25	0.75
5	0.28	0.72
10	0.35	0.65
25	0.41	0.59
50	0.439	0.561
100	0.458	0.542
250	0.4746	0.5254
500	0.4825	0.5175

two different asymptotic expansions for the distribution of Y. If c is large and $p \neq 1/2$, then Y behaves approximately normal as seen in Fig. 2.4. If c is large and $p = 1/2$, then Fig. 2.6 illustrates the approximate half-normal behavior that is proved in Lemma 2.3.2. If c is held fixed and p is extremely close to either 0 or 1, then Y (suitably scaled) has an approximate gamma distribution as seen in Fig. 2.5. This gamma approximation is described in Section 2.3.3.

2.3.1 Large values of c and $p \neq 1/2$

Here we show the behavior of the maximum negative binomial random variate Y when c is large. Separate results will be shown first for $p \neq 1/2$ and then for $p = 1/2$. Roughly speaking, when $p < 1/2$ and c is large, then N_p will tend to be much larger than N_q with high probability, and the second term in the moment generating function of Y given in (2.6) will be negligible. In other words, for large c and $p < 1/2$, the behavior of the maximum negative binomial variate Y will be the same as that of the negative binomial N_p random variable. Conversely, for $p > 1/2$, the random variables Y and N_q will have nearly the same distributions when c is large. The limiting normal behavior of Y in either of these two cases follows that of the usual negative binomial distribution and is detailed more formally in Lemma 2.3.1, below.

We first approximate the mean and variance of Y for large values of c and $p < 1/2$. These moments are

$$\mathrm{E}[\,Y\,] = c(q-p)/p \quad \text{and} \quad \mathrm{Var}[\,Y\,] = cq/p^2$$

plus terms that are $o(c)$ when c is large. Symmetric formulas for these moments occur when $p > 1/2$.

Lemma 2.3.1 *For all fixed* $0 < p < 1/2$, *if* c *grows without bound then the random variable*

$$Z = \{pY - c(q-p)\} \Big/ (cq)^{1/2}$$

has an approximately standard normal distribution.

Proof. Use Lemma 2.2.1 to show that the moment generating function of Z is

$$\begin{aligned} \mathrm{E}[\mathrm{e}^{tZ}] = \exp\Big[-ct(q-p)\Big/(cq)^{1/2}\Big] \\ \times \big\{(\gamma(1-q\gamma)/p)^{-c}\ \Pr[B_c \le q\gamma] \\ + (\gamma(1-p\gamma)/q)^{-c}\ \Pr[B_c \le p\gamma]\big\} \end{aligned}$$

where

$$\gamma = \gamma(t) = \exp[pt/(cq)^{1/2}].$$

For all values of c sufficiently large and some $\epsilon > 0$, we have $p\gamma < 1$ and $q\gamma < 1$ for all $|\, t \,| < \epsilon$ so $\mathrm{E}[\mathrm{e}^{tZ}]$ is well defined in this open interval of t containing 0.

The most important term in the expression for $\mathrm{E}[\mathrm{e}^{tZ}]$ is

$$\Delta = \Delta(t) = \exp\Big[-ct(q-p)\Big/(cq)^{1/2}\Big]\,\big[\gamma(1-q\gamma)/p\big]^{-c}$$

so write

$$\log\Delta = pt(c/q)^{1/2} - c\log(\gamma) - t(cq)^{1/2} - c\log[1 - q(\gamma-1)/p]$$

and expand Δ for large values of c, giving

$$\begin{aligned} \log\Delta &= -t(cq)^{1/2} - c\log[1 - t(q/c)^{1/2} - pt^2/2c + \mathrm{O}(c^{-3/2})] \\ &= t^2/2 + \mathrm{O}(c^{-1/2}). \end{aligned}$$

The two probabilities appearing in the expression for $\mathrm{E}[\mathrm{e}^{tZ}]$ are examined as follows. For all sufficiently large values of c, all $|\, t \,| < \epsilon$, and $0 < p < 1/2$, there exists a δ satisfying $0 < \delta < 1/2$ such that $p\gamma \le 1/2 - \delta$. Then write

$$\begin{aligned} \Pr[\, B_c \le p\gamma \,] &\le \Pr[\, B_c \le 1/2 - \delta \,] \\ &\le \Pr[\, |\, B_c - 1/2 \,| \ge \delta \,] \end{aligned}$$

The random variable B_c has mean 1/2 and variance $[4(2c+1)]^{-1}$. Tchebychev's inequality shows

$$\Pr[\, B_c \le p\gamma \,] \le [4\delta^2(2c+1)]^{-1},$$

demonstrating that $\Pr[B_c \le p\gamma]$ is negligible.

A similar argument proves that $\Pr[B_c \leq q\gamma]$ is very close to one. Ignore this extremely small difference between $\Pr[B_c \leq q\gamma]$ and one to show

$$\mathrm{E}[\,\mathrm{e}^{tZ}\,] = \exp(t^2/2) + R + \mathrm{O}(c^{-1/2}),$$

where the remainder term R satisfies

$$R = \exp[-t(cq)^{1/2}]\,[\gamma(1-p\gamma)/q]^{-c}\ \Pr[B_c \leq p\gamma]$$

and will be shown to be negligibly small.

Write

$$-c\log[\gamma(1-p\gamma)/q] = -c\log(\gamma) - c\log[1 - p(\gamma-1)/q] = \mathrm{O}(c^{1/2})$$

for all $|\,t\,| < \epsilon$ so that

$$\log R = c\log(1-4\delta^2) + \mathrm{O}(c^{1/2}).$$

The leading term and coefficient of c^1 is negative, so R is exponentially small with large values of c. The moment generating function of Z then approaches that of the standard normal distribution completing the proof. ■

2.3.2 Large values of c and $p = 1/2$

A separate set of asymptotic results are needed when $p = 1/2$. The approximate half-normal behavior of the maximum negative binomial distribution with $p = 1/2$ and large values of c can be seen in Fig. 2.6. The folded or half-normal distribution (Stuart and Ord, 1987, p. 117) is that of $|\,Z\,|$, where Z is a standard normal random variable.

In the particular case of $p = q = 1/2$, the moment generating function of the maximum negative binomial distribution given in (2.6) is

$$M_Y(t \mid p = 1/2) \;=\; 2[\exp(t)(2-\exp(t))]^{-c}\,\Pr[B_c \leq \exp(t)/2],$$

from which we show

$$\mathrm{E}[\,Y \mid p = 1/2\,] = 2^{2-2c}\Gamma(2c)/\{\Gamma(c)\}^2$$

$$\mathrm{Var}[\,Y \mid p = 1/2\,] = 2c + \mathrm{E}[\,Y \mid p = 1/2\,] - \{\mathrm{E}[\,Y \mid p = 1/2\,]\}^2$$

for all values of $c > 0$.

When c is large, we have the following approximations from Stirling's formula:

$$\begin{aligned}\mathrm{E}[\,Y \mid p = 1/2\,] &= 2(c/\pi)^{1/2}\{1 - (8c)^{-1} + \mathrm{O}(c^{-2})\}\\ \mathrm{Var}[\,Y \mid p = 1/2\,] &= (2-4/\pi)c + 2(c/\pi)^{1/2} - 1/\pi\\ &\qquad -(\pi c)^{-1/2}/4 + \mathrm{O}(c^{-1}).\end{aligned}$$

Lemma 2.3.2 *For large values of c and $p = 1/2$, the random variable*

$$Z' = (2c)^{-1/2} Y$$

has an approximately half-normal distribution.

Proof. We expand the probability mass function of the maximum negative binomial random variable Y given in (2.4) to approximate the density function $f_{Z'}$ of Z'. That is, define

$$f_{Z'}(z) = (2c)^{1/2} \Pr[\, Y = (2c)^{1/2} z \,],$$

where $(2c)^{1/2}$ is the Jacobian of the transformation from Y to Z'. We restrict attention to values of z that are $O(c^{1/2})$. Take logs and expand all factorials according to Stirling's formula to show that $f_{Z'}$ can be written as

$$\log f_{Z'}(z) = 1 + \log(2/\pi)/2 + [2c + (2c)^{1/2} z - 1/2] \log[1 + (2c)^{-1/2} z]$$

$$-[2c + (2c)^{1/2} z + 1/2] \log[1 + (2c)^{-1/2} z + c^{-1}] + O_p(c^{-1/2}).$$

Next, use $z = O(c^{1/2})$ and expand both logarithms as $\log(1 + \epsilon) = \epsilon - \epsilon^2/2 + O(\epsilon^3)$ showing

$$\log f_{Z'}(z) = \log(2/\pi)/2 - z^2/2$$

plus terms that are $O(c^{-1/2})$ with high probability. This is the logarithm of the density function of the half-normal distribution, completing the proof. ■

2.3.3 Extreme values of p

An approximate gamma distribution for the maximum negative binomial random variable Y is obtained when p is very close to either 0 or 1 and c is held fixed. This behavior can be seen in Fig. 2.5 and will be proved more formally here.

Lemma 2.3.3 *If p is close to zero and c is held fixed, then the random variable*

$$G = pY$$

behaves approximately as the sum of c independent standard exponential random variables.

Proof. The moment generating function of G is

$$\begin{aligned} M_G(t) &= \mathrm{E}\,[\, e^{tG} \,] \\ &= \{q \exp(-pt)/[1 - p\exp(pt)]\}^c \; \Pr[B_c \le p\exp(pt)] \\ &\quad + \{p\exp(-pt)/[1 - q\exp(pt)]\}^c \; \Pr[B_c \le q\exp(pt)], \end{aligned}$$

where B_c is a beta(c, c) random variable with density function f_c defined at (2.5).

For bounded values of t and all p close to zero, we have

$$\Pr[\, B_c \leq p \exp(pt)\,] = \mathrm{O}(p),$$

$$\Pr[\, B_c \leq q \exp(pt)\,] = 1 + \mathrm{O}(p),$$

and

$$\{q \exp(-pt)/[1 - p \exp(pt)]\}^c = 1 + \mathrm{O}(p)$$

so that

$$M_G(t) = \{p \exp(-pt)/[1 - q \exp(pt)]\}^c + \mathrm{O}(p).$$

Then write

$$\exp(-pt) = 1 + \mathrm{O}(p)$$

and

$$\exp(pt) = 1 + pt + \mathrm{O}(p^2)$$

to show

$$\begin{aligned}\{p \exp(-pt)/[1 - q \exp(pt)]\}^c &= \{p[1 + \mathrm{O}(p)]/[p - pt + \mathrm{O}(p^2)]\}^c \\ &= (1 - t)^{-c}\end{aligned}$$

plus terms that tend to zero as $\mathrm{O}(p)$. This is the moment generating function of the sum of c independent standard exponential random variables, completing the proof. ■

Intuitively, when p is small, the Bernoulli sequence $X_1, X_2, \ldots$ will consist mostly of 0's and the normalized times between the rare 1's will have an approximately standard exponential distribution. Similar results hold, by symmetry, for values of p close to one.

2.4 Estimation of p

We consider inference on the Bernoulli population parameter p on the basis of one maximum negative binomial observation y. Throughout we will assume that the value of c is known. A difficulty stems from the lack of identifiability in p and q. Unless we observe the number of successes and failures as well as the total number of trials $Y + 2c$ we are unable to tell if we are estimating p or $q = 1 - p$.

The maximum likelihood estimate of p, denoted by $\widehat{p}$, will be derived with its asymptotic variance. If we know *a priori* that $p < 1/2$, then $\widehat{p}$ has the same asymptotic $(c \to \infty)$ distribution as the maximum likelihood estimate of p when y is sampled from the negative binomial distribution N_p. We extend these results when a sample $y_1, \ldots, y_n$ of maximum negative binomial variates are observed. Section 2.4.3 describes a Bayesian estimate for p.

2.4.1 The likelihood function

The likelihood kernel of the maximum negative binomial distribution

$$l(p) = l(p \mid y) = (pq)^c \, (p^y + q^y)$$

is symmetric about $p = 1/2$ for all values of c and y.

The function $l(p)$ is a polynomial in p of degree $2c + y$. An example of the bimodal shape of l for $c = 3$ is illustrated in Fig. 2.9 for observed values of $y =$

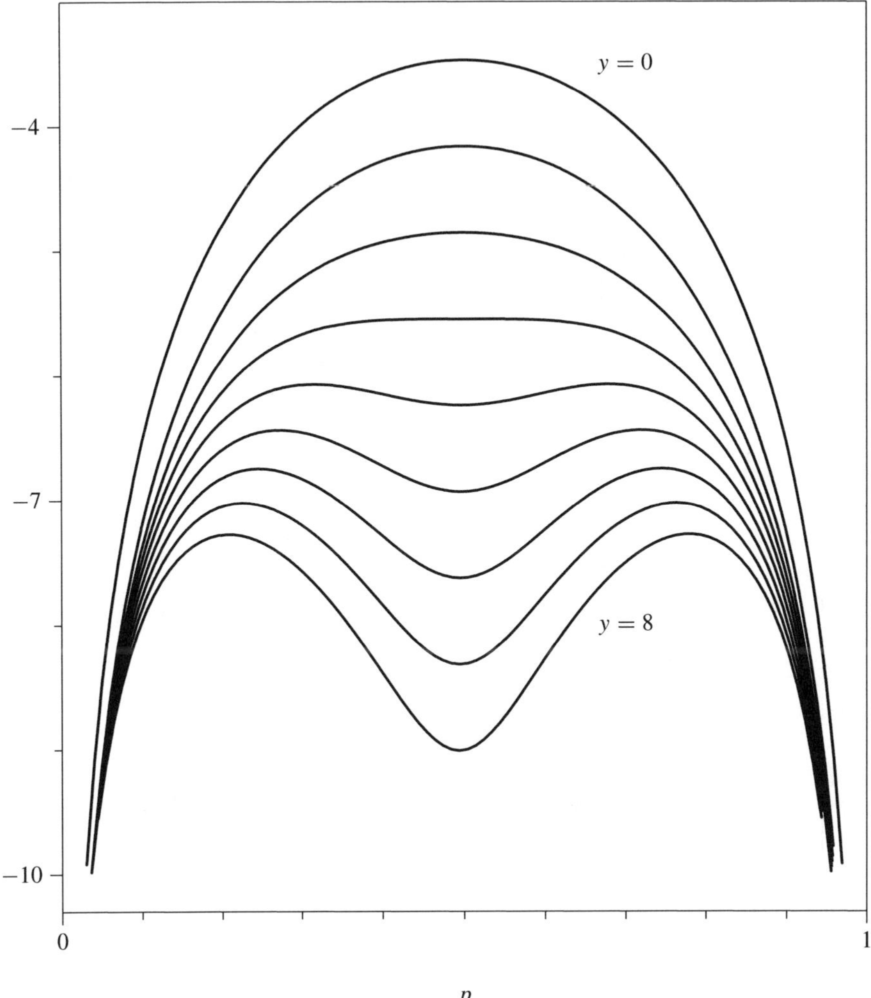

Figure 2.9 The log of the likelihood kernel function $l(p)$ for $c = 3$ and $y = 0, \ldots, 8$.

$0, \dots, 8$. Lemma 2.6.1 in the appendix of Section 2.6 proves that the likelihood kernel function $l(p)$ has a unique mode at $p = 1/2$ if and only if the condition

$$y(y-1) \leq 2c \tag{2.7}$$

holds.

The relation in (2.7) shows that there is a positive probability that the maximum likelihood estimate $\widehat{p}$ of p will equal 1/2. Specifically, Fig. 2.10 plots the

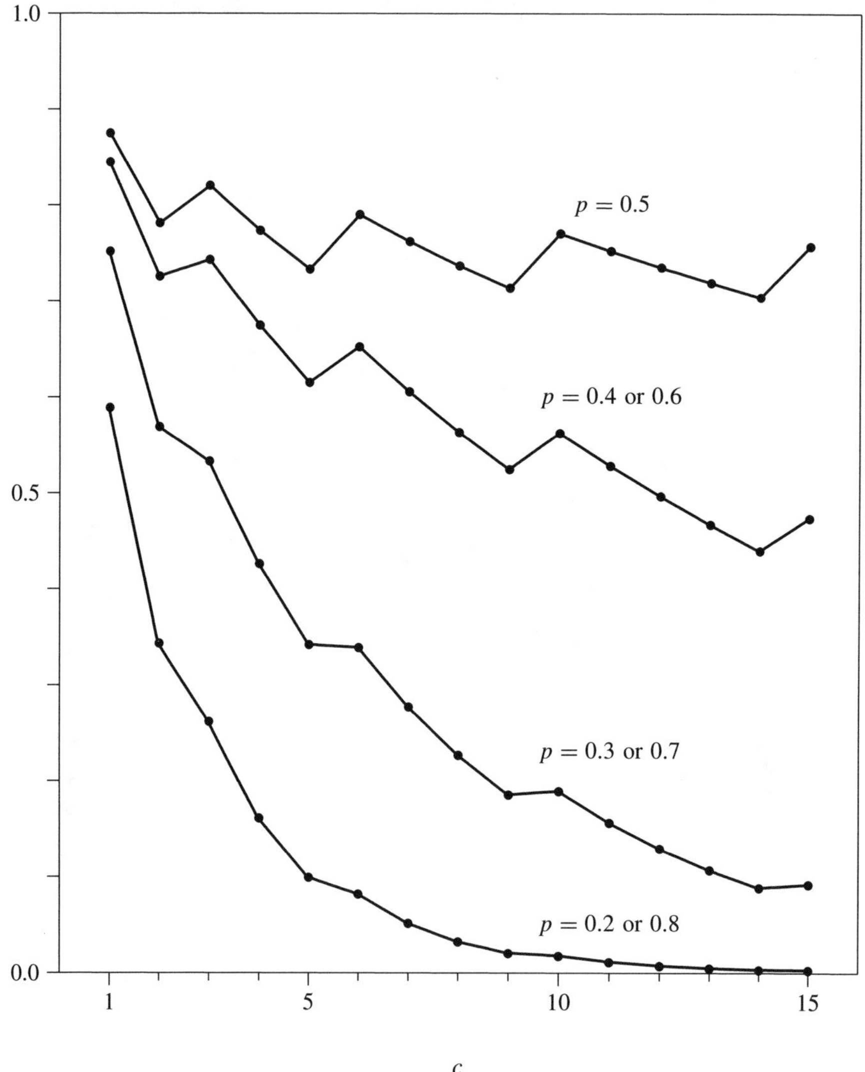

Figure 2.10 The probability that the maximum likelihood estimator $\widehat{p}$ is equal to 1/2 for $c = 1, \dots, 15$. Values of the population parameter p are given.

values of

$$\Pr[\,\widehat{p} = 1/2 \mid c, p\,] = \Pr[\,y(y-1) \le 2c\,]$$

for values of $c = 1, \ldots, 15$ and several values of the population parameter p. These probabilities are generally decreasing with c but are not monotonic because equality in (2.7) does not have integer solutions for y.

It is difficult to statistically distinguish between values of p near 1/2. In Fig. 2.10, we see that up to values of $c = 15$, if p is anywhere between 0.4 and 0.6, then there is at least .5 probability that the maximum likelihood estimated value of p will be 1/2. Much larger values of c are necessary if we want to estimate p near 1/2.

If (2.7) does not hold, then $l(p)$ has two modes symmetric around $p = 1/2$ as illustrated in the example of Fig. 2.9. In other words, if y is small, relative to the value of c, then we estimate the value of p to be 1/2. Conversely, if we observe a relatively large value of y, then the maximum likelihood estimates of p are away from and symmetric about 1/2. Fig. 2.11 plots the maximum likelihood estimate of p for $c = 1, \ldots, 6$ and all possible observations $y = 0, \ldots, 15$.

As a numerical example, suppose $c = 3$ and we observe $y = 3$, then $l(p \mid y = 3)$ has one mode at $\widehat{p} = 1/2$. Similarly, if $c = 3$ and we observe $y = 4$, then $l(p)$ has two equivalent modes at $\widehat{p} = 0.3181$ and 0.6819. The bimodal shape of $l(p)$ with $c = 3$ and $y = 4$ is illustrated in Fig. 2.9.

Unless we are able to observe the Bernoulli sequence $X_1, X_2, \ldots$ and know that the experiment ends with either $X_{Y+2c} = 0$ or $X_{Y+2c} = 1$, we cannot tell if we are estimating p or $1 - p$, on the basis of only the total number of trials $y + 2c$. This problem with identifiability cannot be resolved using maximum likelihood alone. The EM algorithm for this problem, described in Section 2.4.2 , takes the approach of a missing data setting in which we simultaneously estimate the values of p and X_{Y+2c}. A Bayesian approach to this identifiability problem, described in Section 2.4.3, is only useful if the prior distribution of p is not symmetric in p about 1/2.

Before we introduce the EM algorithm in (2.8) and (2.9) below, let us compare the modes of $l(p)$ with those estimates of p assuming negative binomial sampling. The maximum likelihood estimate $\widehat{p}_{N_p}$ of p in the negative binomial distribution of N_p is

$$\widehat{p}_{N_p} = c/(y + 2c)$$

and the estimate $\widehat{p}_{N_q}$ of $p = 1 - q$ in the distribution of N_q is

$$\widehat{p}_{N_q} = (y + c) \,/\, (y + 2c).$$

These estimates are symmetric about $p = 1/2$.

Lemma 2.6.2 in the Appendix shows that when (2.7) does not hold, then $l(p)$ has two equivalent modes that are less extreme (*i.e.* closer to 1/2) than either of the values $\widehat{p}_{N_p}$ and $\widehat{p}_{N_q}$. For the example of $c = 3$ and $y = 4$ illustrated in Fig. 2.9, the local modes of $l(p)$ at 0.3181 and 0.6819 are closer to 1/2 than the corresponding negative binomial estimates $\widehat{p}_{N_p} = 0.3$ and $\widehat{p}_{N_q} = 0.7$.

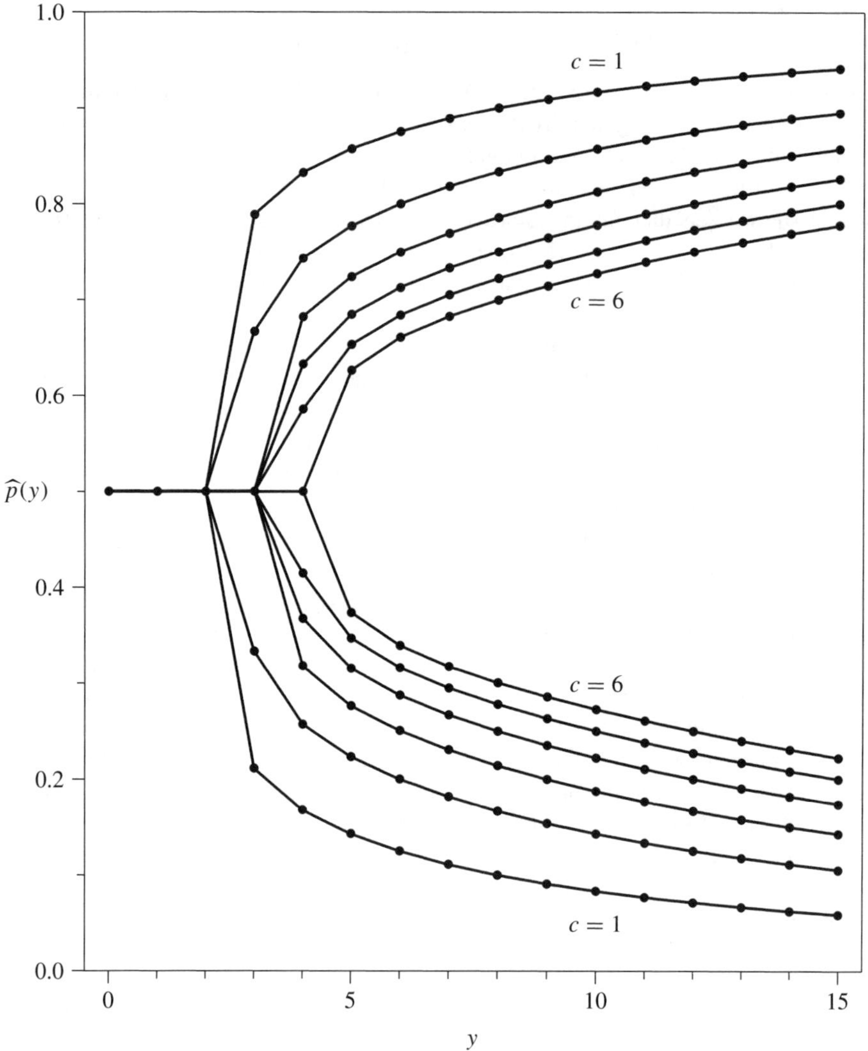

Figure 2.11 The maximum likelihood estimate of p for all $c = 1, \ldots, 6$ and observed value of $y = 0, 1, \ldots, 15$.

This statement about the location of the modes is also confirmed next. We will use the EM algorithm to show that the maximum likelihood estimate of either $\widehat{p}$ or $1 - \widehat{p}$ in the maximum negative binomial distribution is a weighted average of the maximum likelihood estimates of p in the negative binomial distributions of N_p and N_q, respectively.

2.4.2 The EM estimate

Let J denote the indicator of the event of $\{N_p > N_q\}$. That is, $J = 1$ if $X_{Y+2c} = 1$. Similarly, $J = 0$ is the indicator of the event $\{N_p < N_q\}$ or, equivalently, $X_{Y+2c} = 0$. The joint probability of Y and J is proportional to

$$\Pr[\, y,\ j \mid p\,] \propto p^{c+y(1-j)}\, q^{c+jy}.$$

According to the EM method (Dempster, Laird, and Rubin, 1977), the maximum likelihood estimate $\widehat{p}$ of the maximum negative binomial distribution can be obtained as the limit of $(p_k,\ J_k)$, defined by alternating between the equations

$$p_{k+1} = p(J_k) = (1 - J_k)\frac{y+c}{y+2c} + J_k\frac{c}{y+2c} \tag{2.8}$$

and

$$J_{k+1} = J(p_k) = \mathrm{E}[\, J \mid y, p_k\,] = q_k^y \,/ \left(p_k^y + q_k^y\right). \tag{2.9}$$

The estimators $c/(y + 2c)$ and $(y + c)/(y + 2c)$ in (2.8) are the maximum likelihood estimates for parameter p in the negative binomial distributions of N_p and N_q, respectively. The estimate $\widehat{p}$ is then a weighted average of these two estimates, and will be less extreme (that is, closer to $1/2$) than either of these. This statement is presented more formally as Lemma 2.6.2 in Section 2.6.

This EM algorithm is implemented in the R program given in Table 2.4. Section 2.5 includes a numerical example of the EM algorithm in practice and demonstrates how exact confidence intervals for p may be constructed.

Specifically, when (2.7) does not hold, there are two solutions denoted $(p^*,\ J^*)$ and $(1 - p^*,\ 1 - J^*)$ for the EM equations (2.8) and (2.9). When $p^* < 1/2$ then $J^* > 1/2$ and

$$c/(y + 2c) < p^* < 1/2.$$

To show the convergence of the EM sequence $(p_k,\ J_k)$, suppose we start with initial values of $p_0 < 1/2$ and $J_0 > 1/2$. Then $p_{k+1} < 1/2$ and $J_{k+1} > 1/2$ for all successive iterations, so the algorithm will not alternate between p^* and $1 - p^*$.

Using the theorem of Louis (1982), the observed Fisher information is

$$\widehat{I} = -\frac{\partial^2 \log l(\widehat{p})}{\partial p^2} = \frac{y+2c}{\widehat{p}\widehat{q}} - \frac{(1-\widehat{J})\widehat{J}\,y^2}{(\widehat{p}\widehat{q})^2}. \tag{2.10}$$

This relation is symmetric in (p, q) and $(J, 1 - J)$, so it does not matter if $\widehat{J}$ converges to 0 or 1.

When c is very large and we know that $p < 1/2$, then the smaller mode of $l(p)$ has the same asymptotic distribution as the maximum likelihood estimate

$\widehat{p}_{N_p}$ of p when y is sampled from the negative binomial distribution N_p. The proof of Lemma 2.3.1 shows that when c is large and $p < 1/2$, then with high probability N_p will be much larger than N_q. In this case, the maximum negative binomial distribution coincides with the negative binomial distribution of N_p with probability approaching one.

Using the approximation of Bahadur (1960), $1 - \widehat{J}$ estimates

$$\Pr[N_p \geq c] = (4pq)^c/(2\sqrt{c\pi})[(c+1)/(c(q-p)+1)](1+\mathrm{O}(c^{-1})).$$

Since $0 \leq \widehat{J} \leq 1$, the variance of $\widehat{J}$ satisfies

$$\mathrm{Var}[\widehat{J}] \leq \mathrm{E}[\widehat{J}] - \{\mathrm{E}[\widehat{J}]\}^2 = \mathrm{O}[c^{-1/2}(4pq)^c].$$

According to Tchebychev inequality, $\widehat{J}$ converges to one in probability when $p < 1/2$ and c becomes large. Using the Slutsky theorem (Chow and Teicher (1988), pp. 254), we see that for large values of c, the maximum likelihood estimate $\widehat{p}$ has the same asymptotic distribution as $c/(y+2c)$, which is the maximum likelihood estimate for parameter p in the distribution of N_p.

Under N_p negative binomial sampling with $p < 1/2$ and large values of c, the maximum likelihood estimator $c/(y+2c)$ of p has an approximate normal distribution with mean p and variance p^2q/c. For large values of c,

$$c^{1/2}(\widehat{p} - p)/(p^2q)^{1/2}$$

behaves approximately as standard normal. Similarly, $\widehat{I}/c$ converges in probability to $1/(p^2q)$.

In general, let $y_1, \ldots, y_n$ be a random sample from the maximum negative binomial distribution with c known and common p parameter known to be either less than or greater than 1/2. We can use the EM algorithm to obtain the maximum likelihood estimate $\widehat{p}$, alternating between the equations

$$\widehat{p} = \widehat{p}(\widehat{J}_1, \ldots, \widehat{J}_n) = \sum_{i=1}^{n}[(1-\widehat{J}_i)y_i + c] \bigg/ \sum_{i=1}^{n}(y_i + 2c)$$

and

$$\widehat{J}_i = \mathrm{E}[J_i \mid y_i, p = \widehat{p}] = \widehat{q}^{y_i} \big/ \left(\widehat{p}^{y_i} + \widehat{q}^{y_i}\right).$$

The observed Fisher information can be expressed as

$$\widehat{I} = \sum_{i=1}^{n} (y_i + 2c)/(\widehat{p}\,\widehat{q}) - (1-\widehat{J}_i)\,\widehat{J}_i\,{y_i}^2/(\widehat{pq})^2.$$

Lemma 2.4.1 *The maximum likelihood estimate* $\widehat{p}$ *has an asymptotic normal distribution with the mean* p *and variance* $1/\widehat{I}$ *when* n *is large.*

Proof. We restrict our attention to the parameter space of p in $[0, 0.5)$. Suppose that $\widehat{p}_n$ is the smaller maximum likelihood estimate $(0 \le \widehat{p}_n \le 1/2)$. We will first show that with probability equal to one, there is the unique maximum likelihood estimate of $\widehat{p}_n$ in $[0, 0.5)$, so then a standard large sample theory can be applied to show the asymptotic normality of $\widehat{p}_n$ (Lehmann (1983), Sections 6.1–6.3).

The log-likelihood function is written as

$$h(p) = nc \log(pq) + \sum_{i=1}^{n} \log(p^{y_i} + q^{y_i})$$

and the score function is

$$\begin{aligned} \partial h(p)/\partial p &= nc(p^{-1} - q^{-1}) + \sum_i y_i (p^{y_i - 1} - q^{y_i - 1})/[p^{y_i} + q^{y_i}] \\ &= (pq)^{-1} \left[nc(q-p) - p \sum y_i + \sum y_i\, p^{y_i}/(p^{y_i} + q^{y_i}) \right]. \end{aligned}$$

The score function has the unique solution to $\partial h/\partial p = 0$ of p in $[0, 0.5)$ if and only if the function

$$g(p) = nc(q-p) - p \sum y_i + \sum y_i\, p^{y_i}/[p^{y_i} + q^{y_i}]$$

has the unique root in $[0, 0.5)$. The root $p = 1/2$ of $g(p) = 0$ is outside this interval.

The function

$$nc(q-p) - p \sum y_i$$

is linear in p and has the unique zero solution in $[0, 0.5)$.

The function

$$\sum_i y_i\, p^{y_i} / \{p^{y_i} + q^{y_i}\}$$

is positive and strictly increasing in p for $0 \le p < 1/2$. The equation $g(p) = 0$ then has a unique solution in $0 \le p < 1/2$ if and only if

$$\partial g(p)/\partial p \,|_{p=1/2} > 0.$$

We see

$$\partial g(p)/\partial p = -2nc - \sum y_i + \sum y_i^2 (pq)^{y_i - 1}/(p^{y_i} + q^{y_i})$$

so that

$$\partial g(p)/\partial p \,|_{p=1/2} = -2nc - \sum y_i + \sum y_i^2 > 0$$

which is equivalent to

$$n^{-1} \sum y_i^2 - n^{-1} \sum y_i > 2c. \tag{2.11}$$

The expected value and variance derived in Section 2.2.2 show

$$\mathrm{E}[\,Y^2\,] - \mathrm{E}[\,Y\,] > 2c$$

so that with probability one, the inequality (2.11) holds. That is, there is the unique solution to $g(p) = 0$ in $[0, 0.5)$.

Finally, note that there is a unique maximum of the log-likelihood function of $h(p)$ at $p = 0.5$ if and only if

$$n^{-1} \sum_i y_i^2 - n^{-1} \sum_i y_i \leq 2c$$

which simplifies to inequality (2.7) when $n = 1$. ■

2.4.3 A Bayesian estimate of p

A Bayesian estimate for the p parameter on the basis of a single observed value of y may be useful in the maximum negative binomial distribution. Let us assume a beta(α, β) prior distribution on p with density function

$$f(p) = p^{\alpha-1} q^{\beta-1} \Gamma(\alpha+\beta)/\Gamma(\alpha)\Gamma(\beta)$$

for $0 < p < 1$ and parameters $\alpha > 0$ and $\beta > 0$.

The prior mean of p is $\alpha/(\alpha+\beta)$. If $\alpha \neq \beta$, then the beta prior distribution $f(p)$ is asymmetric and can be useful in overcoming the identifiability problem in the estimation of p or $q = 1 - p$.

The posterior density function of p given y

$$f(p \mid y) = \frac{\left(p^{c+y+\alpha-1} q^{c+\beta-1} + p^{c+\alpha-1} q^{c+y+\beta-1}\right) \Gamma(2c+y+\alpha+\beta)}{\Gamma(c+y+\alpha)\Gamma(c+\beta) + \Gamma(c+\alpha)\Gamma(c+y+\beta)}$$

is a weighted average of two beta densities with weights w and $1 - w$, where the weight

$$w = \frac{\Gamma(c+y+\alpha)\Gamma(c+\beta)}{\Gamma(c+y+\alpha)\Gamma(c+\beta) + \Gamma(c+\alpha)\Gamma(c+y+\beta)}$$

satisfies $0 < w < 1$.

The posterior mean of p is

$$\mathrm{E}[\,p \mid y\,] = \frac{c+\alpha+wy}{2c+\alpha+\beta+y}.$$

If $\alpha = \beta$, then the prior and posterior means of p are both equal to 1/2 regardless of the value of y observed. Furthermore, $w(\alpha = \beta) = 1/2$ so the posterior distribution of p can have two equivalent modes, symmetric about 1/2. In other words, a symmetric beta prior distribution on p with mean 1/2 provides no additional benefit in resolution of the identifiability problem. An asymmetric prior distribution will favor one of the two, otherwise equivalent, modes.

2.5 Programs and Numerical Results

This section presents two S-plus/R programs written for fitting and describing the maximum negative binomial distribution. The first of these (`dmnb`) returns the value of the probability mass function for specified values of Y and parameters c and p. This program was used to obtain the ordinates of the plots in Figs. 2.2 through 2.6, for example.

The `EMmnb` program in Table 2.4 obtains the maximum likelihood estimate of p (and $1-p$) using the EM algorithm described in (2.8) and (2.9). This program prints the EM estimates of the indicator J_k, estimating the value of x_{y+2c} that ends the sequence of Bernoulli trials. Each EM iteration includes the value of the gradient, or derivative of the likelihood kernel $l(p)$ at each estimate p_k.

An example of these iterations is given in Table 2.5 for the specific case of $y=7$ and $c=3$. The converged values are $p^*=0.2309$ and $J^*=0.9998$ (or equivalently $p^*=0.7691$ and $J^*=0.0002$). The Fisher information calculated in (2.10) is equal to 73.548 and the approximate standard error of p^* is

$$(73.548)^{-1/2}=0.1166.$$

An exact confidence interval for p can also be obtained for this example. The identifiability issue in this distribution explains why the confidence interval is sometimes expressed as a *pair* of intervals, corresponding to p and $1-p$. These intervals are symmetric about $p=1/2$. The two intervals could be distinct or else might overlap. This phenomenon is illustrated as follows.

Consider the example described above, for which $y=7$ and $c=3$. The exact 90% confidence interval is obtained by solving for values of p in the equations

$$\Pr[\,Y\geq 7\mid c=3,\ p\,]=0.05$$

and

$$\Pr[\,Y\leq 7\mid c=3,\ p\,]=0.05.$$

The first of these two equations has the solutions 0.0660 and 0.9340, which corresponds to the 'outer' endpoints of the interval pair. The second equation has the solutions 0.4500 and 0.5500 corresponding to the 'inner' endpoints of the two intervals. We interpret the solutions of these equations, giving the 90% interval:

$$(0.0660,\ 0.4500)$$

and, equivalently, the corresponding interval:

$$(0.5500,\ 0.9340).$$

If we want greater confidence, then the outer endpoints for the 95% confidence interval for p solves

$$\Pr[\,Y\geq 7\mid c=3,\ p\,]=0.025,$$

giving the outer endpoints 0.0504 and 0.9496.

Table 2.4 R programs to fit the maximum negative binomial distribution.

```
dmnb<-function(y,c,p)
# Maximum negative binomial density function
{
q<-1-p
dmnb<-choose(2*c+y-1, c-1)*(p*q)^c
dmnb<-dmnb*(p^y + q^y)
return(dmnb)
} #-----------------------------------------------------------
EMmnb<-function(y,c)
# EM algorithm for maximum likelihood estimate of
# p parameter in maximum negative binomial distribution
# prints EM iterations, J, information and approx std errors
{
p<-(y+c)/(y+2*c) # starting value for negative binomial
epsilon<-1.0e-7 # small convergence criteria
pk<-0
J<-0
jk<-3/4
print("EM iterations: p, J, score")
while(abs(p-pk)>epsilon) { # EM convergence criteria
pk<-p
p<-((1-jk)*(y+c)+jk*c)/(y+2*c)
jk<-(1-p)^y/(p^y+(1-p)^y)
# gradient of likelihood
grad<-c*p^(c-1)*(1-p)^c-c*p^c*(1-p)^(c-1)
grad<-grad*(p^y + (1-p)^y)
if(y>0)grad<-grad+(p*(1-p))^c*y*(p^(y-1)-(1-p)^(y-1))
print(c(p,jk,grad))
}
# Fisher Information from Louis (1982)
info<-(y+2*c)/(p*(1-p)) + jk*(1-jk)*(y/(p*(1-p)))^2
print("Information") print(info)
# approximate Standard error for valid information
if(info>epsilon) {
info<-1/sqrt(info)
print("Approx Std Error")
print(info)
}
return(p) }
```

Table 2.5 Iterations of EM algorithm for $y = 7$ and $c = 3$ with the R program `EMmnb` in Table 2.4.

Iteration	p_k	J_k	Gradient at p_k
1	0.365	0.9794570	$-.00365519$
2	0.24183	0.9996642	$-.000684964$
3	0.23095	0.9997798	-4.0616×10^{-6}
4	0.2308878	0.999780323	-1.8959×10^{-8}
5	0.2308875182	0.999780326	-8.8383×10^{-11}
6	0.2308875168	0.999780326	-4.1201×10^{-13}

However, for a 95% confidence interval there is no solution to the equation for the inner endpoints

$$\Pr[\, Y \leq 7 \mid c = 3,\ p\,] = 0.025,$$

indicating that the pair exact 95% confidence intervals for p overlap in the center.

2.6 Appendix: The Likelihood Kernel

Lemma 2.6.1 *For nonnegative integers c and y, the likelihood kernel $l(p)$ defined by*

$$l(p) = (pq)^c(p^y + q^y)$$

has a unique maximum at $p = 1/2$ if and only if

$$y(y-1) \leq 2c, \tag{2.12}$$

otherwise $l(p)$ has two maxima symmetric around $p = 1/2$.

Proof. The likelihood kernel $l(p)$ has a unique maximum at $p = 1/2$ if and only if $l''(1/2) \leq 0$, where

$$l''(1/2) = \left(\frac{\partial}{\partial p}\right)^2 l(p)\bigg|_{p=1/2} = 2^{-(2c+y-3)}\,[y(y-1) - 2c].$$

When $y = 0$ or 1, then $l(p)$ has a unique maximum at $p = 1/2$ because $l''(1/2) < 0$. For other values of $y = 2, 3, \ldots,$ the condition $l''(1/2) \leq 0$ is equivalent to the inequality (2.12).

The first derivative of $l'(p)$ of $l(p)$ is

$$l'(p) = \partial\, l(p)/\partial p = 2^{-1}(pq)^{c-1}\,(p-q)\,(p^y - q^y)\,\{y[\xi(p/q) - 1] - 2c\},$$

where $\xi(p/q)$ is the function

$$\xi(t) = \frac{(t+1)(t^y - 1)}{(t-1)(t^y + 1)}.$$

We can verify that $l'(1/2) = 0$. The composite function $\xi(p/q)$ is strictly decreasing in p when $y > 1$, and satisfies

$$\lim_{p \to 1/2} \xi(p/q) = y$$

and

$$\lim_{p \to 1} \xi(p/q) = 1.$$

This shows that the condition $l''(1/2) \leq 0$ implies $l'(p) < 0$, for all $1/2 \leq p \leq 1$.

Conversely, $l''(1/2) > 0$ implies that $l'(1/2 + \epsilon) > 0$ for all positive values of ϵ sufficiently close to zero. Since $l'(1) < 0$ and $\xi(p/q)$ is strictly decreasing in p when $1/2 < p < 1$, then there is a unique solution of the equation $l'(\widehat{p}) = 0$ for some $\widehat{p}$ satisfying $1/2 < \widehat{p} < 1$. Since $l(p)$ is symmetric about $p = 1/2$ and $l'(1/2) = 0$, this completes the proof. ■

The following result shows that the modes of $l(p)$ are less extreme (*i.e.* closer to 1/2) than the maximum likelihood estimates of p in the negative binomial distributions of N_p and N_q. These two estimates are $(y + c)/(y + 2c)$ and $c/(y + 2c)$ respectively.

Lemma 2.6.2 *If* $y(y-1) > 2c$, *then the likelihood kernel* $l(p)$ *has one local maxima at a point* p^*, *satisfying*

$$1/2 < p^* < (y + c)/(y + 2c). \tag{2.13}$$

Proof. Begin by noting that $l(p) = l(1-p)$ is symmetric about $p = 1/2$. A mode at p^*, satisfying (2.13) implies an equivalent mode at $1 - p^*$, satisfying

$$c/(y + 2c) < 1 - p^* < 1/2.$$

Lemma 2.6.1 demonstrates that $l'(1/2) = 0$, and if (2.12) does not hold, then $l''(1/2) > 0$. This implies that $l'(1/2 + \epsilon) > 0$ for all positive values of ϵ sufficiently close to zero. That is, $l(p)$ is a locally increasing function to the right of $p = 1/2$.

It is easy to verify that

$$l'[(y + c)/(y + 2c)] < 0,$$

so $l(p)$ is a locally decreasing function at $p = \widehat{p}_{N_q}$. This demonstrates that the local maximum p^* must satisfy (2.13) according to the uniqueness of the mode demonstrated in Lemma 2.6.1. ■

3

The Maximum Negative Hypergeometric Distribution

An urn contains a known number of balls of two different colors. We describe the random variable counting the smallest number of draws needed in order to observe at least c of both colors when sampling without replacement for a pre-specified value of $c = 1, 2, \ldots$. This distribution is the finite sample analogy to the maximum negative binomial distribution described in Chapter 2. We describe the modes, approximating distributions, and estimation of the contents of the urn.

The motivating examples of this distribution are the same as those of the previous chapter. In Section 2.1.1, Noah needed to sample endangered species with a small number of members. In Section 2.1.2, there are a finite number of patients available to us to screen for genetic abnormalities.

The distribution described in this chapter is mathematically more difficult to work with than the distribution of the previous chapter. Many of the lengthy asymptotic expansions are given in Section 3.5.

3.1 Introduction

In a sequence of independent and identically distributed Bernoulli (p) random variables, the *negative binomial distribution* describes the behavior of the number of failures Y observed before observing c successes, for integer-valued parameter $c \geq 1$. This well-known distribution has probability mass function

$$\Pr[\, Y = y\,] = \binom{c + y - 1}{c - 1} p^c (1 - p)^y \tag{3.1}$$

defined for $y = 0, 1, \ldots$.

Discrete Distributions Daniel Zelterman
 ISBN: 0-470-86888-0 (PPC)

The negative binomial distribution (3.1) is discussed in Section 1.6. In this introductory section, we describe several sampling schemes closely related to the negative binomial. Table 1 in the Preface may also be useful in illustrating the various relations between these distributions.

The *maximum negative binomial distribution* is the distribution of the smallest number of trials needed in order to observe at least c successes and c failures for integer-valued parameter $c \geq 1$. This distribution is motivated by the design of a medical trial in which we want to draw an inference from the Bernoulli parameter p. This example is illustrated in Section 2.1.2 of the previous chapter.

Let Y denote the 'excess' number of trials needed beyond the minimum of $2c$. The probability mass function of the maximum negative binomial distribution is

$$\Pr[\,Y = y\,] = \binom{2c + y - 1}{c - 1}(p^y + q^y)(pq)^c \tag{3.2}$$

for $y = 0, 1, \ldots$ and $q = 1 - p$.

The maximum negative binomial distribution is so-named because it represents the larger of two negative binomial distributions: the number of failures before the cth success is observed and the number of successes until the cth failure is observed.

In the previous chapter, we describe properties of the distribution (3.2). The maximum negative hypergeometric distribution given in (3.7) below and developed in the present chapter is the finite sample analog to the maximum negative binomial distribution (3.2).

The parameters p and $q = 1 - p$ are not identifiable in (3.2). Specifically, the same distribution in (3.2) results when p and q are interchanged. Similarly, it is impossible to distinguish between an inference from p and from $1 - p$ without additional information. In other words, we cannot tell if we are estimating p or q unless we also know how many successes and failures were observed at the point at which we obtained at least c of each. This identifiability problem is presented in Section 2.4 for estimates of the p parameter in the maximum negative hypergeometric distribution.

The *minimum negative binomial* or *riff-shuffle distribution* is the distribution of the smallest number of Bernoulli trials needed in order to observe either c successes or c failures. Clearly, at least c and fewer than $2c$ Bernoulli trials are necessary. The random variable $Y + c$ counts the total number of trials needed until either c successes or c failures are observed for $Y = 0, 1, \ldots, c - 1$. The experiment ends with sample numbered $Y + c$ from the Bernoulli population. Again, a reference to Table 1 in the Preface is useful in demonstrating the relationship between these distributions.

The mass function of the minimum negative binomial distribution is

$$\Pr[\,Y = y\,] = \binom{c + y - 1}{c - 1}\left(p^c q^y + p^y q^c\right) \tag{3.3}$$

for $y = 0, 1, \ldots, c - 1$.

The naming of (3.3) as the minimum negative binomial refers to the smaller of the two dependent negative binomial distributions: the number of failures before the cth success, and the number of successes before the cth failure. This distribution is also discussed in (2.1). In other words, distribution (3.3) says that there will be either c Bernoulli successes and y failures or else c failures and y Bernoulli successes. This distribution is introduced by Uppuluri and Blot (1970) and described in Johnson *et al.* (1992, pp 234–5). Lingappiah (1987) discusses parameter estimation for distribution (2.1).

The three discrete distributions described so far in this chapter are based on sampling from an infinitely large Bernoulli (p) parent population. Each of these distributions also has a finite sample analogy. These will be described next.

The *negative hypergeometric distribution* (Johnson *et al.*, (1992, pp. 239–42)) is the distribution of the number of unsuccessful draws from an urn with two different colored balls until a specified number of successful draws have been obtained. This distribution is also described in Section 1.7.1. If m out of n balls are of the 'successful' type, then the number of unsuccessful draws Y observed before c of the successful types are obtained is

$$\Pr[Y = y] = \binom{c+y-1}{c-1}\binom{n-c-y}{m-c} \Big/ \binom{n}{m} \tag{3.4}$$

with parameters satisfying $1 \leq c \leq m \leq n$ and range $y = 0, 1, \ldots, n-m$. The expected value of Y in (3.4) is $mc/(n-m-1)$.

The negative hypergeometric distribution (3.4) is the finite sample analogy to the negative binomial distribution (3.1). Unlike the negative binomial distribution, the negative hypergeometric distribution has a finite range. The maximum negative hypergeometric distribution described in the following sections is the larger of the two dependent negative hypergeometric distributions .

The *minimum negative hypergeometric distribution* describes the smallest number of urn draws needed in order to observe either c successes or c failures. This distribution is the finite sample analogy to the riff shuffle distribution (2.1). The probability mass function of the minimum negative hypergeometric distribution is

$$\Pr[Y = y] = \left[\binom{m}{c}\binom{n-m}{y} + \binom{m}{y}\binom{n-m}{c}\right] \times \binom{c+y-1}{c-1} \Big/ \left[\binom{c+y}{c}\binom{n}{c+y}\right] \tag{3.5}$$

for $y = 0, 1, \ldots, c-1$.

In Section 3.2, we give the probability mass function of the maximum negative hypergeometric distribution. Section 3.3 details some approximations to this distribution. In Section 3.4, we discuss estimation of the parameter that describes the contents of the urn.

3.2 The Distribution

An urn contains n balls: m of one color; and the remaining $n-m$ of another color. We continue sampling from the urn without replacement until we have observed at least c balls of both colors, for integer parameter $c \geq 1$. Sampling with replacement is the same as sampling from the maximum negative binomial distribution with parameter $p = m/n$. The maximum negative binomial distribution is given in (3.2) and described more fully in Chapter 2.

Let Y denote the random variable counting the number of extra draws needed beyond the minimum $2c$. That is, $Y + 2c$ draws is the smallest number necessary before we have first observed at least c of both colors. All of the Y extra draws from the urn must be of the same color. We will have drawn c of one color and $Y + c$ of the other color at the end of the experiment. We describe the distribution and properties of this random variable in this chapter.

For $k = 1, 2, \ldots$ the kth factorial polynomial is

$$z^{(k)} = z(z-1)\cdots(z-k+1).$$

The *maximum negative hypergeometric distribution* has probability mass function

$$\Pr[Y = y] = \left[m^{(c+y)}(n-m)^{(c)} + m^{(c)}(n-m)^{(c+y)}\right] \times \binom{2c+y-1}{c-1} \Big/ n^{(2c+y)} \qquad (3.6)$$

defined for the range of Y

$$0 \leq y \leq \max\{m-c,\ n-m-c\}.$$

The integer-valued parameters (n, m, c) are constrained to

$$1 \leq c \leq m \leq n \quad \text{and} \quad c \leq n-m.$$

Similarly, we can write

$$\Pr[Y = y] = \left[\binom{m}{c+y}\binom{n-m}{c} + \binom{m}{c}\binom{n-m}{c+y}\right] \times [c/(2c+y)] \Big/ \binom{n}{2c+y} \qquad (3.7)$$

to express the maximum negative hypergeometric distribution (3.6) in terms of binomial coefficients.

The distributions in (3.6) and (3.7) coincide and their values are unchanged when the parameter m is interchanged with $n-m$. This remark illustrates the identifiability problem with the parameters in the maximum negative hypergeometric distribution. A similar identifiability problem occurs with estimation of the p parameter in the maximum negative binomial distribution described in Section 2.4. We describe the estimation of the m parameter for (3.6) and (3.7) in Section 3.4.

Special cases of this distribution are as follows. For general parameter values,

$$\Pr[\,Y = 0\,] = \binom{n-2c}{m-c}\binom{2c}{c} \Big/ \binom{n}{m}.$$

This is the probability that the first $2c$ draws from the urn produce exactly c balls of both colors and no extra draws are necessary.

If $c = m = n/2$, then the maximum negative hypergeometric distribution is degenerate and all of its probability is a point mass at $Y = 0$. In other words, if $c = m = n - m$, then there can be only one possible outcome. In this case, all of the balls in the urn must be drawn before we can observe c balls of both colors.

The special case of $c = m = 1$ with $n \geq 2$ has the form

$$\Pr[\,Y = y \mid m = c = 1\,] = \begin{cases} 2/n & \text{for } y = 0 \\ 1/n & \text{for } y = 1, \ldots, n-2 \end{cases}$$

and zero otherwise.

This is also the form of the distribution for $c = 1$ and $m = n - 1$. The probability of $Y = 0$ is twice as likely as all other outcomes because the event $Y = 0$ occurs when the single 'odd' color appears on either the first or second draw. Values of $Y = 1, \ldots, n-2$ correspond to the single 'odd' color appearing on the third or subsequent draws.

The special case for $c = m$ and $n = 2m + 1$ has mass function

$$\Pr[\,Y = y \mid m = c,\ n = 2c + 1\,] = \begin{cases} (m+1)/(2m+1) & \text{for } y = 0 \\ m/(2m+1) & \text{for } y = 1 \end{cases}$$

and zero otherwise.

This is the distribution of Y for $m = c + 1$ and $n = 2m + 1$. In other words, this represents the distribution of the color of the last ball remaining after all but one have been drawn from the urn. Equivalently, this is also the distribution of the color of the first ball drawn.

3.3 Properties and Approximations

There are five basic shapes that the maximum negative hypergeometric distribution will assume. These are illustrated in Figs. 3.1 through 3.5. In each figure, the limiting maximum negative binomial distribution (3.2) is also presented. This limit can be expressed, more formally, as follows.

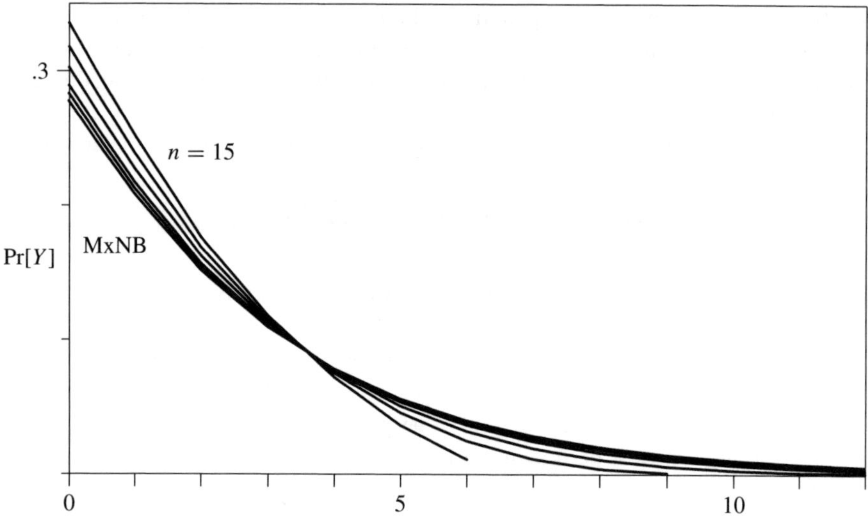

Figure 3.1 The maximum negative hypergeometric distribution for $c = 3$ and $m = .4n$ with values of $n = 15$, 20, 30, 60, and 120. The distribution corresponding to the maximum negative binomial (MxNB) given in (3.2) with parameters $c = 3$ and $p = 0.4$ is the limit when n is large.

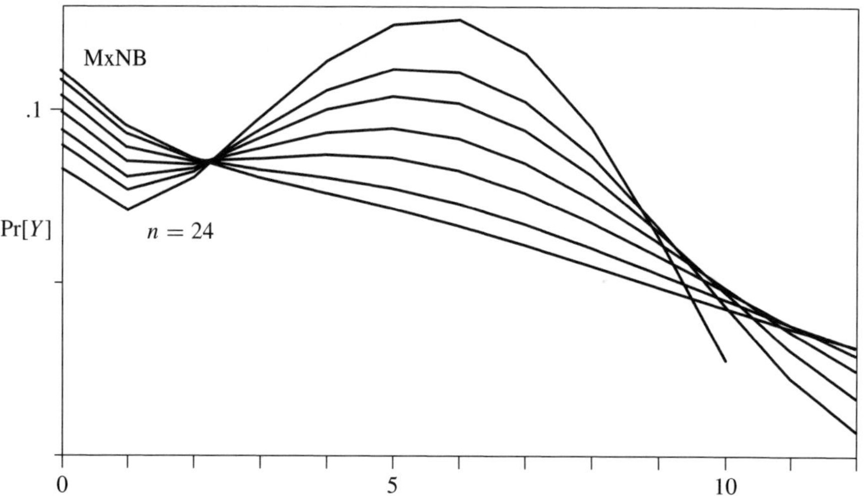

Figure 3.2 The maximum negative hypergeometric distribution for $c = 6$ and $m = n/3$ with $n = 24$, 27, 30, 36, 48, and 96. Examples of the conditions for unimodal distributions are given in Table 3.1. The limiting maximum negative binomial distribution (MxNB) has parameters $c = 6$ and $p = 1/3$.

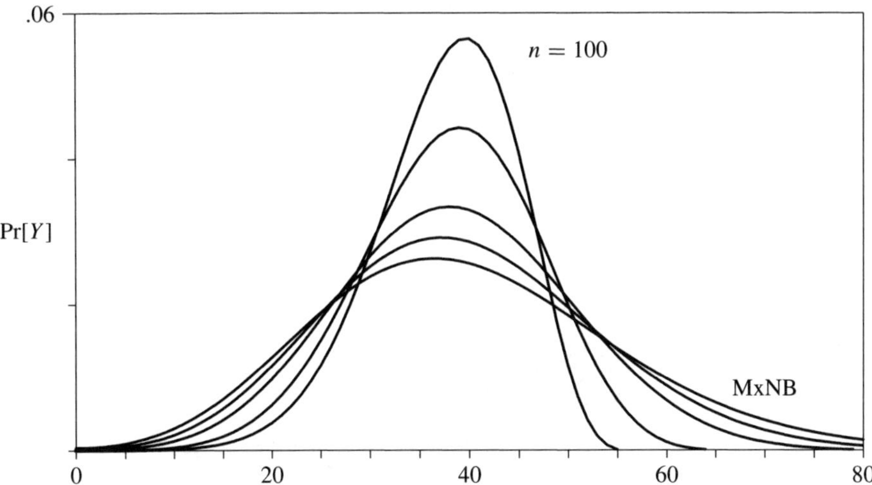

Figure 3.3 The maximum negative hypergeometric distribution for $c = 20$ and $m = n/4$ with $n = 100$, 120, 200, and 400. A normal approximate distribution appears when the (c, m, n) parameters are all large and m/n is not close to zero, one, or 1/2. This is proved in Lemma 3.3.4.

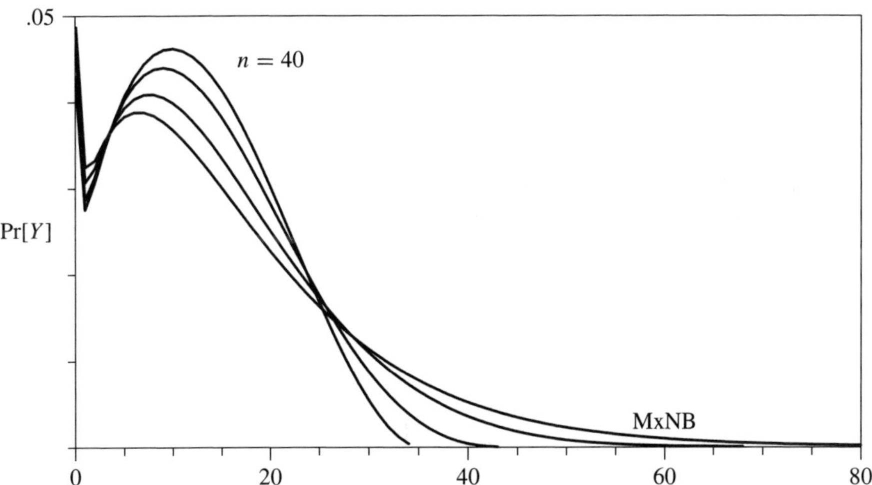

Figure 3.4 The maximum negative hypergeometric distribution for $c = 2$ and $m = n/10$ with $n = 40$, 50, and 100. A gamma-approximate distribution is proved in Lemma 3.3.2 when m is much smaller than n. There is always a local mode at $Y = 0$. The asymptotic maximum negative binomial (MxNB) distribution has parameters $c = 2$ and $p = 1/10$.

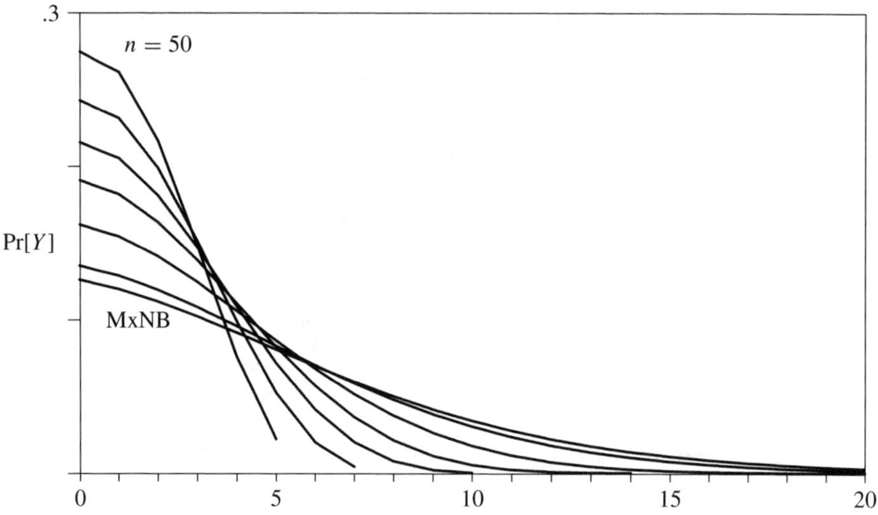

Figure 3.5 The maximum negative hypergeometric distribution for $c = 20$ and $m = n/2$ for $n = 50,\ 54,\ 60,\ 70,\ 100,$ and 300. A half normal approximate distribution appears when c and n are large and $m = n/2$. The limiting distribution is proved in Lemma 3.3.3.

Lemma 3.3.1 *For fixed values of* $c \geq 1$, *let* n *and* m *both grow large such that* $m/n = p$ *for* p *bounded between zero and one. Then, the behavior of the maximum negative hypergeometric random variable* (3.6) *approaches the maximum negative binomial distribution* (3.2) *with parameters c and p.*

Proof. Values of Y remain bounded with high probability under these conditions. In (3.6), we write

$$\begin{aligned} m^{(c+y)}\,(n-m)^{(c)} \Big/ n^{(2c+y)} &\geq (m-c-y)^{c+y}\,(n-m-c)^{c} \Big/ n^{2c+y} \\ &= (m/n)^{c+y}\,[(n-m)/n]^{c} \\ &\qquad \times [1-(c+y)/m]^{c+y}[1-c/(n-m)]^{c} \\ &= p^{c+y}\,q^{c}[1+O_p(n^{-1})], \end{aligned}$$

where $p = m/n$ and $q = 1 - p = (n-m)/n$.

We can also write

$$\begin{aligned} m^{(c+y)}\,(n-m)^{(c)} \Big/ n^{(2c+y)} &\leq m^{c+y}\,(n-m)^{c} \Big/ (n-2c-y)^{2c+y} \\ &= (m/n)^{c+y}\,[(n-m)/n]^{c} \Big/ [1-(2c+y)/n]^{2c+y} \\ &= p^{c+y}\,q^{c}[1+O_p(n^{-1})]. \end{aligned}$$

A similar argument shows

$$m^{(c)}\,(n-m)^{(c+y)} \Big/ n^{(2c+y)} = p^c\,q^{c+y}[1+O_p(n^{-1})],$$

completing the proof. ■

In other words, if m and n are both large, then sampling from the urn without replacement is almost the same as sampling with replacement. Sampling with replacement is the same as sampling from a Bernoulli-parent population yielding the maximum negative binomial distribution (3.2).

Let us describe the basic shapes that this distribution can attain. Figs. 3.1 and 3.2 are similar to Figs. 2.2 and 2.3, respectively, of the maximum negative binomial distribution described in the previous chapter. These pairs of figures show that the maximum negative hypergeometric distribution can follow the same j-shape as the maximum negative binomial distribution or else be bimodal. The modes are described in Section 3.3.1.

If n is large and m/n is not close to zero, one, or 1/2, then Fig. 3.3 shows that the maximum negative hypergeometric distribution has an approximate normal distribution. This limit is stated formally in Section 3.3.4 and the details of the proof are given in Section 3.5.2.

Fig. 3.4 demonstrates another shape for the maximum negative hypergeometric distribution. A gamma approximate distribution is proved in Section 3.3.2. The unusual left tail in this figure occurs because this distribution always has a small local mode at zero. Under the conditions of Lemma 3.3.2, the local mode at $Y=0$ becomes negligible. The modes of this distribution are described in Section 3.3.1.

Fig. 3.5 demonstrates a half-normal approximate shape when n is large and m/n is close to 1/2. This half-normal approximation is stated more formally in Section 3.3.3.

3.3.1 Modes of the distribution

Next, we describe the modes for this distribution. The maximum negative hypergeometric distribution can have either one or two modes. Write

$$\Pr[\,Y=0\,]/\Pr[\,Y=1\,]=(c+1)/c$$

to show that this distribution always has at least one local mode at $Y=0$.

The maximum negative binomial distribution (3.2) also has at least one local mode at $Y=0$ for all values of the parameter p. The local mode of the maximum negative hypergeometric distribution at $Y=0$ is clearly visible in Figs. 3.1, 3.2, 3.4, and 3.5. The local mode at $Y=0$ in Fig. 3.3 is also present but it is very small.

Table 3.1 presents examples of parameter values corresponding to unimodal distributions in (3.7). In general, there will be only one mode at $Y=0$ when m/n is not too far from 1/2. The range of m with unimodal distributions becomes

Table 3.1 Ranges of m parameter that result in unimodal maximum negative hypergeometric distributions for specified values of c and n. Omitted distributions are either degenerate, or the parameter values are invalid.

c	$n = 10$	$n = 50$	$n = 250$
1	Unimodal for all $m = 1, \ldots, n-1$		
2	$3 \le m \le 7$	$9 \le m \le 41$	$38 \le m \le 212$
3	$4 \le m \le 6$	$13 \le m \le 37$	$55 \le m \le 195$
4	$m = 5$	$15 \le m \le 35$	$65 \le m \le 185$
5	—	$16 \le m \le 34$	$73 \le m \le 177$
10	—	$20 \le m \le 30$	$90 \le m \le 160$
15	—	$22 \le m \le 28$	$98 \le m \le 152$
20	—	$24 \le m \le 26$	$103 \le m \le 147$
25	—	—	$106 \le m \le 144$

narrower as c becomes larger when n is fixed. If $m = n/2$, then the distribution is always unimodal.

3.3.2 A gamma approximation

An approximate gamma distribution is illustrated in Fig. 3.4. Under the conditions of the following lemma, the local mode at $Y = 0$ becomes negligible.

Lemma 3.3.2 *For fixed $c \ge 1$, if m grows as $\theta n^{1/2}$ for large n and some $\theta \ge 0$, then $\theta Y/n^{1/2}$ behaves approximately as the sum of c independent standard exponential random variables.*

Proof. Begin at (3.6) and write

$$\binom{2c + y - 1}{c - 1} = \prod_{i=1}^{c-1} (y + 2c - i)/i$$

$$= y^{c-1}(1 + O_p(n^{-1/2}))/\Gamma(c).$$

Define Δ as

$$\Delta = m^{(c)}(n - m)^{(y+c)}/n^{(2c+y)}.$$

Under the conditions of this lemma, the term

$$m^{(c+y)}(n - m)^{(c)}/n^{(2c+y)}$$

is much smaller than Δ and can be ignored.

We have

$$\log \Delta = \sum_{i=0}^{c-1} \log[(m-i)/(n-i)] + \sum_{j=0}^{y+c-1} \log[(n-m-j)/(n-c-j)]$$

$$= c\log[\theta n^{-1/2} + O(n^{-1})] + \sum_{j=0}^{y+c-1} \log[1-(m-c)/(n-c-j)]$$

For ϵ near zero, write

$$\epsilon - \epsilon^2/2 \leq \log(1+\epsilon) \leq \epsilon$$

so that

$$\log \Delta = c\log[\theta n^{-1/2} + O(n^{-1})] - \theta y/n^{1/2} + O_p(y/n)$$

The transformation $X = \theta Y/n^{1/2}$ has Jacobian $n^{1/2}/\theta$ so

$$(n^{1/2}/\theta)\Pr[\,Y\,] = x^{c-1}\mathrm{e}^{-x}/\,\Gamma(c)$$

ignoring terms that tend to zero for large vales of n.

This last expression is the density function of the sum of c independent, standard exponential random variables. ■

When n is large and m grows in proportion to $n^{1/2}$, the m colored balls become relatively rare. The number of draws required to obtain each of these rare balls behaves approximately as independent exponential random variables. The number of draws required to obtain c of these rare balls, then, behaves approximately as the sum of c independent exponential random variables.

3.3.3 A half-normal approximation

The approximate half-normal behavior of the maximum negative hypergeometric distribution is illustrated in Fig. 3.5. If Z has a standard normal distribution, then the distribution of $\mid Z \mid$ is said to be *standard half-normal* or *folded normal*. The density function of the random variable $X = \mid Z \mid$ is

$$(2/\pi)^{1/2}\exp(-x^2/2)$$

for $x \geq 0$ (Stuart and Ord, 1987, p 117).

Lemma 3.3.3 *When n becomes large, if $m = n/2$ and c grows as $n^{1/2}$, then $Y/(2c)^{1/2}$ behaves approximately as a standard half-normal random variable.*

The proof involves expanding all factorials in (3.7) using Stirling's approximation. The details are provided in Section 3.5.1.

3.3.4 A normal approximation

The normal approximation to the maximum negative hypergeometric distribution can be seen in Fig. 3.3. This is proved more formally in Lemma 3.3.4, below. No generality is lost by requiring $m \geq n/2$ because m and $n - m$ can be interchanged to yield the same distribution.

Lemma 3.3.4 *For large values of* n*, suppose* c *grows as* $n^{1/2}$ *and* $m = np$ *for* $1/2 \leq p \leq 1$*. Then* $(Y - \mu)/\sigma$ *behaves approximately as standard normal, where*

$$\mu = c(p - q)/q$$

for $q = 1 - p$ *and*

$$\sigma = (cp)^{1/2}/q.$$

The proof of this lemma is given in Section 3.5.2. The details involve using Stirling's approximation to all of the factorials in (3.7) and expanding these in a two-term Taylor series.

3.4 Estimation

The most practical situation concerning parameter estimation involves estimating the m parameter when c and n are both known. In terms of the original, motivating example drawing inference from the genetic markers in cancer patients, the finite population size n will be known, and the parameter c is chosen by the investigators in order to achieve specified power and significance levels. Noah did not know either m or n but may have had little interest in estimating these parameters. The m parameter describes the composition of the n individuals in the finite-sized patient population available to us. The value of m is known without error if all n subjects are observed.

The estimation of m in this section is made on the basis of a single observation of the random variable Y. We treat the unknown m parameter as continuous-valued rather than as a discrete integer as it has been used in previous sections of this chapter.

The log-likelihood kernel function of m in (3.6) is

$$\Lambda(m) = \log\left[\left(m^{(c)}(n-m)^{(c+y)} + m^{(c+y)}(n-m)^{(c)}\right) \Big/ n^{(2c+y)}\right].$$

The estimator we will describe is the value of m that maximizes Λ, defined for values of m satisfying

$$c \leq m \leq n - c.$$

As a numerical illustration, the function $\Lambda(m)$ is plotted in Fig. 3.6 for $n = 20$ and $c = 3$. Observed values of y are given as $0, 1, \ldots, 7$ in this figure.

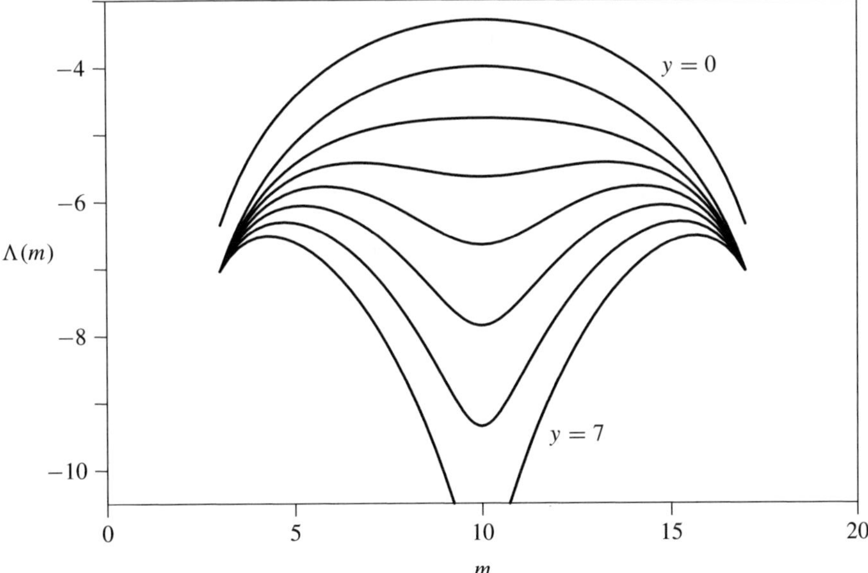

Figure 3.6 The maximum negative hypergeometric log-likelihood kernel function $\Lambda(m)$ for parameter values $n = 20$ and $c = 3$ and observed values $y = 0, \ldots, 7$.

The range of valid values of the m parameter are $3 \le m \le 17$ for the values of c and n in this example. Smaller observed values of $y = 0, 1, 2$ in this example exhibit log-likelihood functions with a single mode corresponding to maximum likelihood estimates of $\widehat{m} = n/2$. For values of $y \ge 3$, the likelihood Λ has two modes, symmetric about $n/2$. These modes are symmetric about $n/2$ because

$$\Lambda(m) = \Lambda(n - m).$$

Intuitively, if the observed value Y is small, then we are inclined to believe that the urn is composed of an equal number of balls of both colors. The exact regions that result in a unimodal likelihood function with $\widehat{m} = n/2$ are plotted in Fig. 3.7 for all values of c up to 20 and n up to 200. The discrete parameter values for c and n are plotted using dots. The dots on these lattice points are connected by lines.

If we observe c of both colored balls in a small number of trials, then this is good statistical evidence of an even balance of the two colors in the population. Conversely, if the observed value of Y is relatively large, then we will estimate an imbalance in the composition of the population. Without the additional knowledge of the number of successes and failures observed we are unable to tell if we are estimating m or $n - m$. This same identifiability issue was also raised in Section 2.4 for the maximum negative binomial distribution.

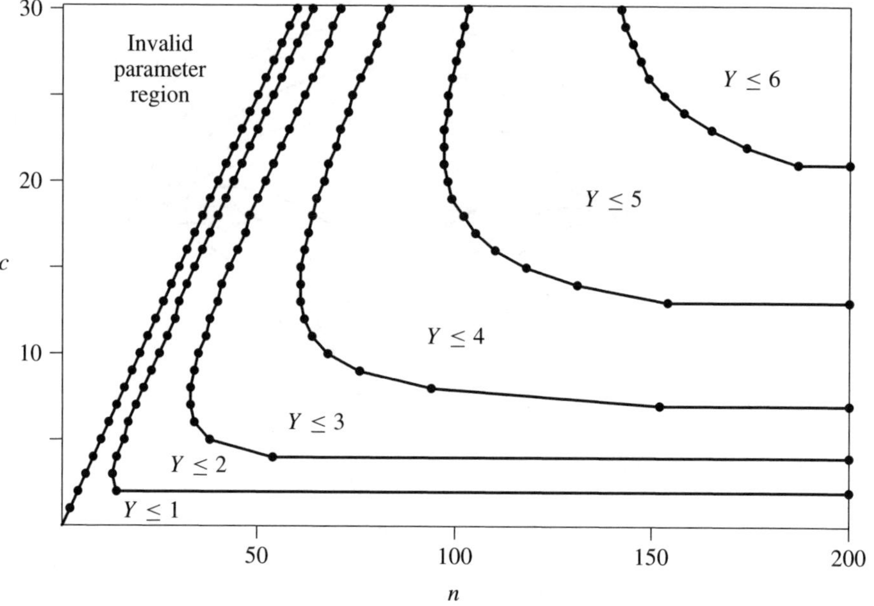

Figure 3.7 Values of the maximum negative hypergeometric random variable Y that exhibit a unimodal likelihood function with maximum at $\widehat{m} = n/2$ for given values of c and n.

More generally, there will be either one mode in the likelihood $\Lambda(m)$ at $\widehat{m} = n/2$ or else two modes, symmetric about $n/2$, depending on the sign of

$$\Lambda''(m) = (\partial/\partial m)^2\, \Lambda(m)$$

evaluated at $m = n/2$. If $\Lambda''(n/2)$ is negative, then there will be one mode of Λ at $n/2$.

In order to examine Λ'', we first need to find expressions for derivatives of factorial polynomials. Useful rules for differentiating factorial polynomials are as follows. For $c \geq 1$,

$$(\partial/\partial m)\, m^{(c)} = m^{(c)} \sum_{i=0}^{c-1} (m-i)^{-1}$$

and for $c \geq 2$,

$$(\partial/\partial m)^2\, m^{(c)} = 2m^{(c)} \sum_{\substack{i=0 \\ i \leq i'}}^{c-1} (m-i)^{-1}(m-i')^{-1}.$$

Use these rules to write

$$
\begin{aligned}
&(\partial/\partial m)\, m^{(c)}(n-m)^{(y+c)} \\
&\quad = m^{(c)}(n-m)^{(y+c)} \left[\sum_{i=0}^{c-1} (m-i)^{-1} - \sum_{j=0}^{y+c-1} (n-m-j)^{-1} \right].
\end{aligned}
$$

This expression shows that the likelihood $\Lambda(m)$ always has a critical value at $m = n/2$. That is,

$$(\partial/\partial m)\Lambda(m)\Big|_{m=n/2} = 0.$$

The critical point of Λ at $m = n/2$ may either be a global maximum or else a local minimum as seen in the example of Fig. 3.6. This distinction depends on the sign of the second derivative Λ'' of Λ.

The second derivative of Λ can be found from

$$
\begin{aligned}
&(\partial/\partial m)^2\, m^{(c)}(n-m)^{(y+c)} = m^{(c)}(n-m)^{(y+c)} \\
&\times \left\{ \left[\sum_{i=0}^{c-1} (m-i)^{-1} - \sum_{j=0}^{y+c-1} (n-m-j)^{-1} \right]^2 \right. \\
&\qquad\qquad \left. - \sum_{i=0}^{c-1} (m-i)^{-2} - \sum_{j=0}^{y+c-1} (n-m-j)^{-2} \right\}.
\end{aligned}
$$

The sign of $\Lambda''(n/2)$ is the same as that of the function

$$\phi(n,c,y) = \sum_{\substack{k=0 \\ k \le k'}}^{y-1} (n/2-c-k)^{-1}(n/2-c-k')^{-1} - \sum_{i=0}^{c-1} (n/2-i)^{-2}.$$

The first summation in ϕ is zero when $y = 0$ or 1. The function ϕ is, then, negative for small values of y demonstrating, that the maximum likelihood estimate of m is $\widehat{m} = n/2$ in these cases. Similarly, ϕ is an increasing function of y and will eventually become positive for larger values of y. This shows that Λ will have two modes for sufficiently large y. These modes are symmetric about $n/2$ because $\Lambda(m) = \Lambda(n-m)$ for all m satisfying

$$c \le m \le n-c.$$

In other words, a small observed value of y leads us to believe that there are an equal number of balls of both colors in the urn and estimate m by $n/2$. Similarly, a large observed value of y relative to c leads us to estimate an imbalance in the composition of the urn.

3.5 Appendix

The details of two proofs are provided here.

3.5.1 The half-normal approximation

The proof of Lemma 3.3.3 is provided here. We assume that $m = n/2$ and $c = n^{1/2}$. The random variable Y is $O_p(n^{1/4})$.

Expand all of the factorials in (3.7) using Stirling's approximation, giving

$$\log \Pr[\, Y = y\,] = -1/2 \log(2\pi) + T_1(c) + T_2(n) + O_p(n^{-1/2}),$$

where

$$\begin{aligned} T_1 &= \log[2c/(2c+y)] - (c+y+1/2)\log(c+y) \\ &\quad - (c+1/2)\log(c) + (2c+y+1/2)\log(2c+y) \end{aligned}$$

contains terms in $O_p(c \log c)$ and

$$\begin{aligned} T_2 &= (n+1)\log(n/2) - (n+1/2)\log(n) \\ &\quad - (n/2 - c + 1/2)\log(n/2 - c) \\ &\quad - (n/2 - c - y + 1/2)\log(n/2 - c - y) \\ &\quad + (n - 2c - y + 1/2)\log(n - 2c - y) \end{aligned}$$

contains terms that are $O_p(n \log n)$.

In all of the following expansions, it is useful to keep in mind that $c = c_n$ is approximately equal to $n^{1/2}$ and $Y = O_p(n^{1/4})$. Write T_1 as

$$\begin{aligned} T_1 &= -\log[(2c+y)/2c] + (2c+y+1/2)\log 2 - 1/2\log(c) \\ &\quad + c\log[(c+y/2)^2/c(c+y)] + (y+1/2)\log[(c+y/2)/(c+y)] \\ &= -\log(1+y/2c) + (2c+y+1/2)\log 2 - 1/2\log(c) \\ &\quad + c\log[1 + y^2/4c(c+y)] + (y+1/2)\log[1 - y/2(c+y)]. \end{aligned}$$

Expand every appearance of

$$\log(1+\epsilon) = \epsilon + O(\epsilon^2)$$

for ϵ near zero to show

$$T_1 = (2c+y+1/2)\log 2 - 1/2\log(c) - y^2/4c + O_p(n^{-1/4}).$$

Similarly, we can write

$$\begin{aligned}T_2 &= (n/2 - c)\log[(n-2c-y)/(n-2c)] + 1/2\ \log[n/(n-2c)]\\ &\quad + y\log[(n-2c-2y)/(n-2c-y)] - (2c+y-1)\log 2\\ &\quad + 1/2\ \log[(n-2c-y)/(n-2c-2y)]\\ &= (n/2-c)\log[1+y^2/O_p(n^2)] + y\log[1-y/O_p(n)]\\ &\quad - (2c+y-1)\log 2 + 1/2\ \log[1+O(c/n)]\\ &\quad + 1/2\ \log[1+y/O_p(n)].\end{aligned}$$

Then write $\log(1+\epsilon) = O(\epsilon)$ for ϵ near zero, giving

$$T_2 = -(2c+y-1)\log 2 + O_p(n^{-1/2}).$$

These expressions for T_1 and T_2 in $\Pr[Y]$ give

$$\log \Pr[\,Y = y\,] = \log 2 - 1/2\log(\pi c) - y^2/4c + O_p(n^{-1/4}).$$

Finally, we note that $(2c)^{1/2}$ is the Jacobian of the transformation $X = Y/(2c)^{1/2}$. Then

$$\log\{(2c)^{1/2}\Pr[\,Y = y\,]\} = 1/2\log(2/\pi) - x^2/2 + O_p(n^{-1/4})$$

is the density of the folded normal distribution, except for terms that tend to zero with high probability. ■

3.5.2 The normal approximate distribution

The details of the proof of Lemma 3.3.4 are given here. Define Ω as

$$\Omega = [c/(2c+y)]\binom{m}{c+y}\binom{n-m}{c}\Big/\binom{n}{2c+y}.$$

The term

$$[c/(2c+y)]\binom{m}{c}\binom{n-m}{c+y}\Big/\binom{n}{2c+y}.$$

in (3.7) is much smaller than Ω and can be ignored under the conditions of this lemma.

Expand all of the factorials in Ω using Stirling's formula, giving

$$\log\Omega = -1/2\log(2\pi) + S_1(n) + S_2(n-c) + S_3(y) + O_p(n^{-1/2})$$

where

$$S_1 = (np+1/2)\ \log(np) + (nq+1/2)\ \log(nq) - (n+1/2)\ \log n$$

corresponds to $m!$, $(n-m)!$, and $n!$;

$$\begin{aligned}S_2 = &(n-2c-y+1/2)\log(n-2c-y)\\ &-(np-c-y+1/2)\log(np-c-y)\\ &-(nq-c+1/2)\log(nq-c)\end{aligned}$$

corresponds to $(n-2c-y)!$, $(m-c-y)!$, and $(n-m-c)!$; and

$$\begin{aligned}S_3 = &\log[c/(2c+y)] + (2c+y+1/2)\log(2c+y)\\ &-(c+y+1/2)\log(c+y)-(c+1/2)\log(c)\end{aligned}$$

corresponds to $c/(2c+y)$, $(2c+y)!$, $(c+y)!$ and $c!$, respectively.

Write out all of the terms in S_1 to show

$$S_1 = np\log p + nq\log q + 1/2\log(npq).$$

We can write S_2 as

$$\begin{aligned}S_2 = &(n-2c-y+1/2)\log n\\ &+(n-2c-y+1/2)\log[1-(2c+y)/n)]\\ &-(np-c-y+1/2)\log(np)\\ &-(n-c-y+1/2)\log[1-(c+y)/np)]\\ &-(nq-c+1/2)\log(nq)-(nq-c+1/2)\log(1-c/n).\end{aligned}$$

Then

$$\begin{aligned}S_1+S_2 = &c\log(pq)+y\log p\\ &+(n-2c-y+1/2)\log[1-(2c+y)/n]\\ &-(np-c-y+1/2)\log[1-(c+y)/np]\\ &-(nq-c+1/2)\log(1-c/nq).\end{aligned}$$

Since

$$(c+y)/n = O_p(n^{-1/2}),$$

we can expand

$$\log(1+\epsilon) = \epsilon - \epsilon^2/2 + O(\epsilon^3)$$

for ϵ near zero to show

$$\begin{aligned}S_1+S_2 = &c\log(pq)+y\log p+(2c+y)^2/2n\\ &-(c+y)^2/2np - c^2/2nq + O_p(n^{-1/2}).\end{aligned}$$

Then write

$$y = \mu + Z\sigma,$$

where Z is a $O_p(1)$ random variable, giving

$$S_1 + S_2 = c\log(pq) + y\log p + [(2c+\mu)^2 pq - (c+\mu)^2 q - c^2 p]/2npq$$
$$+ Z\sigma[(2c+\mu)p - c - \mu]/np + O_p(n^{-1/2}).$$

Substitute $\mu = c(p-q)/q$ to show

$$S_1 + S_2 = c\log(pq) + y\log p + O_p(n^{-1/2}). \tag{3.8}$$

Next write S_3 as

$$S_3 = (c+y)\log[(2c+y)/(c+y)] + (c-1/2)\log[(2c+y)/c)]$$
$$- 1/2\log(c+y).$$

Expand the argument of the first logarithm in S_3 here in a two-term Taylor series, showing

$$\begin{aligned}(2c+y)/(c+y) &= (2c+\mu+Z\sigma)/(c+\mu+Z\sigma)\\ &= [(2c+\mu)/(c+\mu)]\,\{[1+Z\sigma/(2c+\mu)]\,/\,[1+Z\sigma/(c+\mu)]\}\\ &= [(2c+\mu)/(c+\mu)]\\ &\quad\times\{1 - Z\sigma c/[(c+\mu)(2c+\mu)]\\ &\quad + Z^2\sigma^2 c/[(c+\mu)^2(2c+\mu)] + O(n^{-3/4})\}.\end{aligned}$$

Then expand

$$\log(1+\epsilon) = \epsilon - \epsilon^2/2 + O(\epsilon^3)$$

to show

$$\begin{aligned}(c+y)\log[(2c+y)/(c+y)] &= (c+\mu+Z\sigma)\log[(2c+\mu)/(c+\mu)]\\ &\quad - (c+\mu+Z\sigma)\,Z\sigma c/[(c+\mu)(2c+\mu)]\\ &\quad - 1/2\,(Z\sigma c)^2/[2(c+\mu)(2c+\mu)^2]\\ &\quad + Z^2\sigma^2 c/[(c+\mu)(2c+\mu)] + O_p(n^{-1/4}).\end{aligned}$$

Similarly,

$$\begin{aligned}(c-1/2)\log[(2c+y)/c)] &= (c-1/2)\log(2+\mu/c)\\ &\quad + (c-1/2)\log\{1+Z\sigma/(2c+\mu)\}\\ &= (c-1/2)\log(2+\mu/c) + Z\sigma c/(2c+\mu)\\ &\quad - Z^2\sigma^2 c/[2(2c+\mu)^2] + O_p(n^{-1/4})\end{aligned}$$

and

$$\begin{aligned}\log(c+y) &= \log[(c+\mu)(1+Z\sigma/(c+\mu))] \\ &= \log(c+\mu) + O_p(n^{-1/4})\end{aligned}$$

so that

$$\begin{aligned}S_3 = {} & (c+y)\log[(2c+\mu)/(c+\mu)] + (c-1/2)\log[(2c+\mu)/c] \\ & - 1/2\log(c+\mu) - Z^2\sigma^2 c/[2(c+\mu)(2c+\mu)] + O_p(n^{-1/4}).\end{aligned}$$

Substitute values of $\mu = c(p-q)/q$ and $\sigma^2 = cp/q^2$, giving

$$S_3 = (c+y)\log p - \log\sigma + (c-1/2)\log q - Z^2/2 + O_p(n^{-1/4}).$$

This expression, together with the form of $S_1 + S_2$ given at (3.8), shows that

$$\log\Omega = -1/2\log(2\pi) - \log\sigma - Z^2/2 + O_p(n^{-1/4}),$$

demonstrating the approximately standard normal behavior of the random variable $Z = (Y-\mu)/\sigma$.

4

Univariate Discrete Distributions for Use with Twins

The distributions developed in this chapter and the following are motivated by the study of a genetic component for longevity. Is there a gene for long life? How can we detect it and measure its effect? Some of the evidence for a genetic component of longevity comes from the study of the life spans of twins. In this chapter and the following, we examine data on the joint life spans of twin pairs and develop discrete distributions to model the empirical data. There is a large literature on the statistical analysis of paired survival times. Much of the methodology for paired survival times has been developed to accommodate censored data, but there is no censoring in the twin data examined here. Rather than examining the data using survival methods, we will take a nonparametric, permutation approach to demonstrate an association of longevity in the twins and then measure its effect.

As an illustration of the approach we will take, consider a portion of the data that will be examined later in this chapter. Table 4.1 summarizes the life spans of 117 identical female twin pairs born between 1870 and 1880 in Denmark. All of these 234 women have since died, so there is no censoring in the data that we examine. At age 70, there were 146 women still living and 88 had died before attaining this age. The 146 living women were distributed in such a way that 53 of the 117 twin pairs had two living members.

How many twin pairs should we expect to see in which both co-twins are alive at age 70, if there is no association in their life spans? The distribution of the number of pairs in which both co-twins are alive is obtained by randomly matching unrelated living or dead individuals born 70 years earlier into pairs. If we observe

Discrete Distributions Daniel Zelterman
 ISBN: 0-470-86888-0 (PPC)

Table 4.1 Survival of 117 identical female Danish twin pairs born 1870–80 (Hauge *et al.*, 1968).

Age in years	Number of women alive	Number of pairs both alive
30	220	105
35	218	103
40	213	98
45	210	96
50	205	92
55	201	88
60	186	75
65	166	65
70	146	53
75	110	35
80	75	17
85	39	7
90	18	2
95	2	0

many more twin pairs where both are alive than would be expected by this random pairing, then this provides statistical evidence of a positive correlation in their longevity. Of course, twins will probably closely share a similar environment and diet throughout their lives so genetics can only provide a portion of the explanation. We will try to separate the effects of environment from genetics in Section 4.4 by comparing two different genetic types of twins. At that point, we will also explain some of the genetics of twins.

In this chapter and the following, we describe several discrete distributions motivated by the study of longevity in twins. All individuals, both living and dead, at a specified age are randomly paired. The univariate distribution in this chapter, models the number of these twin pairs where both members are still alive at that age. If there is a positive association to longevity in twins, then we would expect to see a statistically large number of twin pairs where both are alive at older ages relative to the number of living individuals. We obtain Poisson and normal approximations to the exact distribution. Odds-ratio parametric models are developed in Section 4.3 to provide a measure of the association of longevity within twin pairs. These models indicate a statistically large number of identical twin pairs where both are alive after age 60 in the cohort of twins born between 1870 and 1880 in Denmark. In Section 4.4, identical twins are contrasted with fraternal twins to separate the genetic and environmental contributions to the similarity in longevity among twins. In that section, we will also explain the genetic differences between these two different types of twins.

In the following chapter, we develop multivariate methods to describe the conditional distribution of twin pairs where both are alive at one age, given the number of pairs where both are alive at a younger age. Multivariate distributions are developed in Chapter 5 to describe the effects of joint longevity to several ages simultaneously.

4.1 Introduction

A controversial issue in demography concerns the existence of a genetic component in human longevity. Fries (1980) gives empirical evidence for a genetic limit to longevity that is invariant to changes in the environment. Mathematical models suggested by Fries' hypothesis are given by Zelterman (1992), Zelterman, Grambsch, Le, *et al.* (1994) and Zelterman and Curtsinger (1995). Critics of this controversial theory include Curtsinger, Fukui, Townsend, and Vaupel (1992), and Schneider and Brody (1983), among others.

Data on twins may yield insight into the role of genetics in determining human longevity. There are many registries of twins throughout the world. In Section 4.4, we look at data on a cohort of twins born in Denmark between 1870 and 1880 (Hauge, *et al.* 1968). The aim of this chapter and the following are to measure the association of longevity within these twin pairs. There were few deaths before age 50 and these were probably due to accidents, illness, and similar causes so we will concentrate on older ages. Twins are likely to be raised together and share a similar environment throughout their lives, so our conclusions are not the final word on the subject.

Several new discrete distributions are developed in this chapter and the following to measure the association of longevity within twin pairs. Suppose there are originally n twin pairs, and $m = m(t)$ denotes the number of individuals still living at age t. When these $2n$ individuals (either living or dead) are randomly paired without replacement, we describe the distribution of the number of these pairs for which both are alive. If longevity has a positive association within twins, then we would expect to see a statistically large number of twin pairs with both co-twins alive at older ages.

Section 4.2 describes the basic distribution and its elementary properties. We obtain Poisson and normal approximations to this distribution and give the details in Section 4.5.2. We describe odds-ratio models in Section 4.3 as a parametric approach to measure the association of longevity within twin pairs. The following chapter develops multivariate distributions to simultaneously model association of longevity to several different ages and the association of within-twin-pair survival to a later age conditional on this association at a younger age.

In Section 4.4, we apply these methods to the Danish Twin Registry. In that section, we will describe the distinction between identical and fraternal twins. The examination of the data shows that many more identical twin pairs are both alive after age 60 than would be found by chance alone. When contrasting identical twins to fraternal twins, the association measure for identical twins is stronger than that for fraternal twins, who share about 50% of their genes. Before we can state these conclusions, let us set up some of the notation and establish the basic methods.

4.2 The Univariate Twins Distribution

Suppose there are n twin pairs and $m = m(t)$ of these $2n$ individuals are alive at age t. The range of values for m is $0, 1, \ldots, 2n$. Similarly, $2n - m$ individuals will have died before attaining age t. Consider the reference distribution in which we randomly match the original $2n$ individuals to form n pairs. We will concentrate on the distribution of the number of pairs for which both individuals are alive. If there is a positive association in longevity, then we would anticipate observing the number of both-alive pairs to be much larger than its expectation if the twin pairs were made up at random.

The distribution of the number of twin pairs, where both are alive, can be obtained from a multinomial distribution with three frequencies:

- $X_1 = X_1(t)$ = number of pairs with both co-twins alive at age t;
- X_2 = number of pairs with one alive, one dead at age t; and
- X_3 = number of pairs, both dead before age t.

The multinomial distribution, in general, is described in Section 1.4.

At first glance, the multinomial distribution in the present application appears to be a two-dimensional random variable. There are two linear constraints, however. One constraint is that there are

$$X_1 + X_2 + X_3 = n$$

twin pairs in all.

The second constraint is the number

$$2X_1 + X_2 = m$$

of individuals alive at age t. We will also condition this number in this chapter and the following.

These two linear constraints demonstrate that the joint distribution of $\{X_1, X_2, X_3\}$ is expressible as a one-dimensional random variable. In particular, we will concentrate on the distribution of X_1, the number of twin pairs who are both alive at a specified age.

The multinomial index is n and the three probabilities are

$$p^2, \ 2p(1-p), \ \text{and} \ (1-p)^2$$

respectively, where $p = p(t)$ denotes the marginal probability that an individual is alive at age t in the cohort.

We want an expression for the conditional distribution of X_1, the number of pairs where both are alive, given $m = 2X_1 + X_2$ individuals alive. Write

$$\Pr[\, X_1 = x \mid 2X_1 + X_2 = m\,] = \Pr[\, X_1 = x \text{ and } X_2 = m - 2x\,] \Big/ \Pr[\, 2X_1 + X_2 = m\,].$$

The numerator of this conditional probability can be written using the multinomial mass function (1.9), giving

$$\begin{aligned}
&\Pr[\, X_1 = x;\ X_2 = m - 2x;\ \text{and } X_3 = n - m + x\,] \\
&\quad = \frac{n!}{x!\,(m-2x)!\,(n-m+x)!}\; p^{2x}\,\{2p(1-p)\}^{m-2x}\,(1-p)^{2(n-m+x)} \\
&\quad = \frac{n!}{x!\,(m-2x)!\,(n-m+x)!}\; 2^{m-2x}\,p^{m}\,(1-p)^{2n-m}.
\end{aligned}$$

Notice that there are no terms in p^x or $(1-p)^x$ in this last expression.

We can then write

$$\Pr[\, X_1 = x \mid 2X_1 + X_2 = m\,] \propto 2^{m-2x} / \{x!\,(m-2x)!\,(n-m+x)!\}, \quad (4.1)$$

ignoring the terms that are not a function of x.

The normalizing constant for this distribution will be determined below. The range of x is

$$\max(0, m-n) \le x \le \lfloor m/2 \rfloor,$$

where $\lfloor y \rfloor$ is the greatest integer in y.

Another derivation of (4.1) is obtained through a reasoning using a permutation argument. The probability that the number of twin pairs, where both are alive, $X_1(m)$ is equal to x is

$$\Pr[\, X_1 = x \mid m, n\,] = 2^{m-2x} \binom{n}{x} \binom{n-x}{m-2x} \Big/ \binom{2n}{m}. \quad (4.2)$$

Intuitively, the terms in (4.2) can be explained as follows. The numerator of (4.2) chooses the x pairs where both are alive, with

$$\binom{n}{x}$$

and

$$\binom{n-x}{m-2x}$$

picks those pairs with only one living twin.

The 2^{m-2x} term permutes the two possible choices of alive/dead within the $m - 2x$ pairs where only one is alive. The denominator

$$\binom{2n}{m}$$

in (4.2) gives the number of ways that m living individuals can be chosen out of the $2n$ total. Notice that (4.1) and (4.2) are not functions of the parameter p.

We can easily verify that (4.1) and (4.2) are the same function of x, up to a multiplicative constant that is only a function of n and m. This demonstrates that distributions (4.1) and (4.2) coincide. We verify that (4.2) sums to unity in Section 4.5.1. In Section 4.3, we develop model (4.1) further to include a measure of association within the twin pairs.

Fig. 4.1 provides a graphical example of the distribution (4.2) for $n = 15$ twin pairs and several different values of m living individuals. This figure illustrates the intuitive relation that more twin pairs, where both are alive, are to be expected when the number of living individuals m increases.

There is a connection here to case-control studies. The study of case-control data often involves a description of the number of concordant or discordant pairs. In this twin data, the number of discordant pairs (one living and one dead) is $X_2 = m - 2X_1$. Similarly, the number of concordant pairs (either both alive or both dead) is $n - m + 2X_1$. The distribution of the number of concordant or discordant pairs, conditional on the number of living individuals m, can then be found using (4.2). The analogy to case-control studies is not complete, however. In our examination of twins, the individuals within each pair are exchangeable. That is, these twins are equivalent and one can be substituted for the other within the same pair. In contrast, a case-control pair is identified as such and differs in

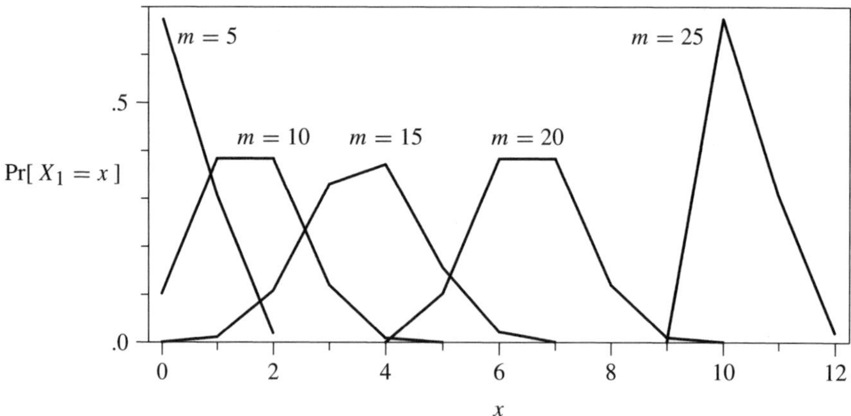

Figure 4.1 The univariate twin distribution (4.2) for $n = 15$ twin pairs and values of m living individuals as given.

terms of their disease state. Exchangeability and models for exchangeable random variables are discussed in Section 7.3.

There is also an analogy to distribution (4.2) using an urn model. Suppose m out of $2n$ balls in an urn are white and the remaining $2n - m$ are red. Imagine drawing balls two at a time, without replacement until the urn is emptied. Let X_1 denote the number of pairs drawn that are both white. The distribution of X_1 is given in (4.2).

We next describe the moments of this distribution. The factorial moments of distribution (4.2) are given in Section 4.5.1. In particular, the expected value of this distribution is

$$\mathrm{E}[\,X_1\,] = \mathrm{E}[\,X_1 \mid m, n\,] = m(m-1)/2(2n-1) \tag{4.3}$$

and the variance is

$$\mathrm{Var}[\,X_1\,] = (\mathrm{E}[\,X_1\,])\,\frac{(2n-m)(2n-m-1)}{(2n-1)(2n-3)}. \tag{4.4}$$

The variance of X_1 is always less than its mean except when both are zero. The ratio $\mathrm{Var}[X_1]/\mathrm{E}[X_1]$ decreases in m, holding n fixed. The variance is zero when m is within one of the extremes of its parameter range; *i.e.*, when $m = 0,\ 1,\ 2n-1$, or $2n$. Similarly, the variance is maximized when $m = n$.

Distribution (4.2) is never symmetric, except in degenerate cases. The third central moment

$$\mathrm{E}[\,X_1 - \mathrm{E}[\,X_1\,]\,]^3 = \mathrm{Var}[\,X_1\,]\,\frac{(2n-2m-1)(2n-2m+1)}{(2n-1)(2n-5)}$$

is always non-negative except when $n = m$.

Let us place distribution (4.2) within two large families of discrete distributions. This distribution is of Ord's Type I. See Ord (1967) or Johnson, Kotz, and Kemp (1992, pp 81–84). Distribution (4.2) is also in the Kemp (1968) family. Its probability generating function $\mathrm{E}[t^{X_1}]$ is expressible as the ratio of two ${}_2F_1$ hypergeometric functions (Johnson, Kotz, and Kemp (1992, pp. 84–91)). The unconditional distribution of $2X_1 + X_2$ at (4.1) is a member of the univariate multinomial distribution (Johnson, Kotz, and Kemp (1992, pp. 460–463)).

Section 4.5.2 describes approximations to distribution (4.2) when n is large. If m^2/n is small, then distribution (4.2) becomes a degenerate point mass at zero. That is, if there are too few living individuals m relative to the number of twin pairs n, then it is unlikely that any two living individuals would appear within the same twin pair.

When m grows in proportion to $n^{1/2}$, then an approximate Poisson distribution is obtained for the number of twin pairs where both are alive X_1. If m grows in proportion to n, then the number of twin pairs where both are alive will have an approximate normal distribution. The details of these approximations are given in Section 4.5.2.

4.3 Measures of Association in Twins

In this section, we describe a parametric model that measures the association of longevity within the twin pairs. Distribution (4.1) considers twins matched at random. The model in this section helps describe the behavior of the number of pairs where both are alive at a given age when there is some degree of association between them. We also want to model the degree of association and draw statistical inference from it. The previous section might be thought of as a model for the null hypothesis of independence in life spans. This section describes a model for a possible alternative hypothesis.

The idea here is to develop a measure of association similar to the way in which the familiar odds ratio is used in 2×2 tables of frequency data. There are many analogies in this model to 2×2 tables, including the way in which we estimate the odds ratio. The development in this section is similar to that of the extended hypergeometric distribution described in Section 1.7.2.

Consider the cells in Fig. 4.2 as representing the four possible states of alive and dead within each twin pair. The distribution described in this section models within-pair association. We use the four probabilities illustrated in the four cells in Fig. 4.2 and develop a generalization of model (4.1). Let $p = p(t)$ denote the marginal probability that a person is alive at age t in the cohort. Both sets of marginal probabilities of this table are equal and the log-odds ratio is θ. The parameter θ will be used to measure the association in longevity between the twin pairs.

The concept of the log-odds ratio does not have the usual interpretation as in a 2×2 table for a matched case-control pair. The alive/dead status of twin

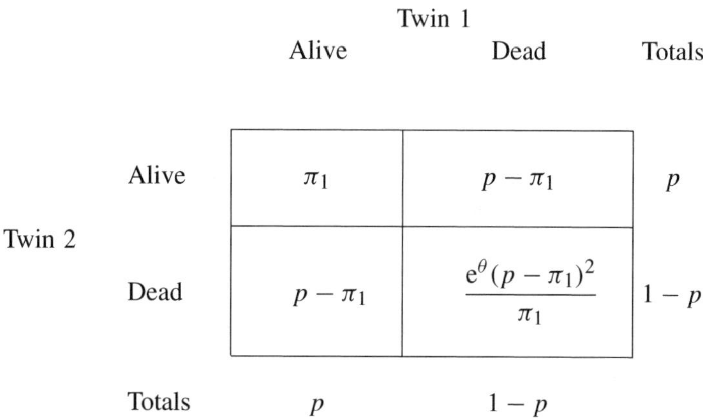

		Twin 1		
		Alive	Dead	Totals
Twin 2	Alive	π_1	$p - \pi_1$	p
	Dead	$p - \pi_1$	$\dfrac{e^{\theta}(p - \pi_1)^2}{\pi_1}$	$1 - p$
	Totals	p	$1 - p$	

Figure 4.2 A model for the probabilities of alive/dead status in twins used in (4.5). The log-odds ratio for this table is θ.

'one' cannot be interpreted as the exposure and the alive/dead status of twin 'two' is not the outcome because the twins are exchangeable within each pair. The exchangeability of co-twins within each pair suggests that we combine the two off-diagonal cells in Fig. 4.2. This combined count was referred to as X_2 in the previous section.

Following the development of the previous section, consider a multinomial distribution with three frequencies:

- X_1 = number of twin pairs, both alive;
- X_2 = number of pairs with one alive, one dead; and
- X_3 = number of pairs, both dead.

The corresponding probabilities for these three multinomial frequencies $\{X_1, X_2, X_3\}$ are denoted by $\{\pi_1, \pi_2, \pi_3\}$, respectively.

The multinomial index is n and the three probabilities are π_1 for the both-alive pairs and

$$\pi_2 = 2(p - \pi_1)$$

is the sum of the probabilities for the two off-diagonal (one alive and one dead) discordant pairs.

Finally,

$$\pi_3 = (p - \pi_1)^2 e^\theta / \pi_1$$

is the probability for the both-dead category in Fig. 4.2.

We can solve the quadratic equation for π_1 giving

$$\pi_1 = p + [2(e^\theta - 1)]^{-1}\{1 - [4p(1-p)e^\theta + (2p-1)^2]^{1/2}\},$$

but this value will not be needed.

As we saw in the derivation of (4.1), we want to describe the conditional distribution of X_1 pairs where both are alive, given that there are $2X_1 + X_2 = m$ living individuals. This conditional distribution satisfies

$$\begin{aligned} &\Pr[\, X_1 = x \mid 2X_1 + X_2 = m \,] \\ &\qquad \propto \Pr[\, X_1 = x \text{ and } 2X_1 + X_2 = m \,] \\ &\qquad = \Pr[\, X_1 = x;\ X_2 = m - 2x; \text{ and } X_3 = n - m + x \,]. \end{aligned}$$

The constant of proportionality here does not depend on the value of x. The multinomial probability of $\{X_1, X_2, X_3\}$ with parameters $\{\pi_1, \pi_2, \pi_3\}$ gives

$$\begin{aligned} &\Pr[\, X_1 = x \mid 2X_1 + X_2 = m \,] \\ &\propto \frac{n!}{x!\,(m-2x)!\,(n-m+x)!}\, \pi_1^x\, [2(p-\pi_1)]^{m-2x}\, [(p-\pi_1)^2 e^\theta/\pi_1]^{n-m+x}. \end{aligned}$$

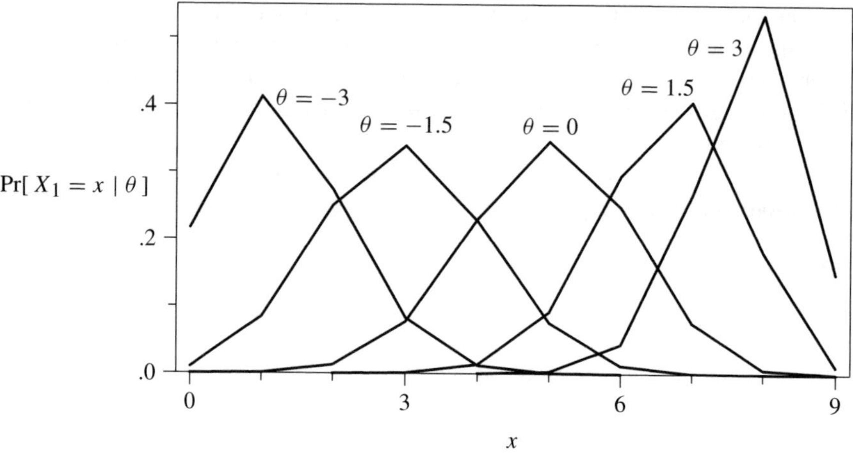

Figure 4.3 The univariate twin distribution (4.5) for $n = 25$ twin pairs with $m = 18$ living individuals and values of the log-odds ratio θ as given.

If we ignore terms that are not a function of x, then the conditional distribution of X_1 given $2X_1 + X_2 = m$ living individuals is proportional to

$$\Pr[X_1 = x \mid 2X_1 + X_2 = m] \propto \frac{2^{m-2x} \exp(\theta x)}{x!\,(m-2x)!\,(n-m+x)!} \tag{4.5}$$

defined for real-valued parameter θ and the same range

$$\max\{0, m-n\} \le x \le \lfloor m/2 \rfloor$$

as in the distributions (4.1) and (4.2).

Intuitively, (4.5) is a weighted distribution in which $\Pr[X_1 = x]$ given at (4.1) is multiplied by the weight $\exp(\theta x)$. The constant of proportionality in (4.5) does not have a simple expression and is a function of (n, m, θ) but not x. When $\theta = 0$, distribution (4.5) reduces to expression (4.1). Although (π_1, π_2, π_3) each depends on the margins in Fig. 4.2, distribution (4.5) is not a function of the marginal probability p.

Distribution (4.5) is a member of the exponential family of distributions (*cf.* Stuart and Ord (1987, Sections 5.47–8)). The maximum likelihood estimate $\widehat{\theta} = \widehat{\theta}(x)$ of θ in (4.5), given a single observed value $X_1 = x$ satisfies the estimating equation

$$\mathrm{E}[X_1 \mid \theta = \widehat{\theta}(x)] = x. \tag{4.6}$$

That is, the maximum likelihood estimator equates the observed and expected values in distribution (4.5) (Fig. 4.3).

The Cramér-Rao inequality shows that the variance of $\widehat{\theta}(x)$ satisfies the approximation

$$\text{Var}\,[\,\widehat{\theta}(X_1)\,] \approx 1\,/\,\text{Var}\,[\,X_1 \mid \widehat{\theta}\,]. \tag{4.7}$$

Distribution (4.5) has many analogies to the extended hypergeometric distribution for a 2×2 table given in Section 1.7.2. Both distributions are known only up to a multiplicative constant. Parameter estimation in the extended hypergeometric distribution also follows (4.6) and (4.7).

The exact $(1-\alpha)\%$ confidence interval $(\theta_1,\, \theta_2)$ of θ after observing $X_1 = x$ is calculated in the following section by solving the pair of equations:

$$\Pr[\, X_1 \geq x \mid \theta_1\,] = \alpha/2$$

and

$$\Pr[\, X_1 \leq x \mid \theta_2\,] = \alpha/2.$$

The SAS program in Table 4.6 can be used to find the maximum likelihood estimate $\widehat{\theta}$ of θ in (4.6) and solve these two equations for the exact $(1-\alpha)\%$ confidence interval of θ. This program was used to obtain all of the computed values in Tables 4.2 and 4.3 in the following section:

Table 4.2 Univariate analysis of $n = 117$ identical (MZ) female Danish twin pairs born 1870–80 (Hauge, *et al.*, 1968).

					Estimate of association		
Age t	Women living m_t	Pairs both alive x	Expected pairs both alive $E[X_1 \mid m_t]$	Exact upper tail	Log odds ratio $\widehat{\theta}$	Exact 95% confidence interval	
30	220	105	103.39	.0488	2.19	−.39	4.37
35	218	103	101.52	.0834	1.80	−.71	3.85
40	213	98	96.90	.2224	1.04	−1.36	2.89
45	210	96	94.18	.0968	1.30	−.61	2.95
50	205	92	89.74	.0731	1.23	−.40	2.71
55	201	88	86.27	.1676	.84	−.75	2.24
60	186	75	73.84	.3430	.35	−.91	1.93
65	166	65	58.78	.0057	1.18	.25	2.13
70	146	53	45.43	.0027	1.17	.32	2.05
75	110	35	25.73	.0005	1.31	.49	2.52
80	75	17	11.91	.0263	.89	−.01	1.79
85	39	7	3.18	.0177	1.36	.09	2.60
90	18	2	.657	.1300	1.47	−.99	3.42
95	2	0	.004	1	—	—	—

Table 4.3 Univariate analysis of $n = 192$ dizygotic (DZ) female–female Danish twin pairs.

Age t	Women living m_t	Pairs both alive x	Expected pairs both alive $E[X_1 \mid m_t]$	Exact upper tail	Estimate of association: Log odds ratio $\widehat{\theta}$	Exact 95% confidence interval	
30	365	174	173.45	.3738	.93	−2.96	3.15
35	352	163	161.30	.1264	1.09	−.73	2.57
40	345	156	154.93	.3017	.57	−1.21	1.97
45	339	150	149.58	.4946	.19	−1.56	1.55
50	330	143	141.74	.3086	.41	−.91	1.55
55	312	129	126.67	.1901	.48	−.51	1.40
60	295	114	113.22	.4477	.12	−.76	.96
65	271	99	95.52	.1499	.41	−.32	1.12
70	234	74	71.18	.2400	.26	−.38	.89
75	184	47	43.96	.2309	.25	−.35	.86
80	122	21	19.27	.3388	.19	−.52	.88
85	68	9	5.94	.1048	.66	−.34	1.61
90	19	0	.446	1	—	—	—
95	6	0	.039	1	—	—	—

4.4 The Danish Twin Registry

We demonstrate the utility of these methods to study longevity in twins born in Denmark between 1870 and 1880 (Hauge, *et al.*, 1968). This data has also been examined by McGue, Vaupel, Holm, and Harvald (1993), Hougaard, Harvald, and Holm (1992), and Anderson, Louis, Holm, and Harvald (1992) using survival models and other methods. We identified $n = 117$ identical (monozygotic or MZ) female twin pairs for whom exact age at death is known for both individuals. Table 4.2 gives the number of living individuals (m) and the number of observed pairs where both are alive X_1 for ages 30 through 95 in five-year intervals. The distinction between MZ and DZ twins will be discussed later in this section. Ages after 85 years will generally be ignored because too few individuals remained alive at that age.

At every age up to 85 years, there are more identical twin pairs where both are alive than the number expected. The expected number of pairs with both co-twins alive is calculated using (4.3) when we randomly match all the women in the cohort into pairs. After age 60, this difference is statistically significant at the 5% level using the upper tail of the exact distribution (4.2). We will ignore data on ages 90 and older because too few individuals remained alive at that age and inference cannot be meaningfully interpreted. After age 60, the estimated log-odds ratios $\widehat{\theta}$ in Table 4.2 are greater than zero at all ages and, except at age 80 years, the exact 95% confidence intervals do not include zero. At younger ages, between age 30 and 60 years, the estimated log-odds ratio is greater than zero, but the exact 95% confidence intervals always cover zero.

At the youngest age, there appears to be a statistically significant relationship. This can be explained by a number of twin pairs who both died at a very early age. These pairs will be explained again in Section 5.6.3.

In summary, the force of longevity within the identical female twin pairs becomes apparent at ages 65 years and later. The univariate inference on the Danish twins indicates that a statistically large number of twin pairs are both alive at older ages than would be expected by chance alone were these individuals matched at random. This univariate analysis is performed marginally, with a separate significance level at each age. The analysis of this data using multivariate models appears in Chapter 5.

The question that remains in this examination of the twin data is how much of this association can be attributed to similarities in the shared environment, upbringing, diet, and so on. Part of this question can be answered by contrasting DZ twins to MZ twins. In MZ or identical twins, a single fertilized egg splits and develops into two individuals with identical genes. Although it is not well understood why this splitting occurs, it does not occur until about ten days after fertilization.

In DZ or fraternal twins, two fertilized eggs develop into two individuals who share approximately 50% of their genetic material. These two DZ individuals could be of opposite sex. We restricted our discussion to female–female DZ pairs in order to provide a good comparison with the MZ pairs who must be of the same sex.

The DZ twins share roughly 50% of their genetic material and MZ twins have identical genes so we may attribute any differences in these two types of twins to the effect of the additional 50% not shared. This reasoning assumes that both types of twins shared similar environmental backgrounds during their lifetimes and only their genetic composition varied. We have no reason to suspect, for example, that female MZ and DZ twins differ in any lifestyle or environmental characteristics that may contribute to human longevity.

The Danish Twin Registry also contains the life span records of 192 female–female DZ twins born between 1870 and 1880. The methodology developed here is also applied to this data set and the results are summarized in Table 4.3, parallel to the data in Table 4.2 for MZ twins. Although Table 4.3 always exhibits more DZ twin pairs where both are alive at older ages than would be expected by chance alone if these DZ twins were randomly matched, this univariate inference indicates that these differences are not statistically significant at any age. In contrast, the MZ twins showed a statistically large number of pairs where both are alive at all ages after 65 years.

The estimated log-odds ratio $\widehat{\theta}$ from the association model (4.5) of Section 4.3 are plotted in Figure 4.4 starting at age 30 and every two years thereafter, separately for the MZ and DZ twins. There were no DZ twins where both were alive after

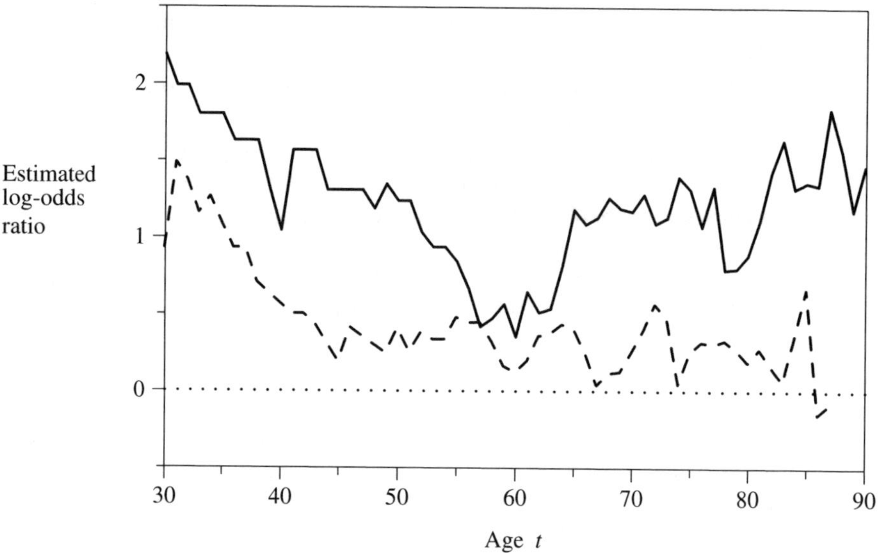

Figure 4.4 Estimated log-odds ratios $\widehat{\theta}(t)$ for the female MZ (solid line) and DZ (dashed) twins for all ages t starting at 30 years.

age 86 and these $\widehat{\theta}$'s cannot be estimated. The estimated log-odds ratios of the MZ twins are about twice as large as those of the DZ twins at every age after 65. Between age 30 and age 65, the estimated log-odds ratios are not significantly different from zero for both MZ and DZ twins.

4.4.1 Estimate of the effect

The examination of the data, so far, demonstrates a high degree of correlation in the joint life spans of MZ twins as measured by the numbers of pairs where both are alive after age 65 years. The question is how large this effect is, in terms of years gained in life span. Let us try to address this question next.

If S is the survival time, then the function

$$\phi(t) = \mathrm{E}[\, S \mid S > t\,]$$

for $t > 0$ is called the *expected residual life*, given that the person has already attained age t. In other words, ϕ describes life expectancy conditional on having already achieved the specified age t.

Let us consider two different estimates of $\phi(t)$ and compare these. The simplest estimator of expected residual life at age t for the data is to average all observed life spans greater than t. That is, the first estimate is

$$\widehat{\phi}_1(t) = \text{Average}\{\text{lifespan} \mid \text{lifespan} > t\}.$$

This estimator is simply the average life span of all persons who lived beyond age t. There is a separate estimator $\widehat{\phi}_1$ for the MZ and the DZ data.

The second estimator is to restrict this average to those individuals whose co-twin is also alive. So define

$$\widehat{\phi}_2(t) = \text{Average}\{\text{lifespan} \mid \text{lifespan} > t \text{ and lifespan of co} - \text{twin} > t\}.$$

If there is no genetic or environmental effect of longevity, then these two estimates should be approximately equal. If there is a genetic effect to longevity, then this should be better estimated by $\widehat{\phi}_2$ because it is more likely to be affecting the life span of the co-twin as well. The estimator $\widehat{\phi}_1$ contains many more unrelated individuals who may or may not possess any beneficial genetic or environmental effects. At great ages t, the estimator $\widehat{\phi}_2$ is more likely to be averaged over those individuals who share the gene and/or environment for longevity, if one exists.

The difference $\widehat{\phi}_2(t) - \widehat{\phi}_1(t)$ is plotted in Fig. 4.5 for all ages t greater than 30 years. A separate line is plotted for the MZ (solid) and DZ (dashed) twin pairs. Up to about age 55, there is negligible difference in $\widehat{\phi}_2 - \widehat{\phi}_1$ for both the MZ and DZ twin pairs. At all ages after 60 years, both sets of differences in Fig. 4.5 are generally positive. The variability of these separate differences increases with age because the respective averages are taken over smaller numbers of living persons.

The DZ twin pairs (dashed line) indicate a positive effect of longevity of approximately a quarter of a year after age 60. The solid line for MZ twins estimates a positive effect of approximately half a year, or perhaps a little more. The

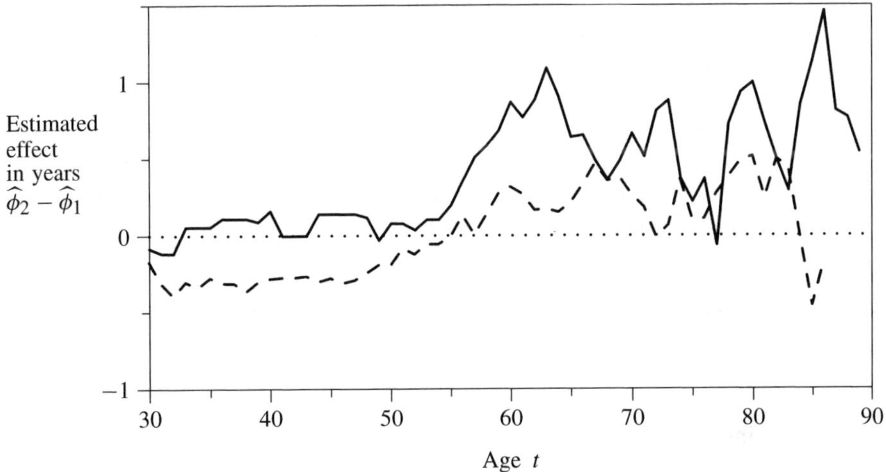

Figure 4.5 Estimated effect of longevity benefit in years measured by $\widehat{\phi}_2(t) - \widehat{\phi}_1(t)$ for the female MZ (solid line) and DZ (dashed) twins for all ages t starting at 30 years.

conclusion of looking at Fig. 4.5 is that the estimated effect of longevity manifests itself in terms of a few additional months of survival, at most.

4.4.2 Approximations

We end the main text of this chapter with a discussion of approximations to distribution (4.1) and (4.2) when the number of twin pairs n is large. The mathematical details of these approximations are given Section 4.5.2. If m^2/n has a finite, nonzero limit, then the number of pairs where both are alive X_1 has an approximate Poisson distribution. If m/n has a nonzero limit, then X_1 has an approximate normal distribution. These two applications are illustrated next.

Table 4.4 provides a portion of the MZ data to illustrate the normal and Poisson approximations to the distribution (4.2). The normal approximations in Table 4.4 match both the mean and variance. The normal significance levels are reasonably close to the exact values if we also include the usual continuity correction. That is, the normal approximate probability of x or more is calculated as $x - 1/2$ or more. Without this correction, the normal significance levels are about half of those of the exact values.

The Poisson approximation is poor at all ages. This poor approximation by the Poisson distribution has several explanations. The Poisson variance is equal to its mean but the variance of distribution (4.2) can be much smaller than its mean. For this reason, the Poisson tail areas appear much larger than the exact tail areas. The problem with the asymptotic Poisson approximation is that it requires m to be on the order of $2n^{1/2}$. Although $n = 117$ is large, $2n^{1/2}$ is 21.6. In other words, only small values of m (relative to n) will have a good Poisson approximation for this data set. At the same time, in the Poisson approximation, the error terms in the asymptotic expansion given in the appendix are $O(m^{-1})$ and require m to be large.

The remainder of this chapter describes some of the mathematical details associated with the distributions given in (4.2) and (4.5). These details include verifying that the distribution given in (4.2) sums to 1 and finding an expression for its moments. Section 4.5.2 demonstrates the Poisson and normal approximate

Table 4.4 Approximate univariate analysis for $n = 117$ identical twin pairs.

Age t	Number living m	Pairs both alive x	$E[X_1]$	$Var[X_1]$	Exact p-value	Approximate significance levels: Poisson	Approximate significance levels: Normal
40	213	98	96.90	.76	.2224	.4690	.2456
60	186	75	73.84	3.10	.3430	.4617	.3539
80	75	17	11.91	5.56	.0263	.0965	.0258

distribution to (4.2). The following chapter develops multivariate distributions to measure whether the genetic effect of longevity appears at just one age or whether it continues to contribute after we condition its effects at earlier ages.

4.5 Appendix

4.5.1 The univariate twins distribution

To show that (4.2) sums to unity, consider the generating polynomial identity

$$(1+z)^{2n} = (1+2z+z^2)^n .$$

This equality holds for all values of z and consequently the coefficients of all of the powers of z must agree on both sides.

Identify the coefficient of z^m on both sides of this equality to show

$$\binom{2n}{m} = \sum_{x}^{\lfloor m/2 \rfloor} \frac{n!\, 2^{m-2x}}{x!\,(m-2x)!\,(n-m+x)!}$$
$$= \sum_x 2^{m-2x} \binom{n}{x} \binom{n-x}{m-2x}.$$

This relation provides the normalizing constant for (4.1) and demonstrates that (4.2) sums to unity. The proof is similar to the Vandermonde theorem used at (1.20) in Section 1.7 to demonstrate that the mass function of the hypergeometric distribution sums to one.

In this Appendix, we will refer to X_1 more simply as X without the '1' subscript.

Moments of distribution (4.2) can be found as follows. For $r = 1, 2, \ldots$ define the factorial polynomial

$$z^{(r)} = z(z-1)\cdots(z-r+1) = z!\,/(z-r)!.$$

The rth factorial moment of distribution (4.2) is

$$\mathrm{E}[\,X^{(r)}\,] = n^{(r)} m^{(2r)}/(2n)^{(2r)}, \tag{4.8}$$

from which we compute the expected value

$$\mathrm{E}[\,X\,] = m(m-1)/2(2n-1)$$

and variance

$$\mathrm{Var}[\,X\,] = \frac{m(m-1)(2n-m)(2n-m-1)}{2(2n-1)^2(2n-3)}$$
$$= \mathrm{E}[\,X\,]\,\frac{(2n-m)(2n-m-1)}{(2n-1)(2n-3)}.$$

The ratio $\text{Var}[X]/\text{E}[X]$ decreases in m, holding n fixed.

The third central moment

$$\text{E}[X - \text{E}[X]]^3 = \text{Var}[X]\frac{(2n-2m-1)(2n-2m+1)}{(2n-1)(2n-5)}$$

is always non-negative except when $n = m$.

The ratio

$$\begin{aligned}\Pr[X = x]/\Pr[X = x-1]\\ &= (m-2x+1)(m-2x+2)/4x(n-m+x)\end{aligned}$$

is strictly decreasing in x, showing that distribution (4.2) is unimodal.

The measure

$$\begin{aligned}\{\Pr[X = x] - \Pr[X = x-1]\} / \Pr[X = x-1]\\ &= [(m+1)(m+2) - x(4n+6)]/[4x^2 + 4x(n-m)] \qquad (4.9)\end{aligned}$$

shows that the modes occur at

$$\tilde{x} = (m+1)(m+2)/(4n+6)$$

and $\tilde{x} - 1$ or within one of $\tilde{x}$ if $\tilde{x}$ is not an integer.

The mean of X is greater than $\tilde{x}$, except in degenerate distributions. The relation at (4.9) also shows this distribution is of Ord's Type I. See Ord (1967) or Johnson, Kotz, and Kemp (1992, pp. 81–84).

The probability generating function of X can be expressed as

$$\text{E}[z^X] = \frac{{}_2F_1[-m/2, (1-m)/2; n-m+1; z]}{{}_2F_1[-m/2, (1-m)/2; n-m+1; 1]},$$

which is the ratio of two ${}_2F_1$ generalized hypergeometric functions. This result also places distribution (4.2) in the Kemp (1968) family (Johnson, Kotz, and Kemp (1992, pp. 84–91)).

4.5.2 Approximating distributions

This appendix describes a degenerate limit and two approximating distributions when n is large.

If m^2/n is very small, then distribution (4.2) becomes degenerate with all of its mass at zero. Specifically,

$$\begin{aligned}\Pr[X = 0] &= 2^m \binom{n}{m} \Big/ \binom{2n}{m}\\ &= \prod_{j=0}^{m-1} 2(n-j)/(2n-j)\\ &> [1 - m/(2n-m)]^m\end{aligned}$$

and

$$\begin{aligned}\log \Pr[\, X = 0\,] &> m \log[1 - m/(2n - m)] \\ &= -m^2/2n + \mathrm{O}(m^2/n).\end{aligned}$$

This last expression tends to zero if m^2 is much smaller than n, showing that $\Pr[X = 0]$ is very close to 1.

When n is large and m grows in proportion to $n^{1/2}$, then an approximate Poisson distribution is obtained. If m grows in proportion to n, then we have a normal limiting distribution. The details of the Poisson and normal approximations are given next.

If m and n are both large such that $m^2/4n$ approaches a finite, nonzero limit denoted by λ, then an approximate Poisson (λ) distribution in (4.2) is obtained. This asymptotic Poisson distribution can be demonstrated by showing that all of the moments of X converge to those of a Poisson variate.

For every $r = 1, 2, \ldots$, from (4.8),

$$\mathrm{E}[\,X^{(r)}\,] = \prod_{j=0}^{r-1} \frac{(n-j)(m-2j)(m-2j-1)}{(2n-2j)(2n-2j-1)} = \lambda^r S_r,$$

where $\lambda = m^2/4n$ and

$$S_r = \prod_{j=0}^{r-1} \{1 - 2j/m\}\{1 - (2j+1)/m\} \,/\, \{1 - (2j+1)/2n\}.$$

Since

$$(1 - 2r/m)^{2r} \le S_r \le (1 - r/n)^{-r},$$

we have $S_r = 1 + \mathrm{O}(m^{-1})$.

This shows that all factorial moments, and more generally, all of the moments of X, agree with those of the Poisson distribution given in (1.11). Following Theorem 4.5.5 of Chung (1974, page 99), for example, X converges to a Poisson random variable in distribution.

We demonstrate next a normal approximate distribution to (4.2) when n is large and m grows in proportion to n. Specifically, for n sufficiently large suppose that

$$m = 2\gamma n \tag{4.10}$$

for some γ satisfying $0 < \gamma < 1$.

Then

$$\mathrm{E}[X] \doteq \gamma^2 n$$

and

$$\mathrm{Var}\,[X] \doteq \gamma^2 (1-\gamma)^2 n.$$

Define the function

$$x = x(z) = \gamma^2 n + \gamma(1-\gamma)n^{1/2} z \tag{4.11}$$

The Jacobian of this transformation is

$$\sigma = \gamma(1-\gamma)n^{1/2}.$$

The first step in demonstrating the normal approximation is to write all factorials in

$$p = p(z) = \sigma \Pr[\, X = x(z)\,] = \frac{2^{m-2x} n!\,(2n-m)!\,m!\,\sigma}{x!\,(m-2x)!\,(n-m+x)!\,(2n)!}$$

using Stirling's formula (1.26).

Define

$$\log p^*(z) = -\frac{1}{2}\log(2\pi) + \frac{1}{2}\log\left[\frac{n(2n-m)m\sigma^2}{x(m-2x)(n-m+x)(2n)}\right]$$

$$+n\log\left[\frac{n(2n-m)^2}{(n-m+x)(2n)^2}\right] + m\log\left[\frac{2m(n-m+x)}{(2n-m)(m-2x)}\right]$$

$$+x\log\left[\frac{(m-2x)^2}{4x(n-m+x)}\right]$$

All of the arguments of factorials in p grow in proportion to n so $\log p$ and $\log p^*$ differ by $\mathrm{O}(n^{-1})$.

Use substitutions (4.10) and (4.11) and set $z=0$ to show

$$\log p^*(z=0) = -\frac{1}{2}\log 2\pi.$$

We next want to expand $\log p^*$ in powers of z about zero. Write

$$\frac{\partial \log p^*}{\partial x} = -(2x)^{-1} + (m-2x)^{-1} - [2(n-m+x)]^{-1} + \log\left[\frac{(m-2x)^2}{4x\,(n-m+x)}\right]$$

and

$$\partial x/\partial z = \sigma = \mathrm{O}(n^{1/2})$$

so that at $z=0$,

$$\frac{\partial \log p^*}{\partial z} = \frac{\partial \log p^*}{\partial x}\frac{\partial x}{\partial z} = \mathrm{O}(n^{-1/2}).$$

Since $x(z)$ is linear in z, at $z=0$ we have

$$\frac{\partial^2 \log p^*}{\partial z^2} = \frac{\partial^2 \log p^*}{\partial x^2}\left(\frac{\partial x}{\partial z}\right)^2 = -1 + \mathrm{O}(n^{-1/2}).$$

The coefficients of higher powers of z in $\log p^*(z)$ are $O(n^{-1/2})$ or smaller so that

$$\log p^*(z) = -\frac{1}{2}\log(2\pi) - z^2/2 + O(n^{-1/2}),$$

demonstrating the approximate standard normal distribution.

4.6 Programs for the Univariate Twins Distribution

These SAS programs fit the distributions of this chapter to the twin data and produce the statistics in Tables 4.2 and 4.3.

```
options linesize=78 center pagesize=59 number nodate;

/*
   Set limits of search to be +/- &limit.
   Increase this value if convergence fails
*/
%let limit=5;

/*
   Log of twin distribution probability, assigned as a function
   n=# of pairs                    m=# living individuals
   k=# of pairs, both alive
*/
%macro twinp(n,m,k);
   (&m - 2*&k)*log(2)                               /* 2^(m-2k)*/
                                                 /*  N choose k */
   + lgamma(&n+1) - lgamma(&n-&k+1) - lgamma(&k+1)
                                              /* N-k choose m-2k */
   + lgamma(&n-&k+1) - lgamma(&m-2*&k+1) - lgamma(&n-&m+&k+1)
                                     /* denominator:  2N choose m*/
   - lgamma(2*&n+1) + lgamma(2*&n-&m+1) + lgamma(&m+1)
%mend twinp;


/*
  Denominator of twin association distribution assigned to &den
*/
%macro denth(n,m,th,den);
   &den=0;
   do jjjjj = max(0,&m-&n) to floor(m/2); /* loop over range */
      &den = &den + exp( jjjjj*&th + %twinp(&n,&m,jjjjj) );
   end;
   drop jjjjj;                        /* delete local variable */
%mend denth;


/*
```

```
    Expected value of association distribution, assigned to &ex
*/
%macro expth(n,m,th,ex);
   &ex=0;
   do jjjjj=max(0,&m-&n) to floor(m/2);   /* loop over range */
      &ex = &ex + jjjjj*exp(jjjjj*&th + %twinp(&n,&m,jjjjj));
   end;
   %denth(&n,&m,&th,dxxxxx);            /*  obtain denominator */
   &ex=&ex/dxxxxx;               /* normalize with denominator */
   drop jjjjj dxxxxx;                /* delete local variables */
%mend expth;


/*
   Upper tail for twin distribution assigned to &tail variable
*/
%macro uptail(n,m,k,th,tail);
   &tail=0;
   do jjjjj=&k to floor(&m/2);/* loop from &k to upper limit */
      &tail = &tail + exp(jjjjj*&th + %twinp(&n,&m,jjjjj));
   end;
   %denth(&n,&m,&th,dxxxxx);            /*  obtain denominator */
   &tail=&tail/dxxxxx;           /* normalize with denominator */
   drop jjjjj dxxxxx;                /* delete local variables */
%mend uptail;


/*
   Lower tail for twin distribution assigned to &tail variable
*/
%macro lotail(n,m,k,th,tail);
   &tail=0;
   do jjjjj=max(0,&m-&n) to &k; /* loop from bottom up to &k */
      &tail = &tail + exp(jjjjj*&th + %twinp(&n,&m,jjjjj));
   end;
   %denth(&n,&m,&th,dxxxxx);            /*  obtain denominator */
   &tail=&tail/dxxxxx;           /* normalize with denominator */
   drop jjjjj dxxxxx;                /* delete local variables */
%mend lotail;


/*
 Find the twin association parameter (th) giving a distribution
  with expected value equal to obs. Interval bisection is used.
  The initial interval for estimation is (-3,+3).  Make this
  wider if the algorithm does not converge.
*/
%macro assoc(n,m,th,obs);
   thlo= -&limit;  thhi= &limit;          /* initial interval */
       /* degenerate model if obs is at extreme of its range */
```

```
   if &obs LE max(0,&m-&n) then thhi=thlo; /* obs is too low */
   if &obs GE floor(&m/2) then thlo=thhi; /* obs is too high */

   do until (abs(thhi-thlo)<1e-6);    /* convergence criteria */
      &th=(thhi+thlo)/2;                   /* examine midpoint */
      %expth(&n,&m,&th,expd);  /* expected value at midpoint */
     /* shrink interval by equating expected value with expv */
      if &obs LE expd then thhi=&th;
      if &obs GE expd then thlo=&th;
   end;
   drop thhi thlo;
%mend assoc;


/*
   Exact 1-&a percent confidence interval of twin association
    parameter
*/
%macro exactci(n,m,k,a,clo,chi);
   thlo= -&limit;  thhi= &limit;           /* initial interval */
       /* degenerate model if obs is at extreme of its range */
   if &k LE max(0,&m-&n) then thhi = thlo; /* obs is too low */
   if &k GE floor(&m/2) then thlo = thhi; /* obs is too high */
   do until (abs(thhi-thlo)<1e-6);    /* convergence criteria */
      &clo=(thhi+thlo)/2;                  /* examine midpoint */
      %uptail(&n,&m,&k,&clo,pt);    /* upper tail at midpoint */
         /* shrink interval by equating upper tail with &a/2 */
      if pt GE &a/2 then thhi=&clo;
      if pt LE &a/2 then thlo=&clo;
   end;
     /* Repeat this for the upper end of confidence interval */
   thlo= -&limit;  thhi= &limit;           /* initial interval */
       /* degenerate model if obs is at extreme of its range */
   if &k LE max(0,&m-&n) then thhi = thlo; /* obs is too low */
   if &k GE floor(&m/2) then thlo = thhi; /* obs is too high */
   do until (abs(thhi-thlo)<1e-6);    /* convergence criteria */
      &chi=(thhi+thlo)/2;                  /* examine midpoint */
      %lotail(&n,&m,&k,&chi,pt);    /* lower tail at midpoint */
         /* shrink interval by equating lower tail with &a/2 */
      if pt LE &a/2 then thhi=&chi;
      if pt GE &a/2 then thlo=&chi;
   end;
   drop thhi thlo;                  /* delete local variables */
%mend exactci;

title1 'The univariate twin distribution';

title2 'Identical MZ Danish twin data';

data MZtwin;
```

```
   input
      age n m x;
   ex = m*(m-1)/(2*(2*n-1));                     /* expected value */
   %uptail(n,m,x,1,uptail); /* probability in the upper tail */
   %lotail(n,m,x,1,lotail);
   %assoc(n,m,thhat,x);       /* maximum likelihood estimate */
   %exactci(n,m,x,.05,clo,chi); /* exact confidence interval */
   label
      age    = 'age in years'
      n      = 'number of twin pairs'
      m      = 'number of living individuals'
      x      = '# of pairs both alive'
      ex     = 'expected value of x'
      uptail= 'probability in upper tail'
      thhat = 'theta hat association' ;
   datalines;
      30  117  220  105
      35  117  218  103
      40  117  213   98
      45  117  210   96
      50  117  205   92
      55  117  201   88
      60  117  186   75
      65  117  166   65
      70  117  146   53
      75  117  110   35
      80  117   75   17
      85  117   39    7
run;

proc print noobs;
  var age m x ex uptail thhat clo chi;
run;

title2 'Fraternal DZ Danish twin data';

data DZtwin;
   input
      age n m x;
   ex = m*(m-1)/(2*(2*n-1));                     /* expected value */
   %uptail(n,m,x,1,uptail); /* probability in the upper tail */
   %assoc(n,m,thhat,x);
   %exactci(n,m,x,.05,clo,chi); /* exact confidence interval */
   label
      age    = 'age in years'
      n      = 'number of twin pairs'
      m      = 'number of living individuals'
      x      = '# of pairs both alive'
      ex     = 'expected value of x'
      uptail= 'probability in upper tail'
```

```
      thhat = 'theta hat association';
   datalines;
      30 192 365 174
      35 192 352 163
      40 192 345 156
      45 192 339 150
      50 192 330 143
      55 192 312 129
      60 192 295 114
      65 192 271  99
      70 192 234  74
      75 192 184  47
      80 192 122  21
      85 192  68   9
run;

proc print noobs;
  var age m x ex uptail thhat clo chi;
run;
```

5

Multivariate Distributions for Twins

We use a large number of pairs both alive as evidence of a positive correlation in the life spans of these twins. In the previous chapter we noted a statistically large number of monozygotic MZ twin pairs, both alive after age 60. This represents the manifestation of a genetic and/or an environmental effect on human longevity. There is little or no evidence of this effect at younger ages provided by our analysis of these data. Does this effect only occur at a relatively short period in life between ages 60 and 65 or does the effect of longevity continue to exert itself at later ages as well? Is there some unobserved life experience that occurs between ages 60 and 65, and are those who successfully meet this challenge destined to live much longer than those who do not? Is the effect of longevity a single event or does it continue to build upon all earlier experiences?

In this chapter, we describe multivariate discrete distributions to answer these questions. Answers are based on measures of the association of longevity in the cohort of female twins born in Denmark between 1870 and 1880. If individuals are matched at random, then a stochastically large number of pairs both alive observed at advanced ages is our evidence of a genetic and/or an environmental effect on longevity. We extend the distributions of the previous chapter to a multivariate setting and derive the simultaneous and conditional distributions of the number of pairs, both alive at two or more different ages. We also propose a semiparametric model of association between two different ages and examine the simultaneous distribution of all twin pairs at all ages.

5.1 Introduction

In Section 5.3, we again look at the cohort of twins born in Denmark between 1870 and 1880. The aim of this chapter is to extend the distributions of the previous

Discrete Distributions Daniel Zelterman
 ISBN: 0-470-86888-0 (PPC)

chapter to provide a multivariate statistical analysis of the Danish twin data at several different ages, both conditionally and simultaneously. As in the previous chapter, our aim is to measure the association of longevity within these twin pairs. A large number of twin pairs with both members alive at an old age is our statistical evidence of a force of longevity. We repeat the caveat that twins are likely raised together and share a similar environment throughout most of their lives, so these conclusions are not the final word on the subject. Nevertheless, a consistent and convincing explanation emerges from the examination of this data that is both intuitive and reasonable. As with the analysis of this data in the previous chapter, we demonstrate statistically significant correlations in life spans between MZ twins. The dizygotic DZ twin pairs, however, have joint life spans that behave as those of randomly paired individuals.

Multivariate discrete distributions are developed here to measure this association. We continue to use the notation of the previous chapter. Suppose there are originally n twin pairs and let $m = m(t)$ denote the number of individuals alive at age t. When these $2n$ individuals (either living or dead) are randomly paired without replacement, we are interested in the distribution of the number of pairs $X = X(m)$ for which both pair members are alive. If longevity has a positive association within twins, then we would expect to see a statistically large number of twin pairs with both individuals alive at older ages.

The marginal distribution of the number of twin pairs, both alive at a given age is

$$\Pr[\, X(m) = k \mid m, n\,] = 2^{m-2k} \binom{n}{k} \binom{n-k}{m-2k} \bigg/ \binom{2n}{m} \tag{5.1}$$

and is described at (4.2) in the previous chapter.

Section 5.2 of the present chapter describes conditional, univariate distributions modeling the number of pairs, both alive at one age, conditional on the data from an earlier age. In Section 5.2.2, we develop a nonparametric measure of association for inference on twin pairs at two different ages. In Section 5.3, we apply these methods to the Danish Twin Registry. We again contrast MZ twins to DZ twins, and compare the measures of association developed in this chapter.

The distributions of Section 5.4 are developed to perform simultaneous multivariate inference on the twin data at several ages. We model the joint survival distribution of twin pairs at several different ages simultaneously. This allows us to obtain a single joint significance level for the entire data given in Tables 5.4 and 5.5.

All of the twin data analyzed up to Section 5.4 has survival times grouped into five-year intervals. The infinitesimal models of Section 5.6 describe methods applicable when every individual's survival time is treated as distinct and belongs to either the longer or shorter lived of her twin pair.

5.2 Conditional Distributions

In Table 4.2, we see that a statistically large number of MZ twin pairs are both alive after age 60. If we condition on the data from one age, are we still going to see this pattern at a later age? Is the effect of longevity a single event or does it continue to repeat its influence on survival at greater ages? We answer these questions using the conditional distributions developed here.

If we condition on the number of twin pairs, both living at age t, then what is the distribution of the number of pairs, both alive at the greater age t'? These conditional distributions are best described by the illustration in Fig. 5.1. At age t, there are m living individuals of the original $2n$. Let m' $(m' \leq m)$ denote the number of individuals alive at age t' $(t' > t)$. Throughout this chapter, primes ($'$) on symbols will always refer to the greater age.

5.2.1 Univariate conditional distribution

Conditional on $X(m) = k$ twin pairs, both alive at age t, the distribution of the number $X(m')$ of twin pairs, both alive at age t' is

$$\Pr[\, X(m') = k' \mid X(m) = k\,] = \sum_j \frac{k!\; 2^{k-k'-j}}{k'!\, j!\, (k-k'-j)!} \binom{m-2k}{m'-k-k'+j} \Big/ \binom{m}{m'} \tag{5.2}$$

where the sum on j is over the number of twin pairs both alive at age t and both dead at age t'.

See Fig. 5.1 to help motivate the functional form of this distribution. The outcome in the three boxes on the right of this figure is conditional on the contents of the three on the left. At age t there are m living people of the original $2n$ and of these, k twin pairs where both are alive. At age t' $(t' > t)$ there are m' $(m' \leq m)$ people alive and k' twin pairs where both are alive. Distribution (5.2) sums over j, the number of twin pairs, where both are alive at age t and both dead at age t'.

The k twin pairs, both alive at age t, can lose none, one, or both of their members by age t'. Specifically, of the k pairs, both alive at the earlier age, k' lose no members, $k - k' - j$ lose one member, and j lose both members. This explains the term

$$\frac{k!}{k'!\, j!\, (k-k'-j)!}$$

in (5.2).

There are two possible choices in each of the $k - k' - j$ twin pairs that were both alive at age t and that lose one member by age t', hence this power of 2 in (5.2). Similarly, in the $m - 2k$ pairs with only one surviving member at age

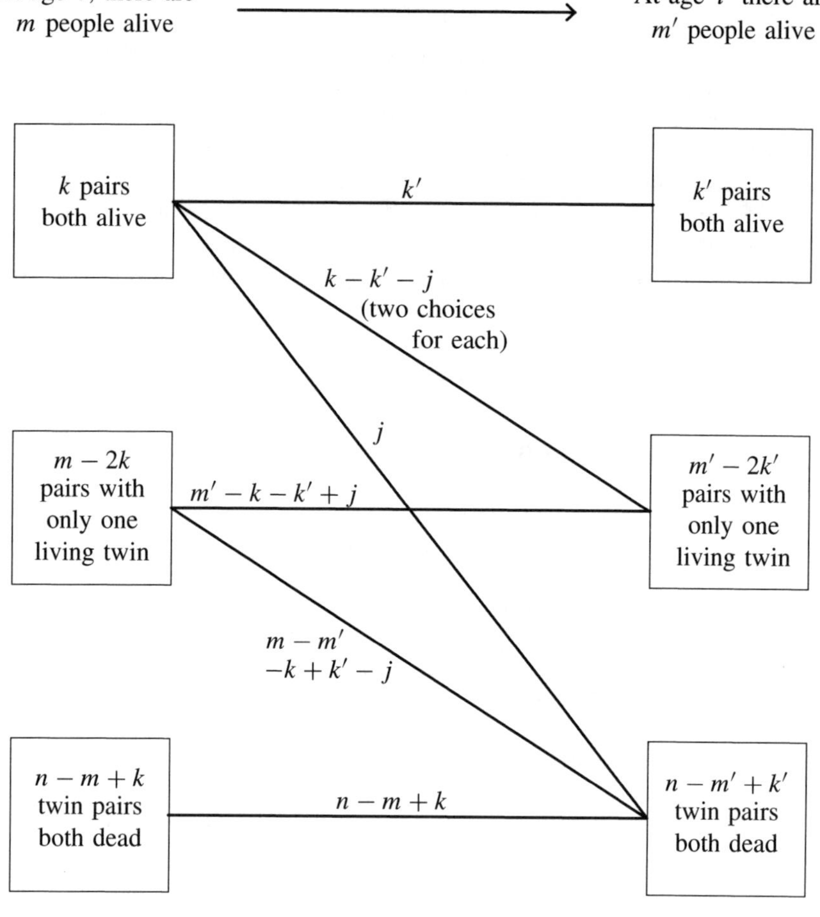

Figure 5.1 Illustration of the notation for the conditional distribution (5.2).

t, this one survivor may or may not live to achieve age t'. This accounts for the binomial coefficient

$$\binom{m-2k}{m'-k-k'+k}$$

in (5.2).

The range of the random variable $X(m')$ (taking values denoted by k' in (5.2)) is

$$\max(0,\ k+m'-m)\ \le\ X(m')\ \le\ \min(\lfloor m'/2 \rfloor,\ k)$$

and the range on j in the summation in (5.2) is

$$\max(0,\ k + k' - m') \ \le\ j\ \le\ \min(k - k',\ m - m' - k + k').$$

The range on $X(m)$ (taking values denoted by k in (5.2)) that we condition on is the same as that of (5.1), namely

$$\max(0, m - n)\ \le\ X(m)\ \le\ \lfloor m/2 \rfloor.$$

The range and the distribution of $X(m')$ in (5.2) does not appear to depend on the number of twin pairs n. The range of $X(m)$ that we condition on does depend on n, however. The ranges of $X(m) = k$, $X(m') = k'$, and j are restricted so that the counts along all paths of Fig. 5.1 and factorials in (5.2) are nonnegative.

Fig. 5.2 plots some examples of the distribution of $X(m')$ given at (5.2) for $m = 60$ and $m' = 30$ living persons, conditional on values of $X(m) = 5, 10, \ldots,$ 30. The largest value possible for $X(m)$ is 30 when $m = 60$. The distribution of $X(m')$ is shifted to the right for larger values of $X(m)$, as we would expect. Larger numbers of pairs, both alive at the earlier age $X(m)$ result in a greater number of both-living pairs $X(m')$ at the greater age as well, all other things involving m and m' remaining equal.

The proof that (5.2) is a valid distribution is similar to the corresponding proof for the hypergeometric distribution given at (1.20) in Section 1.7. To verify that (5.2) sums to unity, we need to identify the coefficient of $z^{m'}$ on both sides

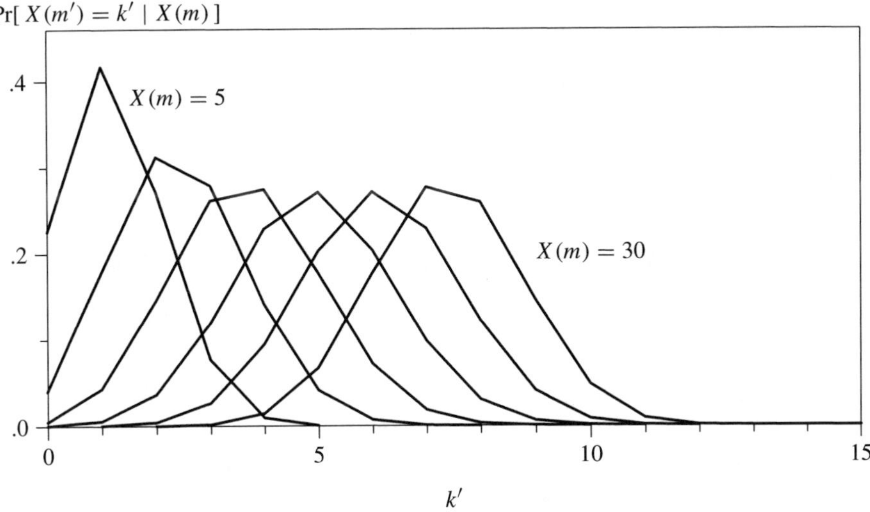

Figure 5.2 The conditional twin distribution (5.2) of pairs, both alive $X(m')$ for $m = 60$ and $m' = 30$ living persons and given values of $X(m) = 5, 10, \ldots, 30$ pairs, both alive at the earlier age.

of the polynomial identity

$$(1 + z)^m = (1 + z)^{m-2k}(1 + 2z + z^2)^k.$$

This proof explains the normalizing binomial coefficient

$$\binom{m}{m'}$$

in the denominator of (5.2).

The conditional factorial moments of $X(m')$ in (5.2) are

$$\mathrm{E}[\, X^{(r)}(m') \mid X(m) = k\,] = k^{(r)} m'^{(2r)}/m^{(2r)}$$

for $r = 1, 2, \ldots$.

In particular, the conditional expected value is

$$\mathrm{E}[\, X(m') \mid X(m) = k\,] = km'(m' - 1)/m(m - 1). \tag{5.3}$$

This expression is consistent with the iterated expectation relationship given by (1.4). That is,

$$\mathrm{E}[\, X(m')\,] = \mathrm{E}[\,\mathrm{E}[\, X(m') \mid X(m)\,]\,]$$

when we refer to the marginal expectation at (4.3) in the previous chapter.

The conditional variance of $X(m')$ given $X(m) = k$ is

$$\mathrm{Var}[\, X(m') \mid X(m) = k\,] = \mathrm{E}[\, X(m') \mid X(m) = k\,] \times$$
$$(m - m')\{\, m + m' - 5 - 2k[2mm' - 3(m + m' - 1)]\}/m^{(4)}.$$

The correlation of $X(m)$ and $X(m')$ is obtained by first writing

$$\begin{aligned}\mathrm{E}[\, X(m)X(m')\,] &= \mathrm{E}[\, X(m)\,\mathrm{E}[\, X(m') \mid X(m)\,]] \\ &= m'^{(2)}/m^{(2)}\mathrm{E}[\, X(m)\,]^2\end{aligned}$$

using iterated expectation (1.4).

The covariance is then

$$\mathrm{Cov}[\, X(m);\; X(m')\,] = m'^{(2)}/m^{(2)}\mathrm{E}[\, X(m)\,]^2 - \mathrm{E}[\, X(m)\,]\,\mathrm{E}[\, X(m')\,].$$

This expression relies only on marginal moments, given at (4.8). After some algebra, we have

$$\mathrm{Cov}[\, X(m);\; X(m')\,] = \frac{m'(m' - 1)(2n - m)(2n - m - 1)}{2(2n - 1)^2(2n - 3)}.$$

This covariance is never negative. The marginal variances of $X(m)$ and $X(m')$ are given at (4.4). The correlation of $X(m')$ and $X(m)$ is then

$$\mathrm{Corr}[\, X(m);\; X(m')\,] = \left[\frac{m'(m' - 1)(2n - m)(2n - m - 1)}{m(m - 1)(2n - m')(2n - m' - 1)}\right]^{1/2}$$

and approaches one when m and m' are close in value.

If we consider drawing pairs of two different colored balls from an urn, the probability distribution of future draws is only a function of the most recent information available. Additional conditional distributions can be obtained from (5.2) using the Markov property of this distribution. In particular, for $m'' \leq m' \leq m$,

$$\Pr[\, X(m'') \mid X(m'),\; X(m)\,] = \Pr[\, X(m'') \mid X(m')\,].$$

Additional multivariate distributions for twins are described in Section 5.4.

5.2.2 Conditional association measure

We next describe a nonparametric model that is used to provide a measure of the association between two different ages in these twin pairs. We want to build a model in which twin pairs that are both alive at age t are more (or perhaps less) likely to jointly survive to age t' relative to the number of deaths that occurred between ages t and t'. The way to do this is to multiply distribution (5.2) by $\exp(k'\tau)$ and provide an appropriate normalizing constant. This factor is used to increase or decrease the likelihood of the path labeled by k' in Fig. 5.1. In model (5.2), k' is the value taken on by the random variable $X(m')$.

The $\tau = \tau(t, t')$ parameter has the interpretation of a log-odds ratio force of longevity pushing the both-alive pairs at age t to make an intact transition to age t'. This distribution continues to condition on the numbers m and m' of living individuals at both ages and the number of twin pairs, both alive at the earlier age $X(m)$.

The distribution of the number $X(m')$ of twin pairs, both alive at age t', conditional on $X(m) = k$ twin pairs, both alive at age t, with association measure $\tau = \tau(t, t')$ is

$$\Pr[\, X(m') = k' \mid X(m) = k;\; \tau\,]$$

$$\propto \exp(k'\tau) \sum_j \frac{k!\; 2^{k-k'-j}}{k'!\; j!\, (k - k' - j)!} \binom{m - 2k}{m' - k - k' + j} \quad (5.4)$$

where the sum on j is over the number of twin pairs both alive at age t and both dead at age t', as in (5.2).

The valid ranges for k', k, and j in (5.4) are the same as those in (5.2). Examples of distribution (5.4) are plotted in Fig. 5.3 for values of τ between -3 and 3. The other parameter values in this plot are fixed at $m = 60$; $m' = 30$; and $X(m) = 25$. Larger values of the τ parameter cause this distribution to shift right toward a larger number of twin pairs $X(m')$, both alive at the greater age t'. The value of $\tau = 0$ in (5.4) yields the conditional distribution at (5.2).

Positive values of τ describe models in which more twin pairs, both alive at the earlier age t continue to be both alive at the later age t'. Similarly, negative values of τ indicate fewer surviving both-alive twin pairs $X(m')$ at age t' than

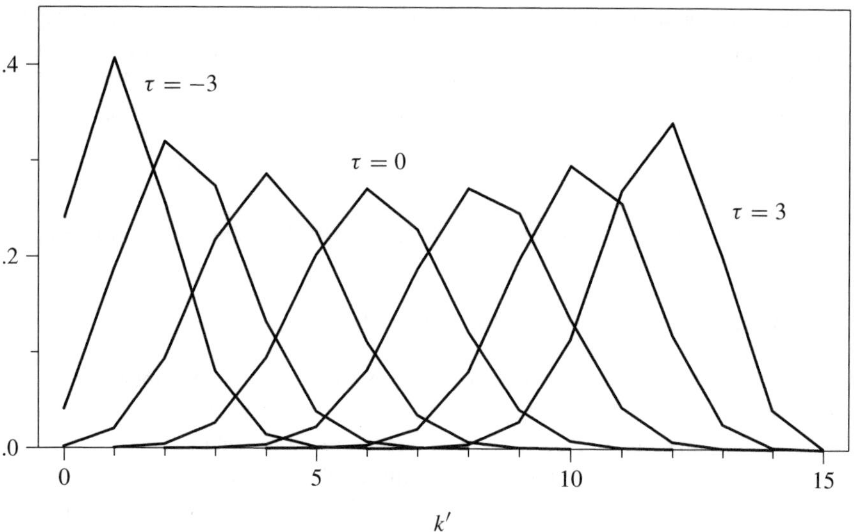

Figure 5.3 The conditional association twin distribution (5.4) of $X(m')$ with $m = 60$ and $m' = 30$ living persons at different ages and $X(m) = 25$ pairs, both alive at an earlier age with association measure $\tau = -3, -2, \ldots, +3$.

would be expected given $X(m)$ pairs, where both are alive at the earlier age. Such a negative correlation for $\tau < 0$ does not have a simple interpretation in practice.

There is no simple expression for the normalizing constant in (5.4) but numerical methods can be used to find the maximum likelihood estimate and exact confidence intervals for τ of (5.4) in Section 5.5. The SAS program to fit this distribution is given in Section 5.7.1.

The distribution at (5.4) is in the standard exponential form (*cf.* Stuart and Ord 1987, Sections 5.47–8). The maximum likelihood estimate $\widehat{\tau}$ of τ satisfies

$$\mathrm{E}[\, X(m') \mid X(m);\ \widehat{\tau}\,] = x(m'),$$

where expectation is taken with respect to distribution (5.4). That is, the maximum likelihood estimate equates the observed value $x(m')$ of $X(m')$ with its expectation, given τ, $X(m)$, m, and m'.

The Cramér-Rao inequality shows that the variance of $\widehat{\tau}(x)$ is approximately equal to

$$\mathrm{Var}\,(\widehat{\tau}) \approx 1\,/\,\mathrm{Var}[\, X(m') \mid X(m);\ \tau = \widehat{\tau}\,].$$

An exact $(1-\alpha)\%$ confidence interval (τ_1, τ_2) for τ can be obtained by solving the equations

$$\Pr[\, X(m') \geq x(m') \mid X(m);\ \tau_1\,] = \alpha/2$$

and

$$\Pr[\, X(m') \leq x(m') \mid X(m);\ \tau_2\,] = \alpha/2.$$

The SAS program to fit the distribution (5.4) is given in Section 5.7.1. This program finds the maximum likelihood estimate $\widehat{\tau}$ of τ and the exact $(1-\alpha)\%$ confidence interval, as just described. This program is also used to provide the summary statistics in Tables 5.1 and 5.2 for the Danish twin data.

5.3 Conditional inference for the Danish twins

We demonstrate the utility of these methods to study longevity in the Danish twins. This data is also examined in the previous chapter using univariate methods. We identified $n = 117$ identical (monozygotic or MZ) female twin pairs for whom exact age at death is known for both individuals. Table 5.1 gives the number of living individuals m and the number of observed MZ pairs where both are alive $X(m)$ for ages 30 through 85 in 5 year intervals. The corresponding Table 5.2 provides the same information for the $n = 192$ DZ twin pairs. A univariate analysis of this data and the comparisons between MZ and DZ twins appears in Section 4.4.

The means and significance levels in Tables 5.1 and 5.2 are all conditional on the numbers of twin pairs, both alive at the previous five-year earlier category. Significance levels are obtained from the conditional distribution (5.2) and the conditional expected counts are given at (5.3). These significance levels are one (upper) tailed. There are no significance levels or estimated values of τ for the youngest ages in Tables 5.1 or 5.2 because there were no earlier ages to condition on. In this analysis, we chose to ignore survival times younger than 30 years.

Significance levels of 1 occur when the observed value of $X(m')$ is equal to the lowest possible value for its valid range, conditional on the information from the previous age group. As a specific example of this, we see in Table 5.1 that between ages 35 and 40 five women died (*i.e.,* $m = 218$ and $m' = 213$). All five of these deaths occurred in different twin pairs that were both alive at age 35. Between these two ages, the number of twin pairs, both alive also decreased by five (*i.e.,* $X(m) = 103$ and $X(m') = 98$). This decrease in $X(\cdot)$ is the largest value possible conditional on the values of m and m'. This results in a significance level of 1. Similarly there is no estimate for τ nor a confidence interval for such extreme data values.

After 60 years, there are always more MZ and DZ pairs, both alive, than would be expected, conditional on all earlier ages. So, for example, more pairs both alive survive to age 70 than would be expected at age 65. Similarly, more pairs jointly survive to age 75 than would be expected at age 70, and so on. The force of longevity within these twin pairs does not express itself at only one age but rather continually reasserts itself on top of all earlier experiences.

At ages 65 and 75, the conditional statistical significance is remarkable with p-values of 0.0036 and 0.0216 respectively for the MZ twins in Table 5.1. The corresponding estimated values of τ are large and their 95% confidence intervals do not include zero. The greatest force for an increased life span appears to occur between ages 60 to 65 and again between ages 70 to 75. The same analysis of DZ twin pairs in Table 5.2 did not reveal any statistically significant comparisons using the conditional distributions described so far in this chapter.

Table 5.1 Conditional inference for $n = 117$ female MZ Danish twin pairs. All inference is conditional on the previous five-year younger age category.

Age	Women living	Pairs both alive	Conditional		Estimated parameter		
			Expected pairs both alive	Univariate statistical significance			
t	m_t	x_t			$\hat{\tau}$	Exact 95% CI	
30	220	105	—	—	—	—	—
35	218	103	103.10	1	—	—	—
40	213	98	98.32	1	—	—	—
45	210	96	95.25	0.2338	1.76	−2.40	4.81
50	205	92	91.47	0.3971	0.92	−3.06	3.37
55	201	88	88.44	1	—	—	—
60	186	75	75.33	0.7209	−0.20	−2.51	1.44
65	166	65	59.70	0.0036	1.56	0.39	2.74
70	146	53	50.24	0.0990	0.83	−0.37	2.00
75	110	35	30.02	0.0216	1.00	0.03	1.99
80	75	17	16.20	0.4412	0.19	−0.87	1.25
85	39	7	4.54	0.0995	0.99	−0.43	2.39

Table 5.2 Conditional inference for $n = 192$ female DZ Danish twin pairs, conditional on the previous five-year younger category.

Age	Women living	Pairs both alive	Conditional		Estimated parameter		
			Expected pairs both alive	Univariate statistical significance			
t	m_t	x_t			$\hat{\tau}$	Exact 95% CI	
30	365	174	—	—	—	—	—
35	352	163	161.81	0.1890	1.11	−1.23	2.83
40	345	156	156.57	1	—	—	—
45	339	150	150.61	1	—	—	—
50	330	143	142.13	0.3146	0.73	−1.62	2.48
55	312	129	127.80	0.2994	0.49	−1.02	1.77
60	295	114	115.30	0.8841	−0.64	−2.90	0.90
65	271	99	96.18	0.1209	0.66	−0.39	1.66
70	234	74	73.77	0.5384	0.04	−0.86	0.89
75	184	47	45.70	0.3861	0.17	−0.60	0.93
80	122	21	20.61	0.5150	0.06	−0.76	0.87
85	68	9	6.48	0.1365	0.70	−0.46	1.84

Estimated transition parameters $\tau_{t-5,t}$ are given in Table 5.1 to describe the association between adjacent five-year ages. The likelihood ratio test for equality of the $\tau_{t-5,t}$, starting at age 65 from the association model (5.4) for MZ twins, is $\chi^2 = 3.80$ (4 d.f.) with a common estimated value of $\widehat{\tau} = 0.8867$. In other words, there is moderate evidence that the force of longevity measured by τ is constant and positive for all ages later in life.

Perhaps unexpected is the lack of many extreme significance levels in Table 5.1 such as are seen in the findings of Section 4.4 in the previous chapter. Only two of the 95% confidence intervals for τ in Table 5.1 do not include the value of 0. In the univariate analysis of this data in Table 4.2, we uncover a larger number of significant relationships between MZ twins. These are not confirmed by the examination in Table 5.1. Perhaps this is due to the relatively short five-year interval span that we condition on in this table. To test this hypothesis let us reexamine the data and separately condition on each of the earlier ages.

Table 5.3 Conditional significance level of Danish twin pairs both surviving to the specified age. The conditioning is on each of several previous age groups, back to age 30.

	Conditioned on years previous						
Age	5	10	15	20	30	40	50
			MZ twins				
45	0.234	0.452	0.503				
50	0.397	0.167	0.284	0.318			
55	1	0.639	0.361	0.471			
60	0.721	0.800	0.679	0.527	0.603		
65	0.004	0.013	0.020	0.015	0.013		
70	0.099	0.003	0.005	0.007	0.004	0.005	
75	0.022	0.007	0.001	0.001	0.001	0.001	
80	0.441	0.127	0.076	0.031	0.035	0.030	0.031
85	0.099	0.089	0.041	0.031	0.020	0.020	0.019
			DZ twins				
45	1	1	0.640				
50	0.315	0.532	0.686	0.398			
55	0.299	0.191	0.287	0.383			
60	0.884	0.629	0.496	0.578	0.506		
65	0.121	0.296	0.207	0.159	0.236		
70	0.538	0.262	0.367	0.296	0.284	0.261	
75	0.386	0.383	0.249	0.303	0.240	0.272	
80	0.515	0.434	0.427	0.354	0.360	0.355	0.346
85	0.136	0.142	0.126	0.126	0.115	0.106	0.111

Table 5.3 lists the conditional significance levels for MZ and DZ twin pairs conditioning on each of the number of pairs, both alive at each of the earlier ages, back to age 30. So, for example, Table 5.3 presents all of the one (upper)-tailed significance levels for the number of twins, both alive at age 65 conditional on each of the numbers, where both are alive at ages 60, 55, and so on, back to age 30.

The DZ twin pairs in Table 5.3 never achieve any remarkable degree of statistical significance at any age conditional on any earlier age. The DZ twin pairs appear no different than the behavior we would expect from two unrelated persons born at the same time. This is also the conclusion reached in the previous chapter.

The MZ twins in Table 5.3 achieve a high degree of statistical significance after age 60, provided we condition on the data from 10 years previous or earlier. In almost every case, there are significantly more MZ twins, both alive after every age greater than 60 than would have been expected 10 years earlier. Our measure of the effect of longevity does not appear before age 65 and its statistically significant effect is only apparent when examined over periods of 10 years or longer intervals.

All of the values of τ corresponding to those in Table 5.3 can be estimated as well. We can estimate τ in (5.4), measuring the conditional effect for a twin pair's survival to each age, given the number of pairs, where both are alive at each of the younger ages. These maximum likelihood estimated values $\widehat{\tau}$ are plotted in Fig. 5.4 for the MZ twins. The one sided significance levels corresponding to the $\widehat{\tau}$ are given in Table 5.3.

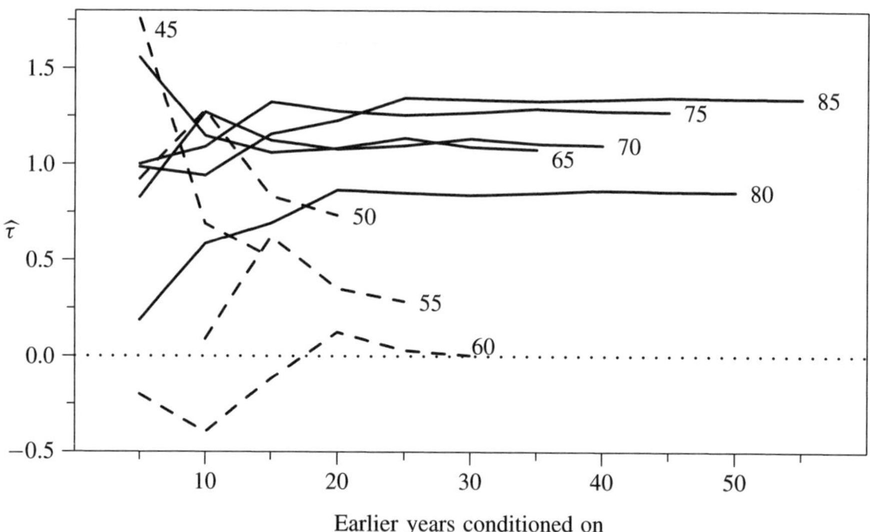

Figure 5.4 The maximum likelihood estimate $\widehat{\tau}$ in (5.4) of the effect of identical, MZ twin pairs both surviving to specified ages conditional on each of the previous five- year age groups. The estimated $\widehat{\tau}$ for ages younger than 60 are plotted in dashed lines to distinguish the pattern seen in older ages.

In Fig. 5.4, for ages younger than 60 years, the $\widehat{\tau}$ of (5.4) show no particular pattern and are plotted in dashed lines to distinguish them from the $\widehat{\tau}$ values corresponding to older ages. The $\widehat{\tau}$ values after age 60 years are all similar in pattern: all are roughly increasing when conditioned on recent previous ages and reach a steady asymptote when we condition on sufficiently earlier ages. These apparent asymptotes for $\widehat{\tau}$ are all in a narrow range between 0.8 and 1.3 for all ages 65 and above. We interpret this to mean that our measure of the force of longevity has a fairly consistent effect. This effect is only measurable after age 60 and only apparent when viewed over sufficiently long time periods of at least 10 years. Longevity is not a single life event, but rather a continuing process that reasserts itself on top of previous experiences. This process has a negligible effect before age 65.

5.4 Simultaneous Multivariate Distributions

We can derive multivariate distributions to model the simultaneous joint distribution of $X(m)$ and $X(m')$ twin pairs, both alive at two different ages. We continue to use the same notation as in the previous sections of this chapter. Specifically, at a younger age, there are m persons who are alive out of n twin pairs. At a later age, there are m' living persons with $m' \leq m$.

The bivariate distribution of $\{X(m),\ X(m')\}$ is obtained writing

$$\Pr[\,X(m),\ X(m')\,] = \Pr[\,X(m') \mid X(m)\,]\ \times\ \Pr[\,X(m)\,]$$

where the marginal distribution $\Pr[\,X(m)\,]$ is given at (5.1) and the conditional distribution $\Pr[\,X(m') \mid X(m)\,]$ appears at (5.2).

In the closed form, the bivariate distribution of $\{X(m),\ X(m')\}$ is

$$\Pr[\,X(m) = k;\ X(m') = k'\,]$$
$$= \sum_j \frac{n!\,2^{m-k-k'-j}}{\begin{array}{c} k'!\,(k-k'-j)!\,j!\,(m'-k-k'+j)! \\ (m-m'-k+k'-j)!\,(n-m+k)! \end{array}} \Bigg/ \frac{(2n)!}{(2n-m)!\,(m-m')!\,m'!} \tag{5.5}$$

where the sum over j and the ranges on (k, k') are the same is as in the distribution (5.2).

The proof that the bivariate distribution of $\{X(m),\ X(m')\}$ sums to one is demonstrated by identifying the coefficient of $y^{m-m'}z^{m'}$ on both sides of the polynomial identity

$$(1+y+z)^{2n} = (1+y^2+z^2+2y+2z+2yz)^n.$$

Fig. 5.5 can be used to help motivate the functional form of the distribution given at (5.5). There are six separate paths in Fig. 5.5 between ages t (middle 3 boxes) and age t' (3 boxes on the right). There are factorials in the denominator

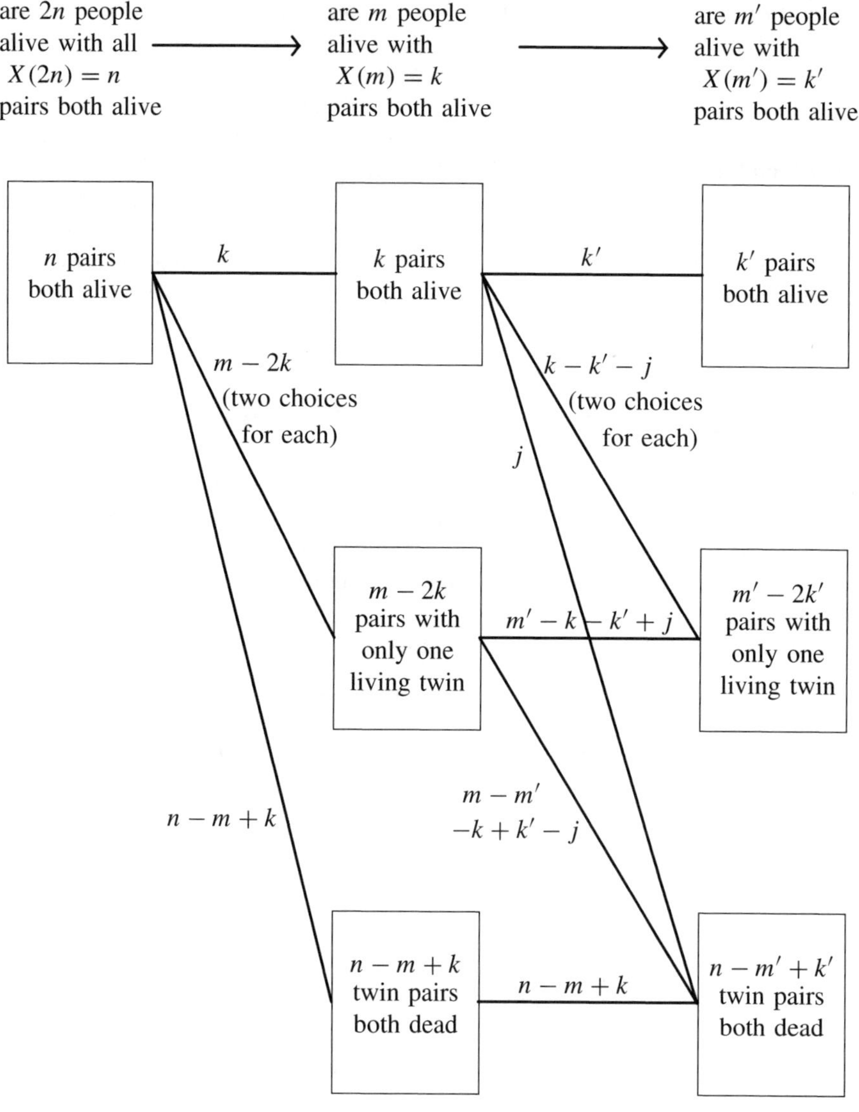

Figure 5.5 Notation for the bivariate distribution (5.5). All individuals die in one of the three age intervals $(0, t)$, (t, t'), (t', ∞). The seven boxes indicate the status of the n twin pairs at ages 0, t, and t'.

for each of these six counts in (5.5). Two paths are identified as each having two choices and the power of 2 in (5.5) is the sum of the counts along these two paths. The normalizing denominator reflects the ages at the time of death of the $2n$ individuals. Specifically, $2n - m$ individuals die in $(0, t)$; $m - m'$ die in (t, t'); and m' die in (t', ∞).

Higher dimensional joint multivariate probability distributions can easily be computed as needed in the data analysis of Section 5.5. For numbers of living individuals

$$m_1 \geq m_2 \geq \cdots \geq m_k > 0$$

at successive ages, the joint distribution of $\{X(m_i)\}$ is

$$\Pr[\, X(m_1), \ldots , X(m_k)\,] = \Pr[\, X(m_1)\,] \prod_{i=2}^{k} \Pr[\, X(m_i) \mid X(m_{i-1})\,]. \tag{5.6}$$

As an example, Table 5.4 in Section 5.5 uses this relation to provide simultaneous inference on up to seven distinct ages. This joint probability distribution depends on expressions for the marginal and conditional distributions given at (5.1) and (5.2), respectively. It does not have a simple mathematical form, but it can be easily evaluated numerically.

Higher dimensional multivariate distributions are motivated by identifying the coefficients in the polynomial identity

$$\left[1 + \sum_i z_i\right]^{2n} = \left[1 + \sum_i z_i^2 + 2 \sum_{i\,i'} z_i z_{i'}\right]^n \tag{5.7}$$

in a similar fashion.

The joint statistical significance of a set of observations $\{x(m_1), \ldots , x(m_k)\}$ requires that we completely enumerate all possible values conditional on $\{m_i\}$ over the range of this joint distribution. This enumeration is equivalent to identifying the appropriate coefficient in the generating polynomial (5.7).

A computational shortcut can be employed in order to obtain exact significance level p-values associated with these multivariate distributions. Let p^0 denote the probability of the observed data. The exact significance level is the sum over all possible outcomes $\{X(m_1), \ldots , X(m_k)\}$ consistent with $\{m_1, \ldots , m_k\}$ having smaller probabilities than p^0. This definition is in keeping with the concept of a two-tailed test in one dimension.

The enumeration algorithm counts outcomes much like an odometer with $X(m_k)$ changing quickly and $X(m_1)$ changing slowly. It is only necessary to include as many terms in (5.6) as are necessary to make this product smaller than p^0. The number of terms necessary determines the intermediate counter in the odometer that is to be advanced. The FORTRAN program that implements this algorithm is given in Section 5.7.2. Table 5.4 includes the number of tables that are enumerated in order to obtain the required significance level using this algorithm.

5.5 Multivariate Examination of the Twins

The conditional analysis of the MZ and DZ twins is given in Tables 5.1 and 5.2. The conditional means and univariate significance levels are conditional on the numbers of twin pairs, both alive at all earlier ages. These significance levels calculated are all one tailed, corresponding to the upper tail in every case. Conditional on all earlier ages, after 60 years, there are always more pairs, both alive than would be expected. That is, the force of longevity within these twin pairs does not express itself at only one age but rather continually reasserts itself on top of all earlier experiences. Multivariate methods provide a broader picture of these data.

The simultaneous significance levels in Table 5.4 are based on the joint probability distribution at the given age and jointly with all earlier ages. The joint probability of all observed MZ frequencies for ages 55 through 85 in Table 5.4 is 1.29×10^{-9}. A complete enumeration for this whole table identified approximately 22 million possible outcomes consistent with the numbers (m's) of all living individuals at each age. This count refers to the number of tables enumerated using the algorithm described in the previous section.

The tail area 0.0026 is the sum over all probabilities smaller than that of the observed table. This is the last value given in the fifth column in Table 5.4 and represents the simultaneous statistical significance level of the whole data set, for ages 55 through 85. The last column in Table 5.4 indicates the number of outcomes that were enumerated to obtain the joint multivariate significance levels. The multivariate statistical examination of the dizygotic or DZ twin pairs is summarized in Table 5.5. None of these significance levels is remarkable.

In summary, the force of longevity within the female MZ twin pairs becomes apparent at ages 65 and later. Both conditional and simultaneous inference on the

Table 5.4 Multivariate analysis of $n = 117$ female MZ Danish twin pairs. Multivariate statistical inference is performed jointly with all of the earlier ages given in this table.

Age t	Number of women alive m_t	Number of pairs both alive $x(m_t)$	Conditional expected pairs both alive	Simultaneous multivariate statistical significance	Number of tables enumerated
55	201	88	88.44	0.2395	17
60	186	75	75.33	0.4088	244
65	166	65	59.70	0.0091	1444
70	146	53	50.24	0.0078	14,744
75	110	35	30.02	0.0020	359,103
80	75	17	16.20	0.0043	3.4×10^6
85	39	7	4.54	0.0026	22×10^6

Table 5.5 Joint multivariate analysis of female DZ Danish twins. Each significance level is performed jointly with all earlier ages.

Age t	Number of women alive m_t	Number of pairs both alive $x(m_t)$	Conditional expected pairs both alive	Joint multivariate statistical significance
55	312	129	127.80	0.3398
60	295	114	115.30	0.3870
65	271	99	96.18	0.2643
70	234	74	73.77	0.4243
75	184	47	45.70	0.5411
80	122	21	20.61	0.6639
85	68	9	6.48	0.5303

Danish twins indicate that a statistically excessive number of twin pairs are both alive at older ages than would be expected by chance alone, were these individuals matched at random. The DZ or fraternal twins, however, have joint life spans that behave as those of two unrelated individuals. This conclusion has been repeated earlier in this chapter and in the previous chapter as well.

5.6 Infinitesimal Multivariate Methods

Instead of dividing the life spans into a few time intervals $(0, t)$, (t, t'), (t', ∞) as in Section 5.2, we now consider the limiting process in which every death time falls into its own unique interval. The result of this arrangement is that there are $2n$ such intervals and each contains only one individual life span. Every individual has a binary classification as to being the first or second of her twin pair to die. The MZ data, given in Table 5.6, consists of an ordered set of binary valued indicators denoted $Y_1, \ldots, Y_{2n}$, whose distribution we describe in this section.

Let $t_1 < \cdots < t_{2n}$ denote the unique ages at time of death for each of the $2n$ individuals. For each $j = 1, \ldots, 2n$, let $Y_j = 1$ if the woman who dies at age t_j is survived by her co-twin and $Y_j = 0$ if she is the longer-lived of her twin pair.

This collection of $2n$ binary indicators is not mutually independent and not identically distributed. For example, we must have $Y_1 = 1$ and $Y_{2n} = 0$ because the shortest lived individual must have a surviving co-twin and the longest lived individual must be the second of her pair to die. These indicators are not independent because the indicators are restricted so that $\sum Y_j = n$.

It is convenient to have a count of the number of twin pairs that have lost at least one member at a given age. For every $j = 2, 3, \ldots, 2n$, let

$$S_j = Y_1 + Y_2 + \cdots + Y_{j-1}$$

Table 5.6 The MZ infinitesimal data Y_j. A value of $Y_j = 1$ means that the j-th youngest woman to die was the first of her co-twin pair and $Y_j = 0$ appears if she was the longer-lived in her pair for $j = 1, \ldots, 2n$. Four pairs are omitted who all died very young. See the description in Section 5.6.3.

										1										2
	1	2	3	4	5	6	7	8	9	0	1	2	3	4	5	6	7	8	9	0
	1	1	1	1	1	1	1	1	1	1	1	1	1	1	1	1	1	1	1	1
20	1	1	1	1	1	1	1	1	1	1	1	1	1	0	1	1	0	1	1	1
40	0	1	0	1	1	0	1	1	1	1	1	0	0	0	0	1	1	0	0	0
60	1	1	1	0	0	1	0	1	0	1	1	0	1	0	1	1	0	1	1	0
80	1	0	0	0	1	1	1	1	0	0	1	1	0	1	1	0	1	1	0	0
100	0	0	0	1	0	1	1	1	0	1	1	0	0	0	0	1	1	1	0	1
120	1	0	0	0	0	1	0	1	0	1	1	1	1	1	1	0	1	0	1	0
140	0	1	0	0	0	0	0	1	1	1	0	0	0	0	0	0	1	0	0	0
160	0	0	0	1	1	0	0	0	1	0	0	0	1	1	1	1	0	0	0	0
180	1	0	0	0	1	0	0	1	0	0	0	0	1	0	0	0	0	0	0	0
200	1	0	0	1	1	0	0	0	0	1	0	0	0	0	0	0	0	0	0	1
220	0	0	0	0	0	0														

denote the number of twin pairs that have lost at least one member, just before time t_j.

We define $S_1 = 0$. Then $n - S_j$ is the number of intact (both alive) twin pairs just before age t_j. The S_j are sums of dependent Bernoulli indicators Y_j. This section describes a small number of distributions useful for modeling the behavior of the S_j. Other models used to describe the distribution of dependent Bernoulli random variables are given in Chapter 7.

5.6.1 Models with no dependence

If there is no association of longevity within each twin pair and all individuals die at ages independently of their co-twin, then we can describe the distribution of the indicators Y_j. The conditional distribution of Y_j, given S_j, is

$$\Pr[\, Y_j = 1 \mid S_j \,] = 2(n - S_j)/(2n - j + 1) \tag{5.8}$$

for $j = 1, \ldots, 2n$.

That is, just before the jth death time t_j there are $2n - j + 1$ living people and of these, $2(n - S_j)$ have a living co-twin. The marginal expectation of Y_j and S_j can be found as follows.

Lemma 5.6.1 *For* $j = 1, \ldots, 2n$

$$\mathrm{E}[\, S_j\,] = [(4n - j)(j - 1)]\,/\,[2(2n - 1)]. \tag{5.9}$$

Proof. With probability one, $S_1 = 0$; $S_2 = 1$; and $S_{2n} = n$, so (5.9) is valid for these cases. The more general proof of this assertion follows by induction for other values of j. In particular, assume (5.9) holds for j. Then write

$$S_{j+1} = S_j + Y_j \tag{5.10}$$

and

$$\begin{aligned} \mathrm{E}[\, S_{j+1}\,] &= \mathrm{E}[\, S_j + Y_j\,] \\ &= \mathrm{E}[\, S_j + \mathrm{E}[Y_j \mid S_j\,]]. \end{aligned}$$

The result follows from (5.8), the induction step (5.9), and algebra to complete the proof. ■

The marginal distribution of Y_j can be found from (5.9) by writing

$$Y_j = S_{j+1} - S_j$$

and

$$\Pr[\, Y_j = 1\,] = \mathrm{E}[\, S_{j+1}\,] - \mathrm{E}[\, S_j\,].$$

Then use the expectation at (5.9) to show the marginal probability

$$\Pr[\, Y_j = 1\,] = (2n - j)/(2n - 1).$$

These probabilities decrease linearly in j, as we would expect.

This completes the discussion of the behavior of Y_j and S_j when there is no association in the life spans of twin pairs.

5.6.2 Models for dependence

In order to include a measure of association in these models, in Section 5.6.3 we fit a variety of models of the form

$$\Pr[\, Y_j = 1 \mid \theta,\ S_j\,] = 2\exp(\theta w_j)(n - S_j)/(2n - j + 1), \tag{5.11}$$

where weights w_j take a variety of functional forms in Table 5.7 to provide semi-parametric models of the dependence of life spans.

A value of $\theta = 0$ in (5.11) returns the model (5.8) of independent life spans in these twin pairs. When all of the w_j are positive, then a negative value of θ is associated with a statistically large number of pairs, both alive at greater ages, as is the case with all of the fitted models in Table 5.7.

Table 5.7 Semiparametric simultaneous models of dependence of longevity for all MZ individuals. The weights w_j are functions of $\phi = (j-1)/2n$. The model indicated by '(*)' is given at (5.15) and the standardized residuals of S_j for this model are plotted in Fig. 5.6.

Weight function w_j		Estimated MLE $\widehat{\theta}$	Estimated $\sigma(\widehat{\theta})$	Wald chi-squared	2× Log-likelihood ratio
Constant	$w_j = 1$	−0.113	.059	3.64	4.42
Increasing	$w = \phi_j$	−0.463	0.159	8.48	10.89
	$\phi^{1/2}$	−0.294	0.107	7.58	9.70
	ϕ^2	−0.670	0.264	6.42	8.15
Decreasing	$1-\phi$	−0.088	0.081	1.19	1.37
	$(1-\phi)^{1/2}$	−0.107	.072	2.24	2.68
	$(1-\phi)^2$	−0.030	0.095	0.10	0.10
Dome shaped	$\phi(1-\phi)$ (*)	−0.995	0.348	8.18	11.04
	$\{\phi(1-\phi\}^{1/2}$	−0.386	0.150	6.67	8.71
	$\{\phi(1-\phi)\}^2$	−5.085	1.691	9.04	12.54

The likelihood function for θ is

$$\Lambda(\theta) = \prod_j \Pr[\,Y_j = 1 \mid S_j,\ \theta\,]^{Y_j}\ \Pr[\,Y_j = 0 \mid S_j,\ \theta\,]^{1-Y_j}.$$

The function $\log \Lambda(\theta)$ is maximized in θ for various choices of w_j and the results are summarized in Table 5.7. The observed information is used to approximate the standard error of this maximum likelihood estimate $\widehat{\theta}$. The Wald chi-squared in this table is

$$[\,\widehat{\theta}\,/\,\text{Est. SE}(\widehat{\theta})\,]^2$$

and the 1 df likelihood ratio test of the hypothesis $\theta = 0$ is

$$2[\,\log \Lambda(\widehat{\theta})\ -\ \log \Lambda(0)\,].$$

In Section 5.6.3, it will also be useful to have expressions for the expected value and variance of S_j using model (5.11). These moments are most easily expressed in recursive form, which, in turn, are also computationally convenient for us.

Begin by writing (5.11) as

$$\Pr[\,Y_j = 1 \mid \theta,\ S_j\,] = \gamma_j(n - S_j) \tag{5.12}$$

where

$$\gamma_j = 2\exp(\theta w_j)/(2n - j + 1).$$

The expected value of S_j under model (5.11) is found in recursive form by writing

$$\mathrm{E}[\,S_{j+1} \mid \theta\,] = \mathrm{E}[\,\mathrm{E}[\,S_{j+1} \mid \theta,\ S_j\,]]$$

using the iterated expectation (1.4).

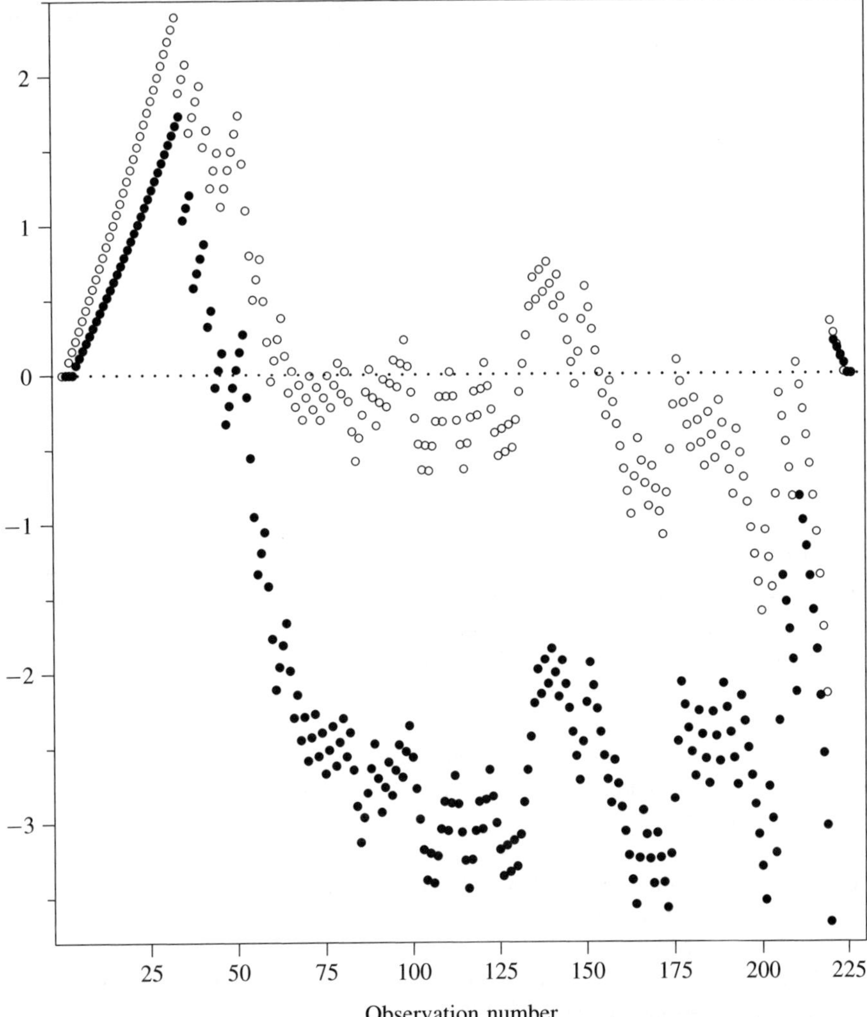

Figure 5.6 Residual plot for the standardized, fitted cumulative sums S_j in the infinitesimal MZ data. The '•' values correspond to the model of no association given in (5.8) and (5.9). The open circles are for fitted model (5.15).

Then use (5.10) and (5.12) to show

$$\begin{aligned} \mathrm{E}[\, S_{j+1} \mid \theta \,] &= \mathrm{E}[\, S_j + \mathrm{E}[\, Y_j \mid S_j \,]\,] \\ &= n\gamma_j + (1 - \gamma_j)\mathrm{E}[\, S_j \mid \theta \,]. \end{aligned} \tag{5.13}$$

This recursive expression (5.13) for the expected value of S_j under model (5.11) is used in Section 5.6.3 to plot the standardized residuals of fitted models in Fig. 5.6.

A similar recursive expression for the variance of S_j is also needed to standardize these residuals. To find this expression, use (1.5) and (5.10) to write

$$\begin{aligned}\text{Var}[\,S_{j+1}\,] &= \text{E}[\text{Var}[\,S_{j+1} \mid S_j\,]] + \text{Var}[\,\text{E}[\,S_{j+1} \mid S_j\,]] \\ &= \text{E}[\,\text{Var}[\,Y_j \mid S_j\,]] + \text{Var}[\,S_j + \text{E}[\,Y_j \mid S_j\,].\end{aligned}$$

Next use (5.12) and some algebra to show

$$\begin{aligned}\text{Var}[\,S_{j+1} \mid \theta\,] = (1 - 2\gamma_j)\text{Var}[\,S_j\,] - \{\gamma_j \text{E}[\,S_j\,]\}^2 \\ + \gamma_j(2\gamma_j n - 1)\text{E}[\,S_j\,] + \gamma_j n(1 - \gamma_j n). \qquad (5.14)\end{aligned}$$

This recursive expression for the variance is used to standardize the residuals of fitted models of S_j in Fig. 5.6.

5.6.3 The infinitesimal data

The MZ data in Table 5.6 omits four twin pairs who all died at very young ages. The statistical examination of the full data is dominated by these huge outliers. The data for the resulting $n = 113$ pairs is modeled here.

A wide variety of choices of the w_j function in (5.11) is listed in Table 5.7. These choices include constant, increasing, decreasing, and dome-shaped functions of j. In every case, the estimated value of θ is negative, indicating that the large probabilities of $Y_j = 1$ and small j appear to be smaller than model (5.8) would anticipate. In other words, the dependence of longevity within these Danish twin pairs results in more pairs remaining intact at greater ages than would appear by chance. These models indicate a significant association and improvement in the fit as indicated by the log-likelihood ratios. All of these models, except those that decrease in j, offer about the same degree of fit and none appears to be clearly better than the others.

The estimated standard deviation of $\widehat{\theta}$ is obtained from the observed information function. All chi-squared tests in Table 5.7 have 1 df.

The standardized residuals of S_j are plotted in Fig. 5.6. The residuals plotted are

$$(S_j - \text{E}[\,S_j])/\{\text{Var}[\,S_j\,]\}^{1/2}.$$

There is an autocorrelation among the S_j and this figure demonstrates patterns of dependence among adjacent residuals.

The '•' marks in Fig. 5.6 correspond to the model (5.8) in which we assume that there is no association in survival time for the MZ twins. In most of the data, this model of S_j represents a poor fit with most of these standardized values taking values of 2 or more standard deviations.

To model association of survival times in the MZ twins, Fig. 5.6 plots the standardized residuals of one of the better fitted models in Table 5.7. The specific model '*' of this table is one of the best fitting of all models examined. This fitted model has the functional form

$$\Pr[\, Y_j = 1 \mid \theta,\ S_j \,] = \frac{2(n - S_j)\exp[\,\theta(j-1)(2n-j+1)/4n^2\,]}{(2n-j+1)}. \tag{5.15}$$

The fitted estimate of θ in this model is $\widehat{\theta} = -.995$, with an estimated standard error of 0.348. A value of $\theta = 0$ in (5.15) returns the original model (5.8) of no association in the twins' survival. The 1 df likelihood ratio test of $\theta = 0$ has a value of 11.04, demonstrating the large improvement that this one parameter model makes over the model of independent survival times.

The expected value and variance for model (5.15) are computed using the recursive expressions (5.13) and (5.14), respectively. The residuals for this model are plotted as $^\circ$ in Fig. 5.6. Except for some of the earliest survival times, this model demonstrates a much better description of the data, with standardized residuals much closer to zero than those of model (5.8).

In general, almost all of the models fitted in Table 5.7 are able to demonstrate a significant improvement over the models (5.8) and (5.9). The negative estimates of θ, in every case demonstrate a positive correlation of life spans in these MZ twin pairs. Additional models for sums of dependent Bernoulli random variables are described in Chapter 7.

5.7 Computer Programs

5.7.1 Conditional distribution and association models in SAS

This program generates the statistics presented in Tables 5.1, 5.2, 5.3 and Fig. 5.4.

```
options linesize=77 nocenter pagesize=59 number nodate nomprint
nomlogic;

/*       Conditional statistical analysis of twins' lifespans

 Conditional statistical analysis of twins' lifespans given
 data from the previous age categories. The upper tail provides
 a univariate, conditional significance level.  For the tau
 measure of association distribution, this program provides:
 maximum likelihood estimate of tau parameter; and the exact
 (1-alpha)% confidence interval.

 Set the limits of searches to be +/- &limit for parameter
 estimates and exact confidence interval endpoints. Increase
 this value if the estimated parameter converges to this value.
 Estimated parameter value will be undefined if the observed
 value is equal to an extreme of its distribution.          */
%let limit = 5;
```

```
/*
  Convergence criteria.  Interval bisection searches stop when
  the interval is smaller than this width
*/
%let epsilon = 1.0e-5;


%macro lfac(k);                                  /* return log of k! */
   lgamma(&k+1)  /* return as a function: no semi-colon here */
%mend lfac;


/* Maximum likelihood estimation of tau, modeling the
 association between two different ages. Find the twin
 association parameter (&tau) giving a distribution with
 expected value equal to &xp.
 Interval bisection is used. The initial interval for
 estimation is +/- &limit. Make this wider if the algorithm
 does not converge.  The algorithm will return undefined tau
 if the observed value of xp is at either of the extremes of
 its range.
     xp  = number of pairs both alive at older age      = X(m')
     mp  = number of living individuals at older age    = m'
     x   = number of pairs both alive at younger age
     m   = number of living individuals at younger age
     tau = ouput, maximum likelihood estimate; undefined for
            extremes of xp or any missing values             */
%macro tauhat(xp,mp,x,m,tau);
   taulo= -&limit;             /* initial estimation interval */
   tauhi= &limit;
   if &x~=. & &m~=. & &xp~=. & &mp~=. then /* if data values
      are not missing and if the observation is not at the
      extremes of its range                                   */
   if (&xp GT max(0,&x+&mp-&m))
         & (&xp LT min(floor(&mp/2),&x)) then
   do until (abs(tauhi-taulo)<&epsilon);     /* convergence? */
      &tau=(tauhi+taulo)/2;                 /* examine midpoint */
      %exptau(&mp,&x,&m,&tau,exx);    /* find expected value */
       /* shrink interval by equating expected value with xp */
      if &xp LE exx then tauhi=&tau;
      if &xp GE exx then taulo=&tau;
   end;
   else &tau = . ;        /* otherwise tau-hat is not defined */
   drop tauhi taulo exx;
%mend tauhat;


/*  Expected value of tau-association distribution conditional
    on an earlier age                                          */
%macro exptau(mp,x,m,tau,ex);
```

```
   &ex=0;                         /* to accumulate expected value */
   exden=0;                      /* to accumulate the denominator */
   if &mp~=. & &x~=.
        & &m~=. & &tau~=. then  /* if no missing values then */
   do kx = max(0,&x+&mp-&m)
         to min(floor(&mp/2),&x);        /* ... loop on range */
      xterm=0;                      /* individual term in the sum */
      %jcond(kx,&mp,&x,&m,xterm);           /* inner summation */
      xterm = xterm * exp(kx*&tau);        /* parameter effect */
      exden = exden + xterm;   /* accumulate the denominator */
      &ex = &ex + kx*xterm;       /* accumulate the numerator */
   end;
      else &ex = . ;
   if &ex~=. & exden~=. then
      if exden > 0 then &ex = &ex / exden;
   drop kx exden xterm;
%mend exptau;


  /* Tau-association distribution conditional on earlier age */
%macro ptau(xp,mp,x,m,tau,prob);
   &prob = . ;                  /* probability returned in &prob */
   ptden = 0 ;                     /* accumulate the denominator */
   if &mp~=. & &x~=. & &m~=. & &tau~=. then/* if not missing */
      do kk = max(0,&x+&mp-&m)
            to min(floor(&mp/2),&x);    /* ... loop on range */
         pterm=0;                  /* individual term in the sum */
         %jcond(kk,&mp,&x,&m,pterm);       /* inner summation */
         pterm = pterm * exp(kk*&tau);   /* parameter effect */
         ptden = ptden + pterm;    /* accumulate denominator */
         if kk=&xp then &prob=pterm;            /* numerator */
      end;
      else &prob = . ;  /* probability is undefined, missing */
   if &prob~=. & ptden~=. then /* if not missing then divide */
      if ptden > 0 then &prob = &prob / ptden;
   drop kk ptden pterm;
%mend ptau;


/* Upper tail of conditional tau association distribution */
%macro ptauhi(xp,mp,x,m,tau,phi);
   &phi = 0 ;                         /* value returned in &phi */
   if &xp~=. & &mp~=. & &x~=. & &m~=. & &tau~=.
         then do;                              /* if not missing */
      do kp = &xp to min(floor(&mp/2),&x);        /* then loop */
         %ptau(kp,&mp,&x,&m,&tau,phixx);  /* one probability */
         &phi=&phi+phixx;        /* accumulate probabilities */
      end;
   end;
      else &phi = . ;
```

```
   drop kp phixx;
%mend ptauhi;


/*  Lower tail of conditional tau association distribution */
%macro ptaulo(xp,mp,x,m,tau,plow);
   &plow = 0 ;                           /* value returned in &plow */
   if &xp~=. & &mp~=. & &x~=. & &m~=. & &tau~=.
            then do;      /* if there are no missing values */
      do kpt = max(0,&x+&mp-&m) to &xp;/* then loop on range */
         %ptau(kpt,&mp,&x,&m,&tau,ploxx); /* one probability */
         &plow = &plow + ploxx;  /* accumulate probabilities */
      end;
   end;
      else &plow = . ;   /* undefined for any missing values */
   drop ploxx kpt;
%mend ptaulo;


/*  Exact 1-&a percent confidence interval of tau association
    parameter                                                */
%macro tauci(kp,mp,k,m,in,a,clo,chi);
   thlo= -&limit;  thhi= &limit;         /* initial interval */
   if &m=. | &k=. | &kp=. | &mp=. | &a=. then do;
      thhi = . ; /* don't estimate if any values are missing */
      thlo= . ;
   end;
       /* degenerate model if kp is at extreme of its range */
   else do;
      if &kp LE max(0,&k+&mp-&m) then thhi = . ;  /* too low */
      if &kp GE min(floor(&mp/2),&k) then thlo =.; /* too hi */
   end;
   if thhi ~= . & thlo ~= . then
      do until (abs(thhi-thlo)<&epsilon);    /* convergence? */
      &clo=(thhi+thlo)/2;                 /* examine midpoint */
      %ptauhi(&kp,&mp,&k,&m,&clo,ptxx);
         /* shrink interval by equating upper tail with &a/2 */
      if ptxx GE &a/2 then thhi=&clo;
      if ptxx LE &a/2 then thlo=&clo;
   end;
     /* Repeat this for the upper end of confidence interval */
   thlo= -&limit;  thhi= &limit;         /* initial interval */
   if &m=. | &k=. | &kp=. | &mp=. | &a=. then do;
      thhi = . ;
      thlo= . ;
   end;
      /* degenerate model if &kp is at extreme of its range */
   else do;
      if &kp LE max(0,&k+&mp-&m) then thhi = . ;  /* too low */
      if &kp GE min(floor(&mp/2),&k) then thlo =.; /* too hi */
```

```
   end;
   if thhi ~= . & thlo ~= . then
      do until (abs(thhi-thlo)<&epsilon);     /* convergence? */
      &chi=(thhi+thlo)/2;                    /* examine midpoint */
      %ptaulo(&kp,&mp,&k,&m,&chi,ptxx); /* lower tail at mid */
         /* shrink interval by equating lower tail with &a/2 */
      if ptxx LE &a/2 then thhi=&chi;
      if ptxx GE &a/2 then thlo=&chi;
   end;
   drop thhi thlo ptxx;              /* delete local variables */
%mend tauci;


/*   Inner summation of the conditional distributions         */
%macro jcond(kp,mp,k,m,tail);
   do jj = max(0,&k+&kp-&mp) to min(&k-&kp,&m-&mp-&k+&kp);
      &tail = &tail + exp( %lfac(&k) + (&k-&kp-jj)*log(2)
         - %lfac(&kp) - %lfac(jj) - %lfac(&k-&kp-jj)
         + %lfac(&m-2*&k) - %lfac(&mp-&k-&kp+jj)
         - %lfac(&m-&mp-&k+&kp-jj)
         - %lfac(&m) + %lfac(&mp) + %lfac(&m-&mp)
      ) ;
   end;
   drop jj;
%mend jcond;


/*  Upper tail of univariate distribution conditional on an
    earlier age
       kp = number of pairs both alive at this age
       mp = number of living individuals at this age
       k  = number of pairs both alive at earlier age
       m  = number of individuals alive at earlier age
       tail= output tail probability, undefined
                 for any missing values
       in = variable used as loop index                      */
%macro cond(kp,mp,k,m,tail,in);
   &tail=0;                        /* initialize the accumulator */
   if (&kp~=.) & (&mp~=.) &
      (&m~=.) & (&k~=.) then do;       /* if not missing then */
      do &in = &kp to min(floor(&mp/2),&k);     /* upper tail */
         %jcond(&in,&mp,&k,&m,&tail);          /* probability */
      end;
   end;
      else &tail = . ;    /* tail is undefined if any missing */
%mend cond;


/* Lower tail of conditional distribution, same args as cond */
%macro lcond(kp,mp,k,m,tail,in);
```

```
   &tail=0;                       /* initialize the accumulator */
   if (&kp~=.) & (&mp~=.) &
      (&m~=.) & (&k~=.) then do;      /* if not missing then */
      do &in = max(0,&kp+&mp-&m) to &kp;        /* lower tail */
         %jcond(&kp,&mp,&k,&m,&tail);          /*  accumulate */
      end;
   end;
      else &tail = . ;   /* tail is undefined if any missing */
%mend lcond;




/* ====================  MZ Twins  ========================= */


title1 'The univariate twin distribution'; title2 'Identical MZ
Danish twin data'; data MZtwin;
   retain prevx1-prevx12 prevm1-prevm12;  /* retain all data */
   array prevx(12) prevx1-prevx12;         /* previous X(m)'s */
   array prevm(12) prevm1-prevm12;            /* previous m's */
   input age n m x;
   prevx(_N_)=x;                      /* save previous X(m)'s */
   prevm(_N_)=m;                         /* save previous m's */
   preva=age;
   if (_N_=1) then output;       /* ignore first observation */
         /* loop backwards over data from all earlier ages */
   if ( _N_ >1 ) then do k=(_N_-1) to 1 by -1;
      prx=prevx(k);              /* X(m) that we condition on */
      prm=prevm(k);                 /* m that we condition on */
                                /* conditional expected value */
      ex = prx*m*(m-1)/(prm*(prm-1));
      %cond(x,m,prx,prm,ctail,i1);  /* cond. upper tail prob */
      %tauhat(x,m,prx,prm,tau);               /* MLE of tau */
      *%tauci(x,m,prx,prm,i1,.05,clo,chi);   /* exact tau CI */
      preva=preva-5;                   /* age we condition on */
      output;                     /* produce a line of output */
   end;
   else do;                    /* ignore the first observation */
      preva=.;                   /* there is no previous data */
      output;                         /* output an empty line */
   end;
   label
      age   = 'age in years'
      n     = 'number of twin pairs'
      m     = 'number of living individuals'
      x     = '# of pairs both alive'
      prx   = '# pairs in previous ages'
      prm   = '# alive in previous ages'
      ex    = 'conditional expected value of x'
      tau   = 'association with previous age'
```

```
      clo   = 'lower confidence on tau'
      chi   = 'upper confidence on tau'
      ctail = 'conditional probability in upper tail' ;
   datalines;
      30  117  220  105
      35  117  218  103
      40  117  213   98
      45  117  210   96
      50  117  205   92
      55  117  201   88
      60  117  186   75
      65  117  166   65
      70  117  146   53
      75  117  110   35
      80  117   75   17
      85  117   39    7
run;

proc print data=MZtwin noobs;
   var age m x tau preva;
*   var age m x ex ctail tau clo chi;
run;

/* ======================  DZ Twins  ====================== */

title2 'Fraternal DZ Danish twin data'; data DZtwin;
   retain prevx1-prevx12 prevm1-prevm12;  /* retain all data */
   array prevx(12) prevx1-prevx12;        /* previous X(m)'s */
   array prevm(12) prevm1-prevm12;           /* previous m's */
   input age n m x;
   prevx(_N_)=x;                     /* save previous X(m)'s */
   prevm(_N_)=m;                        /* save previous m's */
   preva=age;
   if (_N_=1) then output;       /* ignore first observation */
           /* loop backwards over data from all earlier ages */
   if ( _N_ >1 ) then do k=(_N_-1) to 1 by -1;
      prx=prevx(k);                /* X(m) that we condition on */
      prm=prevm(k);                   /* m that we condition on */
                                 /* conditional expected value */
      ex = prx*m*(m-1)/(prm*(prm-1));
      %cond(x,m,prx,prm,ctail,i1); /* conditional upper tail */
      *%tauhat(x,m,prx,prm,tau);                 /* MLE of tau */
      *%tauci(x,m,prx,prm,i1,.05,clo,chi);  /* exact tau CI  */
      preva=preva-5;                   /* age we condition on */
      output;                    /* produce a line of output */
   end;
   else do;                   /* ignore the first observation */
      preva=.;                   /* there is no previous data */
      output;                         /* output an empty line */
   end;
```

```
   label
      age   = 'age in years'
      n     = 'number of twin pairs'
      m     = 'number of living individuals'
      x     = '# of pairs both alive'
      prx   = '# pairs in previous ages'
      prm   = '# alive in previous ages'
      ex    = 'conditional expected value of x'
      tau   = 'association with previous age'
      clo   = 'lower confidence on tau'
      chi   = 'upper confidence on tau'
      ctail = 'conditional probability in upper tail' ;
   datalines;
      30  192  365  174
      35  192  352  163
      40  192  345  156
      45  192  339  150
      50  192  330  143
      55  192  312  129
      60  192  295  114
      65  192  271   99
      70  192  234   74
      75  192  184   47
      80  192  122   21
      85  192   68    9
run;

proc print data=DZtwin noobs;
   var age ctail preva;
run;
```

5.7.2 Fortran program for multivariate inference

Extensive iteration is best performed by a compiled language such as Fortran or C++ rather than an interpreted language such as SAS, R, Basic, or S-plus. Calculation of $\widehat{\tau}$ and its exact $1-\alpha\%$ confidence intervals is not too computationally difficult and can be done in SAS or R. The computation of exact significance levels in Tables 5.4 and 5.5 is computationally intensive and requires a compiled language. Many millions of outcomes needed to be enumerated in order to produce the exact significance levels given in these two tables.

```
!    --- Multivariate probability models for twins ---

! Finds: marginal upper tail probability; conditional
! significance in upper tail given previous age; joint
! statistical two-tailed significance level maximum
! likelihood estimate of tau and exact confidence interval
```

```
!  Uses IMSL routines: dbinom(binomial coefficient),
!  dfac(factorial), dzbren(univarite root of equation),
!  duvmif(univariate minimum)
      USE numerical_libraries       ! invoke numerical library
      implicit none
      common/counts/n,x,m,ix,jx
      integer j,k,m(20),x(20),n,nobs,mo2,up,ix,jx,iparam(7),
     &   maxfn
      double precision p,margin,zero,condit,joint,exact,
     &  rparam(7),lik,tau,one,three,dup,down,tiny,tauup,
     &  taulo,cilo,five,small
      external taulik,tauup,taulo
      data maxfn/100/, small/1.0d-3/, five/5.00d0/
      data zero/0.00d0/, one/1.00d0/, three/3.00d0/
      data tiny/1.0d-6/

      open(unit=10,file='MZfreq.dat')          ! raw data file
      j=1
      read(10,1000,end=20)n
      write(6,1004)n
      do 10 j=1,15
         read(10,1000,end=20)x(j),m(j)
         write(6,1001) m(j),x(j)
   10 continue
   20 continue
      nobs=j-1
!                               marginal, upper tail area p-values
      write(6,1003)
      write(6,1006)
      do 40 j=1,nobs
         p=zero
         mo2=m(j)/2
         do 30 k=x(j),mo2
            p=p+margin(k,m(j),n)
   30       continue
         write(6,1001)m(j),x(j),p
   40 continue
!                                    conditional, upper tail areas
      write(6,1005)
      write(6,1006)
      write(6,1001)m(1),x(1)
      do 60 j=2,nobs
         p=zero
         mo2=m(j)/2
         up=min(mo2,x(j-1))
         do 50 k=x(j),up
            p=p+condit(k,m(j),x(j-1),m(j-1),n)
   50    continue
         write(6,1001)m(j),x(j),p
   60 continue
```

```
!                    joint multivariate significance levels
      do 70 j=1,4
         write(6,1000)
         write(6,1008)(x(k),k=2,1+j)
         write(6,1002)(m(k),k=2,1+j)
         p=exact(x(2),m(2),n,j)
         write(6,1007)p
   70 continue

!    Estimate tau transition between age categories ix and jx
      do 80 ix=1,11
         jx=ix+1
         if(x(ix).EQ.0 .OR. x(jx).EQ.0 .OR. ! quit if invalid
     &        m(ix).EQ.0 .OR. m(jx).EQ.0)stop 9999
         write(6,1000)
         write(6,1000)x(ix),x(jx)
         write(6,1000)m(ix),m(jx)
         if(m(ix)-m(jx) .GT. x(ix)-x(jx)) then   ! tau finite
            call duvmif(taulik, zero, small, five,
     &           tiny, 100, tau)
         else
            write(6,1011)                  ! tau-hat is infinite
            go to 80
         endif
!                                          check for lack of MLE
         if(dabs(tau) .GT. five-small)go to 80
         write(6,1009)tau
!  Find exact 95% confidence interval:  tau +/- 5 is a good
!  starting value for MZ pairs.  Use +/- 2.5 for DZ pairs
         dup=tau+tiny                        ! start up a little
         down=tau-five                        ! start down a lot
         k=maxfn                   ! maximum number of iterations
!                              does this guess bracket a root?
         if(taulo(dup)*taulo(down) .LT. zero) then
            call dzbren(taulo, tiny, tiny, down, dup, k)
            cilo=dup                   ! lower interval endpoint
         else
!                                             if not, don't try
            cilo=tau
         endif
!                 find upper 95% confidence interval endpoint
         dup=tau+five
         down=tau-tiny
         k=maxfn
         if(tauup(dup)*tauup(down) .LT. zero) then
            call dzbren(tauup, tiny, tiny, down, dup, k)
         else
            dup=tau
         endif
         write(6,1010)cilo,dup
```

```
   80 continue
      stop 9999
 1000 format(2i6)
 1001 format(1x,2i5,f12.5)
 1002 format(' Joint multivariate counts: m ',8i5)
 1003 format(/' Marginal upper tail probabilities ')
 1004 format(' Raw data with ',i3, ' twin pairs'
     &   / '     m     x')
 1005 format(/' Conditional upper tail given prior age')
 1006 format('     m     x       p-value')
 1007 format(' Exact joint p-value', 10x, e16.7)
 1008 format(' Joint multivariate counts: x ',8i5)
 1009 format(' Estimated tau: ',f15.6)
 1010 format(' Exact 95% confidence interval ',2f15.6)
 1011 format(' Tau is not finite ')
      end

! -----------------------------------------------------------

      double precision function tauup(tau)

! Function needed to solve for upper 95% confidence interval
!  for tau

      implicit none
      common/counts/n,x,m,ix,jx
      integer nxx,n,x(20),m(20),ix,jx,high,j,k,klow
      double precision tau,zero,condit,den,ao2,lik
      data zero/0.00d0/, ao2/0.025d0/              ! alpha / 2

      den=zero
      tauup=zero
      klow=max(0,x(ix)+m(jx)-m(ix))     ! lower limit of range
      high=m(ix)/2                    ! upper limit of the range
      high=min(x(ix),high)           ! but can't exceed observed
      do 10 j=klow,high              ! loop over the whole range
         den=den      ! accumulate the normalizing denominator
     &      +condit(j,m(jx),x(ix),m(ix),n)*dexp(tau*j)
   10 continue
      do 20 k=klow,x(jx)                        ! sum over lower tail
         lik=condit(k,m(jx),x(ix),m(ix),n)*dexp(tau*k)
         lik=lik/den                  ! probability of this point
         tauup=tauup+lik               ! accumulate probabilities
   20 continue
      tauup=tauup-ao2        ! tail equals alpha/2 at endpoint
      return
      end

!-----------------------------------------------------------
```

```
      double precision function taulo(tau)

! Function needed to solve for lower 95% confidence interval
!  endpoint for tau

      implicit none
      common/counts/n,x,m,ix,jx
      integer nxx,n,x(20),m(20),ix,jx,low,high,j,k
      double precision tau,zero,condit,den,ao2,lik
      data zero/0.00d0/, ao2/0.025d0/                 ! alpha / 2

      taulo=zero
      den=zero
      low=max(0,x(ix)+m(jx)-m(ix))      ! lower limit of range
      high=m(ix)/2                      ! upper limit of range
      high=min(x(ix),high)       ! can't exceed observed value
      do 10 j=low,high
         den=den                       ! accumulate denominator
     &         +condit(j,m(jx),x(ix),m(ix),n)*dexp(tau*j)
   10 continue
      do 20 k=x(jx),high                  ! sum over upper tail
         lik=condit(k,m(jx),x(ix),m(ix),n)*dexp(tau*k)
         lik=lik/den                 ! probability of this event
         taulo=taulo+lik                 ! accumulate upper tail
   20 continue
      taulo=taulo-ao2   ! upper tail equal alpha/2 at endpoint
     return
     end

! -----------------------------------------------------------

      double precision function condit(xp,mp,x,m,n)

!  Conditional probability of xp pairs both alive given
!   mp living individuals and (x,m) at an earlier age

      implicit none
      integer xp,mp,x,m,n,j,jlo,jhi,max,min
      double precision dfac,dbinom,zero,two,term,ff,one
      data zero/0.00d0/, one/1.00d0/, two/2.00d0/

      ff=one             ! calculate x! / xp! to avoid overflow
      do 10 j=xp+1,x
   10 ff=ff*j
      if(x .EQ. xp)ff=one

      jlo=max(0,x+xp-mp)              ! lower range of summation
      jhi=min(x-xp,m-mp-x+xp)         ! upper range of summation
      condit=zero
      do 20 j=jlo,jhi
```

```
         term=ff/(dfac(j)*dfac(x-xp-j))
         term=term*(two**(x-xp-j))
         term=term*dbinom(m-2*x,mp-x-xp+j)
         term=term/dbinom(m,mp)
         condit=condit+term
   20 continue
      return
      end

!------------------------------------------------------------

      double precision function exact(x,m,n,d)

! Exact multivariate significance level of x(1), ... , x(d)
! pairs both alive given m(1), ... ,m(d) living people out
! of n total pairs

      implicit none
      integer x(1),m(1),n,ld,d,j,k(25),items,savek(25)
      double precision p0,term,cum,zero,margin,condit,joint,
     &  item,mod,savep(25)
      logical trace
      data zero/0.00d0/, trace/.FALSE./

      p0=joint(x,m,n,d)
      write(6,1001)p0
      cum=zero
      exact=zero
      items=0
      do 10 j=1,d
   10   savek(j)=-1
      ld=1
      call clear(k,m,n,1,d)
!                           Loop over all possible outcomes in k()
      do 40
         item=margin(k,m,n)
         if(d .LE. 1)go to 30
!                              find the smallest table in the tail
         do 20 ld=2,d
!                                use saved probability if possible
            if(savek(ld) .EQ. k(ld))then
               item=savep(ld)
            else
!                                  otherwise calculate and save it
               item=item
     &              * condit(k(ld),m(ld),k(ld-1),m(ld-1),n)
               savek(ld)=k(ld)
               savek(ld+1)=-1
               savep(ld)=item
            endif
```

```
            if(item .LE. p0)go to 30
   20    continue
         ld=d
!         count tables, accumulate if it is in the tail of p0
   30    items=items+1
         cum=cum+item
         if(item .LE. p0)exact=exact+item
!              periodically print a summary during long runs
!       if(mod(items,250000) .EQ. 0)
!    &       write(6,1004)items,cum,exact
         call incr(k,m,n,d,ld)            ! get the next table
         if(k(1) .LT. 0)exit
   40 continue
      write(6,1002)items           ! number of tables evaluated
 !    write(6,1005)cum          ! check: cumulative probability
      return
 1000 format(' Exact: ',12i5)
 1001 format(' Probability of observed data  ',e15.7)
 1002 format(' Number of tables evaluated    ',i15)
 1004 format(' Exact: items,cum,exact ',i12,3e13.5)
 1005 format(' Exact: cumulative probability ',e15.7)
      end

! -----------------------------------------------------------

      subroutine incr(k,m,n,d,ld)

!  Increment the counters in k(1), ... ,k(d) looping over all
!    possible outcomes of twin pairs both alive

      implicit none
      integer k(1),m(1),n,ld,d,j,up,min,i

      j=ld
      do 10 i=1,d+1
         up=m(j)/2                      ! upper limit on j-th age
         if(j .GT. 1)up=min(up,k(j-1))
         k(j)=k(j)+1                         ! increment j-th age
         if((k(j) .LE. up) .AND. (j .LT. d))
    &       call clear(k,m,n,j+1,d)        ! reset later ages
         if(k(j) .LE. up)return   ! done if below upper limit
         k(j)=-1                ! bogus values indicate the end
         j=j-1                          ! back up to previous age
         if(j .LE. 0)return    ! done if we backed up too far
   10 continue
      stop 940             ! error - this can't happen normally
      end

! -----------------------------------------------------------
```

```
      double precision function joint(x,m,n,d)

! Joint probability of x(1), ... , x(d) twin pairs both
! given m(1), ... , m(d) living people out of n total pairs

      implicit none
      integer d,x(1),m(1),n,j
      double precision margin,condit

      joint=margin(x(1),m(1),n)  ! marginal probability of 1st
      if(d .LE. 1)return
      do 10 j=2,d                ! times conditional prob of others
         joint=joint*condit(x(j),m(j),x(j-1),m(j-1),n)
   10 continue
      return
      end

! -----------------------------------------------------------

      double precision function taulik(tau)

!  Log likelihood for tau parameter modeling transition
! between ages ix (earlier, conditioned on) and jx (later)

      implicit none
      common/counts/n,x,m,ix,jx
      integer nxx,n,x(20),m(20),ix,jx,low,high,j
      double precision tau,lik,zero,condit,den
      data zero/0.00d0/

      lik=condit(x(jx),m(jx),x(ix),m(ix),n)
      lik=lik*dexp(tau*x(jx))                        ! numerator
      den=zero
      low=max(0,x(ix)+m(jx)-m(ix))                 ! lower range
      high=m(ix)/2                                 ! upper range
      high=min(x(ix),high)
      do 10 j=low,high                    ! accumulate denominator
         den=den+condit(j,m(jx),x(ix),m(ix),n)*dexp(tau*j)
   10 continue
      lik=dlog(lik)-dlog(den)                     ! log-likelihood
      taulik=-lik       ! minimize the negative log-likelihood
      return
      end

! ---------------------------------------------------------

      subroutine clear(k,m,n,first,d)

!  Reset values of counters in k(first, ... ,d) to their
!  lowest possible values
```

```
      implicit none
      integer k(1),m(1),n,first,d,j,max
      logical trace
      data trace/.FALSE./

      do 10 j=first,d
         k(j)=max(0,m(1)-n)
         if(j .GT. 1)k(j)=max(0,k(j-1)+m(j)-m(j-1))
   10 continue
      return
      end

! -----------------------------------------------------------
```

6

Frequency Models for Family Disease Clusters

We have all heard about how some traits run in families. Such characteristics might include musical ability, good looks, or longevity. Undesirable characteristics might include serious health problems or perhaps bad luck. In many epidemiologic studies, the first indication of an environmental or genetic contribution to a disease is the way in which the diseased cases cluster within the same family units. The concept of clustering is different from incidence. These separate concepts are compared in Section 6.1. The basic unit of analysis is a family or a litter that is composed of an arbitrary number of members. In terms of the urn model, a family can be thought of as sampling a handful of balls from an urn.

A variety of different sampling distributions are employed in collecting data of this type. Each of these sampling schemes will be illustrated with a numerical example. One method called ascertainment sampling can lead to a large bias unless we can correct for it. Ascertainment bias is described and the appropriate sampling distribution is demonstrated in Section 6.2.2.

In this chapter, we will assume that all individuals are exchangeable, except for their disease status. This assumption is used to provide an exact test of the initial hypothesis of no familial link with the disease, conditional on the number of diseased cases and the distribution of the sizes of the various family units. Several numerical examples with real data are examined in Section 6.3 and illustrate these methods.

Chapters 7 and 8 describe some parametric generalizations of binomial sampling models to provide measures of the effect size of the disease clustering. Several models for clustering appear in those chapters. Briefly then, the present chapter can be thought of as describing the null hypothesis of no familial link with the disease status. Chapters 7 and 8 provide models for possible alternative hypotheses in

Discrete Distributions Daniel Zelterman
 ISBN: 0-470-86888-0 (PPC)

which the diseased individuals do not occur at random among the various families. Chapter 9 considers examples that take covariates into account.

6.1 Introduction

The role of genetics and environment in epidemiology has a rich history and much of the work done in this field takes the form of the recording of disease cases within the same family. For years, researchers have attempted to sort out the role of inherited mutations by recording the incidence of disease within families. Several recent examples include: Li, Fraumeni, Mulvihill *et al.* (1988); Goldar, Cannon-albright, Oliphant *et al.* (1993); Wingo, Lee, Ory *et al.* (1993); Claus (1995); and Shattuck, Oliphant, McClure *et al.* (1997). The currently ongoing STAR clinical trial (NSABP, 1999) seeks to modify the risk patterns in sisters of breast cancer victims, as another example. More generally, one often wishes to know whether cancer occurs more frequently in some families than others. That is to say, whether the diseased cases cluster within conditionally observed family units whose risks may not be homogeneous. This question represents the primary step in the process of identifying susceptibility alleles and determining the extent to which these inherited mutations are associated with the development and progression of a genetically based disease such as cancer.

This and the following two chapters are concerned with the multivariate binary outcome indication of occurance or nonoccurance of disease among family members. The analysis of correlated binary data has seen considerable research advances in the past decade and we can only cite a few of the many works. Generalized estimating equations (GEE) are developed in Liang and Zeger (1986) to allow for specification of mean and variance structures of models that can be applied to binary valued data, in particular, as in Lipsitz, Laird, and Harrington (1991); Liang, Zeger, and Qaqish (1992); Commenges, Jacqmin, Letenneur, and Van Dujin (1995); Commenges and Abel (1996); Waller and Zelterman (1997); and O'Hara Hines (1998). New models for sums of dependent Bernoulli data are developed in the following two chapters.

Given a specified family history of disease, Berry, Parmigiani, Sanchez *et al.* (1997) use Bayesian methods to quantify the risks associated with an unaffected family member. Britton (1997) proposes a test to detect within-family clustering of infected individuals for the susceptible-infective-removed epidemic model. Recent work in modeling the risk of disease as a function of family histories based on logistic regression include: Pregibon (1984); Wong and Mason (1985); Bonney (1987); Piegorsch and Casella (1996); Bedrick and Hill (1996); Betensky and Whittemore (1996); FitzGerald and Knuiman (1998) and Ten Have, Kunselman, Pulkstenis, and Landis (1998). Grimson (1993) and Grimson and Oden (1996) derived probability models that examine the frequencies of families with no cases.

In the previous two chapters, we restrict our attention to twins, that is to say, families all of size two. In Section 6.2, we generalize those methods to include combinations of families of arbitrary sizes and derive the exact probability of a given set of disease cluster frequencies. We assume that all possible reorganizations of individuals into family units are equally likely, provided that we maintain the same distribution of the sizes of the various families and the number of disease cases in the sample.

Section 6.2 develops models assuming that all individuals are independent and exchangeable across sampled families. The exact likelihood measures how the healthy and diseased individuals randomly arrange themselves within these homogeneous families. The distribution of cases within families under this null hypothesis is explained in Section 6.2. The distribution of cases in these triangular-shaped tables depends on the number of cases observed in the sample as well as the distribution of observed family sizes.

The exact method described in Section 6.2.1 tests this null hypothesis against an unspecified alternative. Pesarin (2001) suggests that an unspecified alternative hypothesis associated with data of this type motivates the use of exact tests. The relatively sparse nature of the data also provides motivation for the use of exact tests. Exact methods can also be efficient in many settings where the alternative hypothesis is restricted or does not have a parametric form.

In Section 6.2.1, we describe an algorithm for enumerating all possible sample realizations to obtain the exact significance level of an observed set of frequencies. Mathematical shortcuts are identified to facilitate this computation.

Section 6.2.2 addresses the bias introduced by ascertainment sampling such as that used in the collection of the data in Table 6.2. Section 6.3 examines several datasets using these examples. Parametric forms for useful alternative hypotheses are given in Chapter 7. Chapter 9 describes examples that include covariates.

6.1.1 Examples

The data of Table 6.1 is given by Liang, Zeger, and Qaqish (1992) and lists the frequency of interstitial pulmonary fibrosis (IPF) in 203 siblings of 100 chronic obstructive pulmonary disease (COPD) patients. COPD is an impairment of lung function, especially with regard to ventilation. In COPD, the lungs fail to close adequately when exhaling. COPD typically arises in heavy smokers and in long-term asthmatics.

IPF is a general name for a wide range of lung disorders. It is marked by scarring of the lung tissues and may arise from a number of unrelated causes. It may have a genetic basis. IPF often appears after radiation exposure (for cancer, for example) and is sometimes drug related.

The 60 cases of IPF summarized in Table 6.1 are distributed among 100 families that vary in size between one and six siblings in addition to the proband with COPD. There were no families of size five in this dataset.

The methods we develop in Section 6.2.1 are an exact statistical test of the random distribution of the 60 cases of IPF based on the way in which they present within the same familial units. A statistically significant result from such a test indicates that some individuals are at greater or lowered risk of IPF because of

Table 6.1 The observed frequencies of 60 cases of IPF among 203 siblings in 100 families with a COPD patient (Liang, Zeger, and Qaqish 1992).

Number of siblings	Number of families	Number of cases	Number of affected siblings i						
n	f_n	m_n	0	1	2	3	4	5	6
1	48	12	36	12					
2	23	9	15	7	1				
3	17	19	5	7	3	2			
4	7	5	3	3	1	0	0		
6	5	15	1	0	1	1	1	0	1
Totals	100	60							

Table 6.2 Frequencies of 31 cases of childhood cancer in the siblings of 24 probands (Li, Fraumeni *et al.* 1988).

Number of siblings	Number of families	Number of cases	Number of affected siblings i				
n	f_n	m_n	0	1	2	3	4+
0	1	0	1				
1	2	0	2	0			
2	8	10	1	4	3		
3	4	7	0	2	1	1	
4	2	2	0	2	0	0	0
5	1	1	0	1	0	0	0
6	1	1	0	1	0	0	0
7	1	1	0	1	0	0	0
8	3	6	0	1	1	1	0
9	1	3	0	0	0	1	0
Totals	24	31					

genetic or environmental risk factors at the family or individual level that are not presented in this dataset. We develop methods for calculating the expected frequencies for this data under a variety of models in this chapter and the two that follow.

A second example is summarized in Table 6.2. This table describes the distribution of 31 cases of childhood cancer among members of 24 families. Li, Fraumeni *et al.* (1988) use the high incidence of cancer in siblings of childhood cancer victims to describe evidence of a genetic disorder. The authors of that study examined the Cancer Family Registry of the Epidemiology Branches of the U.S. National

Cancer Institute for families with the Li–Fraumeni syndrome. Eligibility for entry into their study was limited to families with at least three close relatives in whom cancer was documented by review of the available relevant records.

The researchers of this study first identified the initial cases (referred to as the *proband*) and then examined their siblings. Using this sampling method, every family will have at least one case. The data in Table 6.2 omits the proband and summarizes childhood cancer among the siblings of the proband. Their report includes cancer incidence among more distant relatives, but we will not examine that additional data here.

A third example is a random sample of families in Brazil reported by Sastry (1997). Table 6.3 summarizes a survey of deaths of children in northeast Brazil. This area of Brazil is poorer and less developed than the rest of the country and has a corresponding higher incidence of infant mortality. The data was extracted from a household survey as part of the Demography and Health Survey. The multilevel survey used a cluster-sampling scheme that selected many families from a relatively small number of communities. Maternity histories were collected on women aged 15 to 44 over a 3-month period in 1986. This table counts the frequencies of 430 childhood deaths in 2946 families of sizes up to eight children.

In our fourth example, Smith and Pike (1976) describe a survey of 40 households, also in northeast Brazil. All members of these households were serologically tested for *Trypanosoma cruzi* (*T. cruzi*). This infectious disease is associated with Chagas cardiomyopathy, often leading to premature death. A summary of the frequencies of household sizes and the distribution of 57 cases of *T. cruzi* is given in Table 6.4. Subsequent analyses of this data using a variety of statistical measures appear in Grimson and Oden (1996).

The fifth example is a laboratory study from Paul (1982) and represents a complete census in which all pedigrees have been included even if they contained no

Table 6.3 The frequency of childhood deaths in Brazilian families (Sastry 1997).

Number of siblings	Number of families	Number of deaths	Number of affected siblings i							
n	f_n	m_n	0	1	2	3	4	5	6	7+
1	267	12	255	12						
2	285	48	239	44	2					
3	202	80	143	41	15	3				
4	110	54	69	30	9	2	0			
5	104	103	43	34	15	9	3	0		
6	50	67	15	18	8	5	3	0	1	
7	21	38	4	4	7	4	2	0	0	0
8	12	28	1	2	4	3	1	1	0	0
Totals	2946	430								

Table 6.4 Distribution of 57 cases of *T. cruzi* in 40 Brazilian households (Smith and Pike 1976; Grimson and Oden 1996).

Number of members n	Number of households f_n	Number of cases m_n	Number of affected household members i							
			0	1	2	3	4	5	6	7+
1	1	0	1	0						
2	8	8	2	4	2					
3	13	11	5	5	3	0				
4	5	5	2	1	2	0	0			
5	5	9	2	1	0	1	0	1		
6	4	17	0	0	1	0	1	1	1	
7	1	1	0	1	0	0	0	0	0	0
8	1	3	0	0	0	1	0	0	0	0
9	1	1	0	1	0	0	0	0	0	0
13	1	2	0	0	1	0	0	0	0	0
Totals	40	57								

affected individuals. In such experiments, researchers expose pregnant laboratory animals to one of several concentrations of known toxic substances. The subsequent litters born to these mothers are examined for stillbirths, birth defects, or other malformations. The data is given in Table 9.5. This example is typical of many laboratory teratology and toxicity experiments in which all subjects are recorded and accounted for. This example and those including covariates are described in Chapter 9.

6.1.2 Sampling methods employed

These examples illustrate that a variety of sampling schemes are often incorporated in the collection of data of this type. Let us restate these different methods and make their distinction clear. The statistical examination of these examples is given in more detail in Section 6.3.

The data of Table 6.1 was sampled using cases of one disease (COPD) to identify families whose members have a different disease (IPF). The proband with COPD was used to bring the family to the attention of the researchers, who then examined their siblings for IPF.

Our presentation of the childhood cancer data in Table 6.2 is restricted to the siblings of the proband with the probands omitted. This second example identifies families through members with the same disease creating a bias towards families with more cases. In other words, the researchers of the study first identified the initial cases (proband) and then examined their siblings.

This type of sampling results in a bias in this data towards families with more cases. A family with two children with cancer, for example, has two potential probands, and such a family is twice as likely to be sampled as a family with only one child with cancer. Such a sample is said to exhibit a *length bias*. We identify the appropriate sampling distribution for examining this type of data in Section 6.2.2.

In the *T. cruzi* example summarized in Table 6.4, the sampling unit is a household that might include unrelated individuals. This is in contrast to the examples considered so far, in which the sampling unit is a set of siblings. Nevertheless, the *T. cruzi* example is an illustration of the effects of contagion for individuals living in environmental proximity.

The laboratory studies of teratology examined in Chapter 9 represent a complete census. All individuals in all litters were included whether they contained a birth defect or not.

The methods developed in the present chapter are applicable to all of these sampling schemes.

6.1.3 Incidence and clustering

Before we proceed with the analysis of this type of data, let us make the distinction between the separate concepts of *incidence* and *clustering*. We say that a sample exhibits high incidence if there are many more diseased cases in the sample than in the unsampled population. In contrast, this chapter and those following are concerned with tests and models for clustering. We say that clustering is present when many diseased cases occur in a relatively small number of the families sampled. A cartoon illustration of these two separate concepts is given in Fig. 6.1.

Two examples already presented will demonstrate the separate concepts of incidence and clustering. The incidence of 60 cases of IPF in Table 6.1 represents an unusually large number in a sample of 203 children, for example, but this is not of particular concern to us in the present work. Our study of clustering, on the other hand, is how these 60 cases are distributed among the 100 families of various sizes. The question we want to address is: Do these 60 cases appear randomly distributed among the various families, or do an unusually large number of cases tend to occur in a small number of families?

As another example of these two separate concepts, Li, Fraumeni *et al.* (1988) are widely cited as having discovered a genetic-based risk factor for childhood cancer. The evidence they provide is the unusually high incidence of 31 cases appearing among the siblings of probands in the 24 families that they identified. In contrast, our examination of their data given in Table 6.2 does not reveal significant departures from a random distribution of these cases across the families ($p =$ .3101), using the exact test procedure described in Section 6.2.1. That is, their data exhibits high incidence but no clustering of cases.

It is generally not too difficult to verify that the disease incidence in a sample is higher than that of the general population. This hypothesis is indicative of a

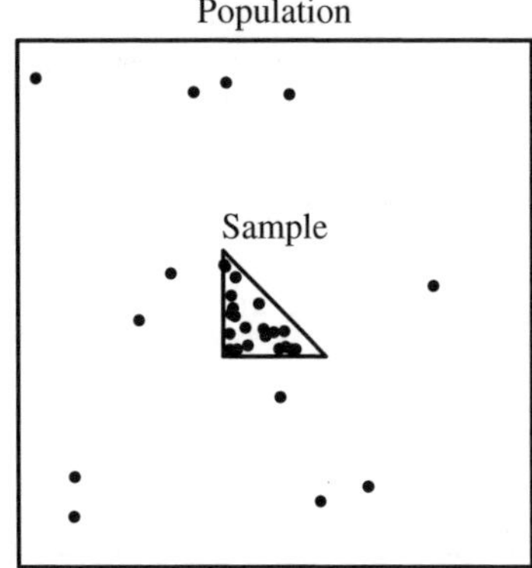

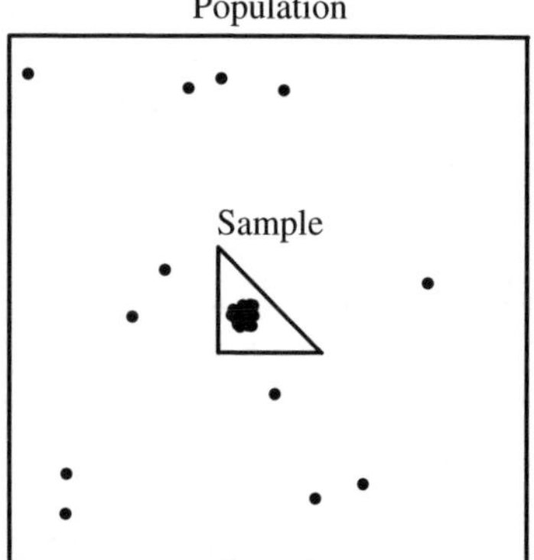

Figure 6.1 Two cartoon illustrations contrasting the concepts of incidence and clustering. The dots represent diseased cases.

possibly unmeasured risk factor that is present in the sampled families at a higher rate than among those in the surrounding reference population.

Clustering among the sampled families suggests that there are additional risk factors that vary across sampled families and family members. The appearance of clustering suggests that these additional risk factors are not the same across the sampled families.

The analysis of family-level data should then be examined in two stages. The first stage is to test whether the incidence is higher than the surrounding population. This hypothesis tests whether there are risk factors identified by the sampling mechanism. A test of clustering asks whether there are additional unmeasured risk factors among the sampled families, often prompting further examination.

6.2 Exact Inference Under Homogeneous Risk

In this chapter, we describe the distribution of frequencies in triangular tables, such as the examples illustrated in the previous section. The joint distribution of the frequencies is a multivariate discrete distribution. This distribution will condition on the number of cases observed in the sample and the distribution of sizes of the families sampled.

Let f_n denote the number of sampled families of size n for each $n = 1, 2, \ldots, I$. Each f_n represents the row-sum of the frequencies in each of the examples presented in the previous section. There are then $N = \sum n\, f_n$ sampled individuals in the data.

Let m denote the number of individuals who have the disease of interest (cases), and let the remaining $N - m$ subjects be otherwise healthy. The aim of this section is to describe the probability distribution of how these m affected individuals arrange themselves within the various sized families. In this section, we assume that all N individuals are independent and identically distributed across the various families. A more general setting is detailed in Section 6.5.2 to account for the effects of individual-level covariates.

In terms of balls sampled from an urn, we begin with N balls: m of one color and the remaining $N - m$ of a different color. We reach in and draw out a handful of balls, without replacement. Each handful represents a different family. We record each (handful) draw in terms of its size and composition. The process ends when the urn is emptied. In this section, we describe the joint distribution of the composition of frequencies conditional on the sizes of the various urn draws.

In the following two chapters, we demonstrate methods for modeling statistical dependency among family members. Briefly then, the model in the present chapter corresponds to the null hypothesis that the disease status of all individuals is independent of all other members of the same family. Models for different possible alternative hypotheses of within-family dependence are given in the Chapter 7.

Let the random variable X_{ni} denote the number of families of size n having i $(i = 0, 1, \ldots, n)$ diseased members. Four numerical examples of such triangular shaped tables of frequencies are given in Section 6.1.1 at the beginning of this chapter. The nonnegative integer-valued random variables $\boldsymbol{X} = \{X_{ni}\}$ are constrained by

$$\sum_{i=0}^{n} X_{ni} = f_n; \tag{6.1}$$

the number of families of size n for each $n = 1, 2, \ldots, I$; and

$$\sum_{n} \sum_{i} i\, X_{ni} = m \tag{6.2}$$

affected individuals. In Section 6.2.1, we give an algorithm for generating all possible sets of nonnegative integers $\{x_{ni}\}$ that satisfy these conditions.

The joint probability of observing the frequencies $\boldsymbol{x} = \{x_{ni}\}$, given $\boldsymbol{f} = \{f_n\}$ and m is

$$\Pr[\boldsymbol{X} = \boldsymbol{x} \mid \boldsymbol{f}, m] = \prod_{n=1}^{I} \left[f_n! \prod_{i=0}^{n} \binom{n}{i}^{x_{ni}} \Big/ x_{ni}! \right] \Big/ \binom{N}{m}. \tag{6.3}$$

The proof that these probabilities sum to one, and the moments of this multivariate discrete distribution, are given in Section 6.5.1. That section also motivates the functional form of this distribution. If all families are of size $n = 2$, then distribution (6.3) reduces to the twins distribution given at (4.2).

Section 6.5.2 shows that a generalization of (6.3) that includes covariates measured on individuals leads to the same partial likelihood as that of proportional hazards in the analysis of survival data. A similar conclusion is reached by the methods of Li, Yang, and Schwartz (1998). The examples in Chapter 9 include covariates measured at the family or animal litter level.

The (marginal) expected value of each frequency X_{ni} in (6.3) is

$$\mathrm{E}[X_{ni}] = f_n \binom{n}{i}\binom{N-n}{m-i} \Big/ \binom{N}{m} = f_n \binom{m}{i}\binom{N-m}{n-i} \Big/ \binom{N}{n} \qquad (6.4)$$

for inequalities $i \le m \le N$ and $i \le n \le N$, for which the various binomial coefficients are defined.

The expected counts in (6.4) follow constraints (6.1) and (6.2) when the X_{ni} are replaced by their expectations in these expressions. The expected value of X_{ni} in (6.4) is f_n times the probability mass of a hypergeometric distribution with mean mn/N. The hypergeometric distribution is discussed in Section 1.7.

The model for the expected value of X_{ni} given by Ekholm, Smith, and McDonald (1995) in their 'homogeneous model' is f_n times the binomial mass function:

$$\mathrm{E}[X_{ni}] = f_n \binom{n}{i} p^i (1-p)^{n-i}, \qquad (6.5)$$

where $p = m/N$ is the proportion of diseased cases in the sample.

When p is not very close to 0 or 1, then models (6.4) and (6.5) should be very close in value. The expected values of the counts in the IPF/COPD data are given in Table 6.5 using (6.4). These values are in close agreement with those given in Table 1 of Ekholm *et al.* using (6.5). The deviance for the IPF/COPD data is 23.15 using model (6.4) and 22.55 using model (6.5), both with 15 df. The point here is not to show that one model fits significantly better than the other, but rather to show how close these two fitted models are to each other. In Section 6.3, the models (6.4) and (6.5) are fitted to each of the examples of the previous section.

Table 6.5 The expected frequencies for the IPF/COPD data of Table 6.1 under the model of homogeneous risk using (6.4).

			Number of affected siblings i						
n	f_n	E M_n	0	1	2	3	4	5	6
1	48	14.19	33.81	14.19					
2	23	13.60	11.39	9.63	1.99				
3	17	15.07	5.91	7.54	3.13	0.423			
4	7	8.28	1.70	2.92	1.83	0.499	0.050		
6	5	8.87	0.59	1.54	1.64	0.905	0.274	0.0433	0.00277
Totals	100	60							

6.2.1 Enumeration algorithm

This section outlines an enumeration algorithm that facilitates the computation of the exact significance level for a given table of data. The FORTRAN program to implement this procedure is given in Section 6.6 at the end of this chapter.

The exact significance level or p-value for a given dataset is the sum of the probability (6.3) over all possible outcomes that are at most as likely as that of the observed data. This sum is over all outcomes whose values of N, m and $\boldsymbol{f}$ are the same as those of the observed data.

Let M_n denote the total number of diseased cases that occur in all families of size n. The M_n do not have an important interpretation by themselves, but are useful in describing a complete enumeration of all possible frequencies and outcomes in distribution (6.3). The M_n satisfies

$$M_n = \sum_i^n i\, X_{ni}$$

for each $n = 1, \ldots, I$ and

$$\sum M_n = m.$$

The $\boldsymbol{M} = \{M_n : n = 1, \ldots, I\}$ have a joint multivariate hypergeometric distribution with probability mass function

$$\Pr[\, \boldsymbol{M} = \boldsymbol{m} \mid \boldsymbol{f},\, m\,] = m!(N-m)! \prod_n (nf_n)! \Big/ N! \prod_n m_n!(nf_n - m_n)! \qquad (6.6)$$

for values $\boldsymbol{m} = \{m_n\}$ subject to $\sum m_n = m$ and $0 \le m_n \le nf_n$.

The expected value of M_n is $m\, nf_n/N$. The observed values m_n of M_n for the IPF data are given in Table 6.1 and their expected values are given in Table 6.5.

If we restrict our attention to families all of size n, then the conditional distribution of $\boldsymbol{X}_n = \{X_{ni} : i = 0, \ldots, n\}$, given f_n and m_n is

$$\Pr[\, \boldsymbol{X}_n = \boldsymbol{x}_n \mid f_n, m_n\,] \;=\; f_n! \prod_{i=0}^{n} \left[\binom{n}{i}^{x_{ni}} \Big/ x_{ni}! \right] \Big/ \binom{nf_n}{m_n}. \qquad (6.7)$$

Useful properties of distribution (6.7), including moments, are similar to those of (6.3) and are given in Section 6.5. The special case of (6.7) for twins (that is, families all of size $n = 2$) is described in Chapter 4.

The first routine needed is one that generates all possible outcomes of the multinomial distribution. This outermost level of the algorithm allocates all possible arrangements of the m cases into families of size $n = 1, \ldots, I$ according to the multinomial enumeration. Each step in the algorithm systematically generates every possible vector $\boldsymbol{m} = \{m_n\}$ with $\sum m_n = m$ excluding any step where $m_n > nf_n$. (If $m_n > nf_n$, then there are more cases than people among families of size n).

At the inner level, the algorithm conditions on the m_n cases distributed among the f_n families of size n. For each family size $n = 1, \ldots, I$, the algorithm again uses the multinomial generator to produce all possible counts $\boldsymbol{X}_n = \{x_{ni}\}$ in (6.7), subject to $\sum_i x_{ni} = f_n$ and $\sum_i i\, x_{ni} = m_n$.

Many steps of the inner level of the algorithm may be omitted, resulting in considerable savings in computing time. Let p^0 denote the probability of the observed table from (6.3) and let $\sum^*$ denote the sum over those values $\boldsymbol{X}$ for which $\Pr[\boldsymbol{X}] > p^0$. The exact significance level for the observed table is then equal to

$$1 - \sum_{\boldsymbol{X}}^{*} \Pr[\,\boldsymbol{X} \mid m, N\,] = 1 - \sum_{\boldsymbol{M}} \sum_{\boldsymbol{X}}^{*} \Pr[\,\boldsymbol{M} \mid f, N\,] \Pr[\,\boldsymbol{X} \mid \boldsymbol{M}\,].$$

If $\Pr[\boldsymbol{M}]$ at (6.6) is smaller than the probability p^0 of the observed frequency table, then it is not necessary to further enumerate all possible tables X_{ni} that comprise the complete distribution in the inner levels of the algorithm.

6.2.2 Ascertainment sampling

Epidemiologists and geneticists have long known that there may be a bias when estimating incidence from data of the type described here, depending on how the families are introduced to the sampling process. It is often through a single affected individual, called the *proband*, that the family is brought to the attention of the epidemiologist. If a family has two affected siblings, for example, then these two potential probands make the family twice as likely to appear in the sample as a family with only one case. See Lange (1997, Section 2.6) or Elandt-Johnson (1971, Chapter 17) for more details and methods related to the estimation of incidence when this form of weighted sampling is employed. Elston and Sobel (1979) identify other relevant types of sampling distributions encountered in the collection of data of this type.

Distribution (6.3) does not take into account the distribution of family disease frequencies when ascertainment sampling has taken place. Consider then, a weighted distribution in which the probability that a family is sampled is proportional to the number of affected siblings in the family. Under such a weighted sampling scheme, the following proposition is proved in Section 6.5.3:

Proposition 6.2.1 *The ascertainment weighted distribution of the frequencies X_{ni} in (6.3) with all probands omitted is the same as the unweighted distribution of $X_{n-1\,i-1}$.*

If the population exhibits unclustered, randomly distributed cases, then we can omit the proband from every family and treat the remaining individuals as an unclustered sample. The bias that ascertainment sampling introduces is an increase in the number of cases in the sample but does not alter the distribution of these cases in the sample, except to ensure that every family has at least one case. As discussed in Section 6.1.3, disease clustering is to be distinguished from measures of incidence that ascertainment methods seek to correct for. An example of this proposition in practice is the exact analysis of the childhood cancer data in Table 6.2. After omitting the probands, this data is well explained by model (6.3). This analysis is given in Section 6.3.2. Examples of other types of weighted sampling appear in Chapter 8.

6.3 Numerical Examples

The examples of Section 6.1.1 are examined here. A summary of the deviances and chi-squared values for these examples is given here using both the hypergeometric and binomial models given at (6.4) and (6.5), respectively. The exact methods of Section 6.2.1 are also given provided the computing effort is reasonable.

The relatively sparse nature of the frequency data is an indication that the usual chi-squared approximations for the deviance and χ^2 may not hold. In several instances, there are huge differences in the values of these two statistics. The usual asymptotic equivalence of these two statistics also fails to hold in sparse data such as that examined here. Furthermore, the presence of a large number of zero frequencies often adds some ambiguity to the determination of the number of degrees of freedom for a given dataset.

Zelterman (1987) shows that other test statistics may be appropriate when working with such data. When working with this type of sparse frequency data, the general conclusion of Haberman (1977) is that the difference of the deviances of two nested models should behave approximately as chi-squared despite the nonasymptotic behavior of the individual deviances. These deviance differences are used to compare models in Chapter 7.

6.3.1 IPF in COPD families

The exact probability of observing the data in Table 6.1 is 1.4×10^{-10}, conditional on $m = 60$ cases of IPF in $N = 203$ siblings and family size frequencies $f_1 = 48, \ldots, f_6 = 5$ using distribution (6.3). The exact statistical significance of this data is .00883 (Table 6.6). This is the sum of the probabilities of all (approximately 10^{10}) tables consistent with $\boldsymbol{f}, m$ having smaller values of (6.3). A Monte Carlo p-value of .00848 with 10^7 simulated replications was also obtained. Other summary statistics for this data are given in Table 6.6.

These extreme significance levels provide strong evidence that IPF does not occur at random in these 100 families. The expected counts for the model (6.4) are given in Table 6.5. The source of the lack of fit in this examination of the data is the presence of the remarkable outlier: $x_{66} = 1$. Almost all of the value of the $\chi^2 = 373.23$ given in Table 6.6 can be traced to this single family of size 6 with all members exhibiting IPF. An extremely small expected count (.00277) is anticipated in this category and one occurred in the data. This is clear evidence of a cluster in one family. Several models for disease clustering are proposed for this data in the following chapter and have a much better fit.

Table 6.6 Exact significance levels, deviance, chi-squared goodness-of-fit statistics for the IPF/COPD dataset. The hypergeometric model is given at (6.4); the binomial model is given at (6.5).

Sample size	Exact p-value	Fitted model	χ^2	Deviance
$N = 203$	0.00883	Hypergeometric	373.23	23.15
$m = 60$		Binomial	312.30	22.55

Table 6.7 Summary statistics for the childhood cancer example.

Sample size	Exact p-value	Fitted model	χ^2	Deviance
$N = 89$	0.3108	Hypergeometric	30.04	28.40
$m = 31$		Binomial	29.61	28.45

6.3.2 Childhood cancer syndrome

The exact significance of the data in Table 6.2 is 0.3108, indicating that the cancer cases are randomly distributed across the various families. This illustrates an application of the proposal given in Section 6.2.2. Specifically, ascertainment sampling was employed by the authors of this dataset. After omitting the probands, the remaining cancer cases appear independently distributed across family members. This nonsignificant p-value is evidence of homogeneity of cancer risk across the various families. There is little evidence of an unmeasured covariate in the data that can further explain the differing cancer rates among these families.

The complete enumeration, as described in Section 6.2.1, involved evaluating 171 million tables. The FORTRAN program given in Section 6.6 took a few minutes on a laptop computer.

Fig. 6.2 presents a bubble plot of the standardized chi-squared residuals `StResChi` for the hypergeometric mean. The model, these residuals, and this plot are all obtained using the SAS program given in Section 8.9.

The chi-squared residual is

$$(\text{observed} - \text{expected})/\text{expected}^{1/2}.$$

The `StResChi` residuals are further normalized to take into account variances of the estimated parameters by the GENMOD procedure in SAS.

The areas of the bubbles in Fig. 6.2 are proportional to the sizes of the families. There are no outstanding residuals in this plot, confirming that the model of homogeneous risk fits the data well. The line of residuals along the bottom of this figure corresponds to observed zero frequencies whose residuals are all negative because their expected counts must be positive. These are connected with a dotted

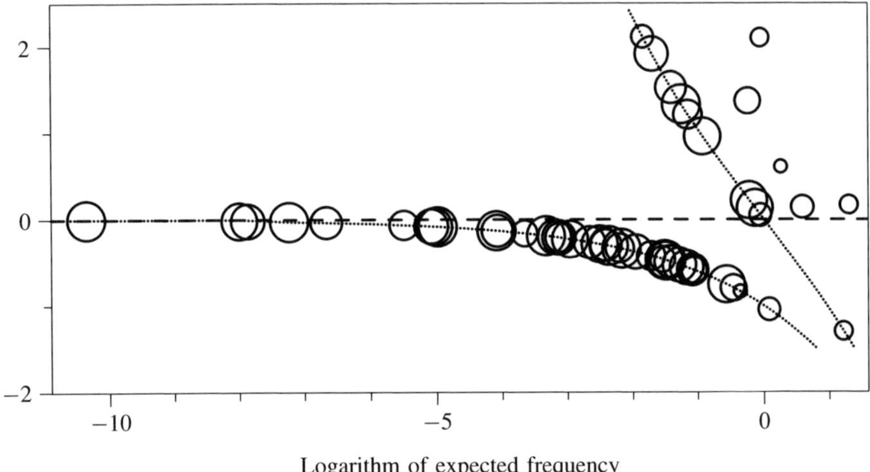

Figure 6.2 Bubble plot of the chi-squared residuals for the childhood cancer data plotted against log-fitted value for model (6.4). Bubble areas are proportional to the family sizes. Zero frequencies have residuals along the lower dotted line and frequencies equal to one have residuals along the upper dotted line.

line. Similarly, the several observed frequencies equal to one fall along the upper dotted line indicated in this figure.

Smaller sized families had greater expected frequencies because there were more small-sized families in the sample. The small bubbles corresponding to these small-sized families appear at the right side of the figure.

The statistical analysis of this data by Li *et al.* was to compare the incidence of cancer among sampled members of this dataset to the overall population. The conclusion that makes their work so remarkable is that the incidence of childhood cancer in these families is so much higher than that of the overall population. This comparison makes use of the ascertainment methods that are designed to estimate the incidence under this type of sampling. The relevant references are given in Section 6.2.2.

6.3.3 Childhood mortality in Brazil

The data of Table 6.3 summarizes a survey of deaths of children in northeast Brazil, as reported by Sastry (1997). The summary statistics for this data are given in Table 6.8. The huge value of $\chi^2 = 2362$ shows that the childhood death data of Table 6.3 does not follow the model (6.3) of homogeneous risk. The counts in this data are too large for us to obtain an exact p-value, but a simulation showed that the significance level must be smaller than 10^{-7}.

The lack of fit can be traced to several unusual frequencies that are indicated in Table 6.9. There are several observed frequencies that are much larger than

Table 6.8 Summary statistics for the Brazilian children dataset.

Sample size	Simulated p-value	Fitted model	χ^2	Deviance
$N = 2946$	$<10^{-7}$	Hypergeometric	2362	151.04
$m = 430$		Binomial	2300	152.10

Table 6.9 Unusually large frequencies in the Brazilian family data are given by + and counts much smaller than expected are denoted with a −.

			Number of affected siblings i							
n	f_n	m_n	0	1	2	3	4	5	6	7+
1	267	12	255	12−						
2	285	48	239	44−	2					
3	202	80	143	41	15	3				
4	110	54	69	30	9	2	0			
5	104	103	43	34	15	9+	3+	0		
6	50	67	15	18	8	5	3+	0	1+	
7	21	38	4	4	7	4	2+	0	0	0
8	12	28	1	2	4	3	1	1+	0	0
Totals	2946	430								

expected and two others that are too small. The large outliers, as is also the case in Table 6.1, correspond to those large families with many events. It is not clear whether children in large families are at greater risk or else parents who lose a child are more likely to have another.

There are also observed frequencies that are much smaller than expected in families with only one or two children. In such small families, the few children may receive better care, and this probably results in many fewer deaths than would be expected. As a result, the incidence of mortality appears to be correlated with the size of the family involved. There are methods for dependent family clusters given in Section 8.3 that provide a better summary for this dataset.

6.3.4 Household *T. cruzi* infections

The frequency data for this example appears in Table 6.4. In this example, the sampling unit is a household that might include unrelated individuals. Grimson (1993) argues whether to include the $f_1 = 1$ household of size 1. In our examination of the data, such observations contribute to the analysis.

There are several remarkable outliers in this data. Among the largest of these are the three single households of sizes five and six with five or more affected

Table 6.10 Summary statistics for the *T. cruzi* dataset.

Sample size	Simulated p-value	Fitted model	χ^2	Deviance
$N = 162$	7.5×10^{-4}	Hypergeometric	250.48	51.43
$m = 57$		Binomial	217.31	50.28

members. These three households contribute 174.9 or 80% to the value of the $\chi^2 = 217.3$ for the binomial model (Table 6.10). All of the expected counts are so small that the single household of size 13 must represent an outlier no matter how many affected members it has. The simulated significance level for this data is 7.5×10^{-4}, based on 10^7 replicated frequency tables.

The usual concept of degrees of freedom is not justified in this example. Families of size 13 could have $0, \ldots, 13$ affected members or 14 possible outcomes. Ordinarily, this would account for 13 df, allowing for us to lose 1 df by conditioning on the number of families of this size. In this data, however, there is only one family with 13 members and it seems unreasonable for this single observation to contribute 13 df.

The best analysis we can offer at present is to identify outliers in this data and simulate the significance level. A better approach is to compare nested models to the binomial and then evaluate the contribution of a small number of parameters. This approach is described in Section 7.4, in which the *T. cruzi* data is examined again.

6.4 Conclusions

In this chapter, we have described a general approach to the statistical examination of data summarizing frequencies of events that are recorded within family units. A variety of sampling methods are commonly employed in the collection of family data and may result in biases that have to be corrected. Data of this type is often collected and used to measure disease incidence. Our methods, in contrast, are useful to assess homogeneity of disease risk across families. The lack of homogeneity might be attributed to as yet unmeasured covariates. We can test homogeneity using exact or asymptotic (χ^2) methods and then identify positive or negative outlying frequencies in the observed data. Several methods for modeling the nonhomogeneous risk across families are given in the following chapter.

The separate concepts of incidence and clustering can be measured and are discussed in Section 6.1.3. The epidemiologist may be interested in whether the disease rate is greater among the sampled families as compared to the surrounding population. There are standard methods for performing this test. The methods described in this chapter are concerned with the test of homogeneity of risk among the sampled families. This homogeneity test would be used as a starting point in a search for possibly unmeasured environmental or genetic covariates.

This suggests that statistical modeling and testing should be performed in two stages: Firstly, to compare the sampled families to the overall population, and secondly, to see if there might be additional factors that might be useful in assessing the risk of disease. The methods of Section 8.3 describe a way to combine these separate tests into one model for the Brazilian childhood deaths summarized in Section 6.3.3 and Table 6.3.

All the models described in this chapter can be fitted in SAS. The SAS program is given in Section 8.9 for the childhood cancer data as an example. This program fits the hypergeometric and binomial models given at (6.4) and (6.5), respectively. The deviance and chi-squared goodness-of-fit statistics are computed in the GENMOD procedure. The expected frequencies are produced as well as the bubble plot of chi-squared normalized residuals given here in Fig. 6.2. The program is given in the following chapter because it also fits a number of models for disease clustering that are described in that chapter.

The program used to obtain the exact significance levels was written in FORTRAN. The source code is given in Section 6.6. This program implements the exact enumeration algorithm described in Section 6.2.1.

The additional appendix sections that follow provide the mathematical details of the family disease cluster distribution (6.3) and the other concepts described in this chapter. This distribution may be thought of as the null hypothesis of no disease clustering among the sampled families. The following two chapters discuss several possible alternative hypotheses of dependence in the disease status among sampled families.

6.5 Appendix: Mathematical Details

6.5.1 The distribution of family frequencies

The proof that the probability distribution given at (6.3) sums to one, subject to the constraints of (6.1) and (6.2), follows the same line of reasoning used in Section 1.7 to show that the probabilities of the hypergeometric distribution sum to one. The idea behind the proof, in the present case, is to identify the coefficients of z^m on both sides of the generating polynomial

$$\begin{aligned}(1+z)^N &= (1+z)^{f_1}\,(1+z)^{2f_2}\,\cdots\,(1+z)^{If_I}\\ &= (1+z)^{f_1}(1+2z+z^2)^{f_2}\,\cdots\,\left[(1+z)^I\right]^{f_I},\end{aligned} \tag{6.8}$$

where f_n are the number of families of size n ($i = 1, \ldots, I$) and $N = \sum nf_n$ is the total number of subjects in the sample.

The assumption of exchangeability of the N individuals in the study is the same as freely choosing the powers of z on both sides of equation (6.8). This polynomial identity is valid for all values of z. The coefficients of every power of z must agree on both sides of this identity. The coefficient of z^m on the left-hand side of (6.8) provides the normalizing denominator for distribution (6.3).

Identifying the coefficient on the right side of (6.8) is the same as summing over all valid outcomes in the family frequency distribution (6.3). This summation on the right side of (6.8) is the same task required to obtain the exact statistical significance level. In Section 6.2.1, a mathematical shortcut is introduced that greatly simplifies this computation.

Factorial moments of distribution (6.3) can be expressed as follows: for $r = 1, 2, \ldots$, define the factorial polynomial

$$z^{(r)} = z(z-1)\cdots(z-r+1)$$

and $z^{(0)} = 1$.

The (marginal) factorial moments of a single frequency X_{ni} in distribution (6.3) are

$$\mathrm{E}[\,X_{ni}^{(r)}\,] = \mathrm{E}[\,X_{ni}^{(r)} \mid N,\ m,\ f_n\,] = f_n^{(r)} \binom{n}{i}^r \binom{N-rn}{m-ri} \bigg/ \binom{N}{m} \tag{6.9}$$

for values of $n,\ i,\ r$ and parameters $(N,\ m,\ f_n)$ for which this expression is meaningful.

In particular, the expected value of X_{ni}

$$\mathrm{E}[\,X_{ni}\,] = f_n \binom{n}{i}\binom{N-n}{m-i} \bigg/ \binom{N}{m} = f_n \binom{m}{i}\binom{N-m}{n-i} \bigg/ \binom{N}{n}$$

is also given at (6.4).

The variance of X_{ni} is

$$\mathrm{Var}[\,X_{ni}\,] = f_n \binom{n}{i} \bigg/ \binom{N}{m}^2 \left\{ f_n \binom{n}{i} \left[\binom{N-2n}{m-2i}\binom{N}{m} - \binom{N-n}{m-i}^2 \right] \right.$$
$$\left. + \binom{N}{m} \left[\binom{N-n}{m-i} - \binom{n}{i}\binom{N-2n}{m-2i} \right] \right\}.$$

Multivariate, joint factorial moments of distribution (6.3) are given as follows. Let $\{r_{ni}\}$ denote a set of nonnegative integers and define

$$r_{n+} = \sum_i r_{ni}.$$

The joint factorial product moments of the frequencies $\boldsymbol{X} = \{X_{ni}\}$ are

$$\mathrm{E}\left[\prod_n \prod_i^n X_{ni}^{(r_{ni})}\right] = \prod_n \left[f_n^{(r_{n+})} \prod_i \binom{n}{i}^{r_{ni}} \right] \binom{N - \sum n r_{ni}}{m - \sum i r_{ni}} \bigg/ \binom{N}{m}$$

If only one r_{ni} is positive, then this expression reduces to the corresponding statement for a marginal frequency X_{ni} given at (6.9).

As an example of these joint moments, we have

$$\mathrm{E}[\,X_{n0}\,X_{n'0}\,] = f_n f_{n'} \binom{N-n-n'}{m} \Big/ \binom{N}{m}.$$

The covariance between the frequencies X_{n0} and $X_{n'0}$ of families of sizes $n \neq n'$ with no cases is then

$$\begin{aligned} &\mathrm{Cov}[\,X_{n0};\,X_{n'0}\,] \\ &= f_n\, f_{n'} \left[\binom{N-n-n'}{m}\binom{N}{m} - \binom{N-n}{m}\binom{N-n'}{m} \right] \Big/ \binom{N}{m}^2 . \end{aligned}$$

We can write

$$\begin{aligned} &\binom{N-n}{m}\binom{N-n'}{m} \Big/ \binom{N-n-n'}{m}\binom{N}{m} \\ &\qquad = \prod_{t=0}^{m-1} [(N-n-t)(N-n'-t)] \,/\, [(N-n-n'-t)(N-t)] \\ &\qquad = \prod_{t} [1 + nn'/(N-n-n'-t)(N-t)] \;>\; 1 \end{aligned}$$

to show that this covariance is negative.

6.5.2 A model for covariates

The generalization of (6.8) to account for covariates measured at the individual level is described here. Let $\boldsymbol{u}_k$ denote a vector of covariate values measured on the kth individual for $k = 1, \ldots, N$ and let δ_k denote a binary valued variable indicating their diseased status ($\delta_k = 1$) or not ($\delta_k = 0$). We then have $\sum \delta_k = m$ cases in the sample.

Suppose the relative risk of disease for the kth individual is expressible as

$$\theta_k = \exp(\boldsymbol{u}_k' \boldsymbol{\beta})$$

for regression coefficients $\boldsymbol{\beta}$ to be determined by maximizing the partial likelihood, described as follows.

The numerator of the partial likelihood for $\boldsymbol{\beta}$ is

$$\prod_{k}^{N} \{\theta_k(\boldsymbol{\beta})\}^{\delta_k}$$

and the denominator (by analogy to (6.8)) is the coefficient of z^m in the generating polynomial

$$\prod_k^N (1 + \theta_k z) \,.$$

This partial likelihood is identical to that of the model for proportional hazards regression in survival analysis. An algorithm to calculate this partial likelihood exactly is given by Gail, Lubin, and Rubinstein (1981). The analogy between (6.3) and survival analysis is that those individuals who are disease-free ($\delta = 0$) are considered censored and may develop the disease at some later date. Those who have the disease ($\delta = 1$) are treated as though they became diseased at the time of the survey.

6.5.3 Ascertainment sampling

The proof of the Proposition in Section 6.2.2 for the weighted ascertainment sampling uses a generating polynomial, as in (6.8). The unweighted generating polynomial for distribution (6.7) with all families of size i is $(1 + z)^i$. That is, distribution (6.7) is obtained by identifying the coefficient of z^{m_i} on both sides of the identity

$$\{(1+z)^n\}^{f_n} = \left\{1 + \binom{n}{1} z + \binom{n}{2} z^2 + \cdots z^n\right\}^{f_n} .$$

The generating polynomial in which the probability of ascertainment is proportional to the number of affected individuals is then

$$\sum_i i \binom{n}{i} z^i .$$

This polynomial can also be written as

$$\sum_{i=0}^{n} i \binom{n}{i} z^i = nz(1+z)^{n-1} .$$

The polynomial on the right-hand side corresponds to removing the proband and yields the same distribution as in (6.7) for a family of size $n - 1$. In other words, the weighted distribution of cluster frequencies X_{ni} is the same as that of the unweighted distribution of $X_{n-1\,i-1}$ after omitting the proband. An example of this property in practice is the analysis of the data in Table 6.2 in which all probands have been removed.

6.6 Program for Exact Test of Homogeneity

The family frequency models given in (6.4) and (6.5) can be fitted using the GENMOD procedure in SAS. The bubble plot of Fig. 6.2 was produced using the

GPLOT procedure. The program in Section 8.9 fits these models to the childhood cancer data of Table 6.2. The program to fit these models is not given here, but rather, at the end of the following chapter because it also fits a number of models for several alternative hypotheses of disease clustering that are developed in that chapter.

The FORTRAN program given here provides an exact p-value for the test of significance of the null hypothesis model of no disease clustering. The algorithm implemented in this program is described in Section 6.2.1.

```
!       Exact test of disease clustering for family members

      implicit none
      double precision zero,const,thisp,dexp,p,stat(20)
      integer maxfac,n(50),m(20),k,sib,aff,freq,oldsib,i,ns,
     &   minsize,naff,nsibs,nfam,jcases,fm(20,20),j,maxsize
      logical done
      double precision fac(8000),fac0(8001)  ! factorial table
      equivalence (fac(1),fac0(2))     ! define zero subscript
      common/factab/fac0
      data maxfac/8000/, zero/0.000d0/, fm/400*0/

!          build table of log factorials with a zero subscript
      fac0(1)=zero                     ! log of zero factorial
      do 10 j=1,maxfac
         const=j           ! convert integer to double precision
         fac(j)=fac(j-1)+ dlog(const)        ! add to previous
   10 continue

!       read frequency data, build frequency matrix table -fm-
      open(10,file='family.dat')                  ! input file
      write(6,1001)                           ! print headings
      oldsib=-1         ! group family sizes together in output
      maxsize=1                    ! find largest sized family
      do 20 j=1,10000000                        ! read forever
        read(10,*,end=40,err=30)sib,aff,freq     ! list format
      if(sib .GT. 20)go to 30
      if(aff .GT. 19)go to 30
        fm(aff+1,sib)=freq          ! build frequency table
        if(sib .GT. maxsize)maxsize=sib  ! largest family size
        if(sib .NE. oldsib)write(6,*)            ! skip a line
        oldsib=sib
        write(6,1000)sib,aff,freq      ! echo the data read in
   20 continue
   30 if(j.EQ. j)then                ! input error processing
         write(6,1003)sib,aff,freq              ! print message
         stop 9876                                 ! terminate
      endif
   40 write(6,1000)                        ! done reading data
```

```
!                                Find marginal totals from fm
      call build(fm,m,1,maxsize,nfam,nsibs,naff,const)
!                           Probability of the observed table
      call prob(fm,1,maxsize,const,p)
      write(6,1002)p
!         Generate test statistics, expected values under null
      call test(fm,m,1,maxsize,stat,ns,naff,nsibs,.true.)
!            Enumerate all possible tables for exact tail area
      call enum(nsibs,naff,nfam,m,maxsize,stat,const,p)

      stop 9999
1000  format(5x,3i15)
1001  format(17x,'Family frequency data read in:'/
     &  t18,'Sibs       Affected       Frequency  ')
1002  format(t14,'Probability of this table:  ',e15.7)
1003  format(///' INVALID DATA:',3i10/' Terminating ')
      end

!-------------------------------------------------------------

      subroutine enum(nsibs,naff,nfam,m,maxsize,refstat,
     &    const,p0)

!      Enumerate all possible outcomes consistent with margins

      implicit none
      logical done(20),alldone
      double precision stat(20),refstat(20),p,ptail,const,
     &  psum,p0,dsqrt,one,dabs,zero,dcase,pasum,proba
      integer freq(20,20),m(20),maxsize,level,j,naff,nsibs,
     &  nfam,lnfam,lnsibs,lnaff,lm(20),alloc(20),per,mod,
     &  ncase,rem(20)
      data one/1.00d0/, zero/0.00d0/
      data per/1000000/  ! how often output tables are printed

!         OUTER LOOP: allocate cases to various sized families
      alldone=.true.
      psum=zero
      pasum=zero
      ncase=0
      dcase=zero
   10 call cmulte(alloc,naff,maxsize,alldone) ! allocate cases
      if(alldone .OR.
     &      (alloc(maxsize) .GT. maxsize*m(maxsize)))then
         write(6,1002)p0,psum,ptail,dcase      ! final message
         return                                     ! all done
      endif
!         alloc(i) cases in families of size i: Is this valid?
      do 20 j=1,maxsize
         if(alloc(j) .GT. j*m(j))go to 10  ! is count too big?
```

```
  20 continue                 ! find hypergeometric probability
     call pralloc(alloc,m,maxsize,naff,nsibs,proba)
     pasum=pasum+proba
!                Shortcut: If proba < p0 then skip inner loop
     if(proba .LE. p0)then
        psum=psum+proba          ! accumulate total probability
        ptail=ptail+proba      ! accumulate probability in tail
        go to 10              ! go back to skip past inner loop
     endif

! INNER LOOP: generate family frequencies with these
! allocations of cases to families of various sizes
     level=maxsize
  40 done(level)=.true.
  50 call cfe(m(level),alloc(level),level,
    &   freq(1,level),done(level))
!                     go up one level when done at this level
  60 if(.NOT. done(level))go to 70! if not done at this level
     if(level .GE. maxsize)go to 10    ! return to outer loop
     level=level+1                           ! go to next level
     go to 50          ! and go to the start of the inner loop
  70 level=level-1                         ! down to next level
     if(level .GE. 1)go to 40        ! go to top of inner loop
     ncase=ncase+1   ! number of cases evaluated (in integer)
     dcase=dcase+one    ! number of cases in double precision
     call prob(freq,1,maxsize,const,p)      ! find probability
     psum=psum+p                   ! accumulate total probability
     if(p .LE. p0)ptail=ptail+p        ! accumulate tail area
                               ! periodically print out tables
     if(mod(ncase,per).EQ.0)then
        write(6,1001)ncase,(alloc(j),j=1,maxsize)
        call out(freq,m,nsibs,naff,nfam,1,maxsize)
        write(6,1002)p,psum,ptail,dcase
     endif
     level=1                              ! continue inner loop
     go to 50                        ! go to top of inner loop

1001 format(/' ENUM:ncase: ',i14,' alloc: ',15i3)
1002 format(/' Prob of this table:',e16.8,
    &   4x, ' Cumulative prob: ',e16.8, /
    &        ' Tail probability:  ',e16.8,
    &   4x, ' Case number:     ',e16.8)
     end

!------------------------------------------------------------

     subroutine test(fm,m,first,last,stat,ns,
    &    naff,nsibs,trace)

!    Compute test statistics for the set of family
```

```
!      frequencies in -fm-. If -trace- then print them out

      implicit none
      double precision fac(8000),fac0(8001)
      equivalence (fac(1),fac0(2))
      common/factab/fac0
      integer first,last,m(1),fm(20,20),naff,nsibs,ns,j,i,
     & ia,ib,ic,nssave
      double precision stat(1),zero,one,two,dexp,dlog,be,
     & binp,sbe,he,she,fmij,dble,eps,chi1,chi2,dsqrt
      logical trace
      data zero/0.0d0/, one/1.0d0/, two/2.0d0/, eps/1.0d-9/
      data nssave/5/

      if(trace)write(6,1000)                        ! print heading
      ns=nssave
      do 10 j=1,ns
         stat(j)=zero                  ! initialize test statistics
   10 continue
      binp=dble(naff)/dble(nsibs)                   ! binomial p MLE
!         be=binomial expectation
!        he=hypergeometric expectation
      write(6,1001)
      do 100 j=first,last
         if(m(j) .LE. 0)go to 100
         sbe=zero
         she=zero
         do 80 i=1,j+1
            ia=i-1
            be=dexp(fac(j)-fac(ia)-fac(j-ia))*m(j)
            he=be
            if(ia .GT. 0)be=be*binp**ia
            if(ia .LT. j)be=be*(one-binp)**(j-ia)
            do 30 ib=1,j
               ic=ib-1
               he=he/(nsibs-ic)
               if(ic .LT. ia)then
                  he=he*(naff-ic)
               else
                  he=he*(nsibs-naff+ib-j)
               endif
   30       continue
            fmij=dble(fm(i,j))
!                                          two chi-squared residuals
            chi1=zero
            chi2=zero
            if(be .GT. eps)chi1=(fmij-be)/dsqrt(be)
            if(he .GT. eps)chi2=(fmij-he)/dsqrt(he)
            if(trace)write(6,1001)j,ia,fm(i,j),be,he,chi1,chi2
            sbe=sbe+be
```

```
            she=she+he
!                                   test statistics:  deviance
            if(fmij .GT. eps)then
               if(be .GT. eps)
     &            stat(1)=stat(1)+fmij*dlog(fmij/be)
               if(he .GT. eps)
     &            stat(2)=stat(2)+fmij*dlog(fmij/he)
            endif
                                         ! Pearson chi-squared
            if(be .GT. eps)stat(3)=stat(3)+(fmij-be)**2/be
            if(he .GT. eps)stat(4)=stat(4)+(fmij-he)**2/he
                                        ! exact log-likelihood
            stat(ns)=stat(ns)+fmij*(fac(ia)+fac(j-ia))
   80    continue
         if(trace)write(6,1002)m(j),sbe,she
         if(trace)write(6,1001)
  100 continue
      stat(1)=stat(1)*two
      stat(2)=stat(2)*two
      if(trace)write(6,1003)(stat(j),j=1,ns)
      return

1000 format(/t20,'Test Statistics for Family Clusters',
    &  //,t31,'Obs''d',t42,'Expectations:',4x,
    &    'Chi Residuals',/
    &  t14,'# sibs   # aff    freq     Bin.        Hyp.',
    &  '    Bin.    Hyp.')
1001 format(7x,3i9,2f11.5,2f8.2)
1002 format(t14,'Totals:',t26,i9,2f11.5)
1003 format(t14,'Deviance:',     t35,2f11.5,/,
    &       t14,'Chi-squared:',  t35,2f11.5,/,
    &       t14,'Log-likelihood',t35,f11.5)
      end

!---------------------------------------------------------------

      subroutine build(fm,m,first,last,nfam,nsibs,naff,const)

!     Find marginal totals from -fm- and build the constant
!     part of the likelihood

!    fm(i,j)= # of families with j sibs,
!                   (i-1) of whom are affected
!    m(j)   = # of families with j sibs
!    nfam   = # number of families
!    nsibs  = # of siblings
!    naff   = # of affected sibs
!    const  = constant part of the log-likelihood

      implicit none
```

```
      integer fm(20,20),naff,nfams,nsibs,first,last,i,j,
     &    m(20),fmij,nfam
      double precision const,zero
      double precision fac(8000),fac0(8001)
      equivalence (fac(1),fac0(2))
      common/factab/fac0
      data zero/0.0000d0/

      nfam=0
      nsibs=0
      naff=0
      const=zero
      do 20 j=first,last
         m(j)=0
         do 10 i=1,j+1
            fmij=fm(i,j)
            naff=naff+(i-1)*fmij                ! number of cases
            m(j)=m(j)+fmij          ! # of families of this size
 10      continue
         const=const+fac(j)*m(j)+fac(m(j))
         nfam=nfam+m(j)                     ! total # of families
         nsibs=nsibs+j*m(j)                 ! total # of siblings
 20   continue
      const=const-fac(nsibs)
      const=const+fac(naff)+fac(nsibs-naff)
      return
      end

!------------------------------------------------------------

      subroutine prob(fm,first,last,const,p)

!    Evaluate the probability of the table -fm-

      implicit none
      integer fm(20,20),first,last,i,j,jj,nsibs,jp,max0
      double precision zero,const,p,dexp,lminf,slf
      double precision fac(8000),fac0(8001)
      equivalence (fac(1),fac0(2))
      common/factab/fac0
      data zero/0.00d0/
      data lminf/-708.75d0/  ! log of smallest positive d.p. #

      slf=const                ! constant part of the likelihood
      do 20 j=first,last
         do 10 i=1,j+1                    ! sums of log factorials
            slf=slf - (fac(i-1)+fac(j-i+1))*fm(i,j)
            slf=slf - fac(fm(i,j))
 10      continue
 20   continue
```

```
!     Is the probability positive or zero in double precision?
      p=zero
      if(slf .GT. lminf)p=dexp(slf)
      return
      end

!-------------------------------------------------------------------

      subroutine out(freq,m,nsibs,naff,nfam,first,last)

! Print a table of frequencies and check it for
! inconsistencies in the marginal sums or other errors

      implicit none
      logical error
      integer freq(20,20),m(20),nsibs,naff,nfam,i,j,
     &    first,last,csibs,cfam,caff,cm(20)

      csibs=0
      cfam=0
      caff=0
      error=.FALSE.
      write(6,1001)nsibs,naff,nfam
      error = error .OR. (nsibs .LT. 0)
      error = error .OR. (naff .LT. 0)
      error = error .OR. (nfam .LT. 0)
      do 30 j=first,last
         cm(j)=0
         write(6,1006)m(j),(freq(i,j),i=1,j+1)
         error = error .OR. (m(j) .LT. 0)
         do 20 i=1,j+1
            cfam=cfam+freq(i,j)
            cm(j)=cm(j)+freq(i,j)
            caff=caff+(i-1)*freq(i,j)
            error=error .OR. (freq(i,j) .LT. 0)! negative freq
   20    continue
   30 continue
!                                 Check for inconsistencies, errors
      if(error)go to 900
      if(caff .NE. naff)go to 900
      if(cfam .NE. nfam)go to 900
      do 50 j=first,last
         if(cm(j) .NE. m(j))go to 900
   50 continue
      return
!                                                   ERROR processing
  900 write(6,1000)
      write(6,1001)csibs,caff,cfam
      write(6,1006)(cm(j),j=first,last)
      stop 8888
```

```
1000 format(' OUT: error detected',3i5)
1001 format(/1x,i5,' sibs',i8,' affected',i8,' families')
1006 format(1x,20i4)
     end

!-----------------------------------------------------------

      subroutine cfe(n,m,i,x,done)

!   Enumerate all possible cluster frequencies for n families
!   all of size i with m infected individuals.  x(j) is the
!   number of families with j-1 infected individuals.
!   Done signifies the start and end of the sequence.

     implicit none
     logical done
     integer x(1),m,n,i,j,k,sn,sm,ip1

     ip1=i+1                                ! index: i plus one
!                        test for valid input parameter values
     if(i .LT. 1)stop 440
     if(m .LT. 0)stop 441
     if(m .GT. i*n)stop 442
!      Special case in which only one outcome is possible: m=i*n
     if(m .EQ. i*n)then
        done=.NOT. done
        do 10 j=1,i
  10    x(j)=0
        x(ip1)=n                  ! all individuals are affected
        return
     endif
!                                          Special case: n=0 or 1
     if(n .LE. 1)then
        done=.NOT. done
        do 20 j=1,ip1
  20    x(j)=0
        if(m .GT. i)stop 443
        x(m+1)=n
        return
     endif
!                               Special cases:  m=0 or 1; or i=1
     if(i .EQ. 1 .OR. m .LE. 1)then
        done=.NOT. done
        do 30 j=1,ip1
  30    x(j)=0
        x(1)=n-m
        x(2)=m
        return
     endif
```

```
      if(done)then                   ! Initialize the general case
         j=m/n                                      ! integer divide
         j=j+1                                           ! plus one
         if(j .GT. i)stop 444            ! Error: m is too large
         do 40 k=1,ip1
 40      x(k)=0
         x(j+1)=m-(j-1)*n  ! two smallest possible frequencies
         x(j)=j*n-m
         done=.FALSE.
         return
      endif
!                   otherwise update existing frequencies in x
 50   j=3
 60   x(j)=x(j)+1                               ! increase odometer
      sn=n               ! How many frequencies are already used?
      sm=m
      do 70 k=3,ip1
         sn=sn-x(k)              ! number of families left to us
         sm=sm-(k-1)*x(k)           ! number of cases left to us
 70   continue
!                 Are a valid number of frequencies available?
      if((0 .LE. sm) .AND. (sm .LE. sn))then
         x(2)=sm      ! two smallest frequencies are determined
         x(1)=sn-sm
         return
      endif
      if((0 .LE. sn) .AND. (sn .LT. sm))go to 50
      x(j)=0                                ! reset odometer column
      j=j+1                       ! go to next column of odometer
      if(j .LE. ip1)go to 60
      done=.TRUE.                    ! when we run out of columns
      return
      end

!------------------------------------------------------------

      subroutine pralloc(alloc,m,maxsize,naff,nsibs,proba)

!  Multivariate hypergeometric probability of an
!  allocation -alloc-  of cases

      implicit none
      integer m(1),alloc(1),maxsize,naff,nsibs,i,j
      double precision proba,dexp,lminf
      double precision fac(8000),fac0(8001)
      equivalence (fac(1),fac0(2))
      common/factab/fac0
!           log of smallest positive double precision number
      data lminf/-708.75d0/
```

```
      proba=fac(naff)+fac(nsibs-naff)-fac(nsibs)
      do 10 j=1,maxsize
         proba=proba+fac(j*m(j))
         proba=proba-fac(alloc(j))
         proba=proba-fac(j*m(j)-alloc(j))
   10 continue
      if(proba .LT. lminf)proba=lminf
      proba=dexp(proba)
      return
      end

!-----------------------------------------------------------

      subroutine cmulte(n,m,k,done)

!  On successive calls, generate the complete multinomial
!  outcomes in k categories with sample size m into
!  vector n(). DONE signifies completion of the task or
!  initialization on input.

      implicit none
      integer i,j,k,m,n(1),sum
      logical done

      if(k .EQ. 1)then          ! special case for one category
         n(1)=m
         done=.not.done
         return
      endif
      if(m .EQ. 0)then         ! special case: zero sample size
         done=.NOT. done
         do 10 j=1,k
   10    n(j)=0
         return
      endif
      if(done)go to 500                  ! is this an initial call?
      j=2                              ! initial category to update
  100 n(j)=n(j)+1        ! generate next vector in the sequence
      sum=0                               ! find the cumulative sum
      do 200 i=j,k
  200 sum=sum+n(i)
      if(sum .GT. m)go to 300              ! is anything left over?
      n(1)=m-sum                  ! n(1) is what ever is left over
      return
  300 n(j)=0                                   ! clear this column
      j=j+1                         ! carry over to the next column
      if(j .LE. k)go to 100                 ! run out of columns?
      done=.TRUE.                    ! done when we run off the end
      return
```

```
500 do 600 i=2,k      ! initialize on the first call to cmulte
600 n(I)=0
    n(1)=m                  ! all counts in the first category
    done=.FALSE.    ! set flag to signify unfinished sequence
    return
    end
```

7

Sums of Dependent Bernoulli's and Disease Clusters

This chapter develops discrete distributions that describe the behavior of a sum of dependent Bernoulli random variables. These distributions are motivated by the manner in which multiple individuals with a disease appear to cluster within the same family. This chapter builds models that represent possible alternative hypotheses to those models of Chapter 6.

Chapter 6 develops a method to test the null hypothesis that diseased cases appear in various sized families, independently of the health status of other family members. This null hypothesis is that every member of every family has the same risk of disease. In this present chapter, we explore several different methods for modeling the dependence of disease status among members of the same family. These models describe the behavior of sums of dependent Bernoulli random variables. In Chapter 9, we apply these methods to the problem of modeling birth defects in litters of laboratory animals in teratology experiments.

7.1 Introduction

Much is known about the behavior of the binomial distributed sum of independent Bernoulli random variables. Considerably less has been written about the distribution in which there is dependence among the binary valued Bernoulli indicators. In this chapter, we develop several models for sums of Bernoulli counts that are not independent.

The data in Table 7.1 is given by Liang *et al.* (1992). This table summarizes the frequencies of $m = 60$ individuals with IPF among the $N = 203$ children in 100 families. This example is discussed in greater detail in Section 6.3.1. The

Discrete Distributions Daniel Zelterman
 ISBN: 0-470-86888-0 (PPC)

Table 7.1 Frequencies $\{X_{ni}\}$ of $m = 60$ cases of IPF in 100 families. Source: Liang *et al.* (1992).

Number of siblings	Number of families	Number of cases	Number of affected siblings i						
n	f_n	m_n	0	1	2	3	4	5	6
1	48	12	36	12					
2	23	9	15	7	1				
3	17	19	5	7	3	2			
4	7	5	3	3	1	0	0		
6	5	15	1	0	1	1	1	0	1
Totals	100	60							

frequencies in Table 7.1 describe the distribution of IPF cases within the 100 families.

In each row of this table, there are f_n families of size n ($n = 1, \ldots, 6$). The number of cases in each row is m_n and there is a total of $\sum m_n = m = 60$ cases in the whole dataset. The statistical analysis of this data in Chapter 6 conditions on the number of cases m but not the individual number of cases m_n in families of size n.

Each of the individuals in every family can be described by Bernoulli distributed indicators of their IPF status. A genetic or environmental component of IPF may induce dependence among members of the same family. Models of such dependence with covariate effects are described in Chapter 9.

Chapter 6 develops a model of the expected frequencies for family data such as that in Table 7.1. The assumption in Chapter 6 is that all family members in families of all sizes have the same disease risk. The frequency X_{ni} is the number of families of size n with i affected members. The (marginal) expected value of each frequency X_{ni} given in (6.3) is

$$\mathrm{E}[\,X_{ni}\,] = f_n \binom{n}{i}\binom{N-n}{m-i} \Big/ \binom{N}{m} = f_n \binom{m}{i}\binom{N-m}{n-i} \Big/ \binom{N}{n} \tag{7.1}$$

for inequalities $i \leq m \leq N$ and $i \leq n \leq N$ for which the various binomial coefficients are defined.

Model (7.1) specifies that the frequencies in any one row are proportional to the probabilities of a hypergeometric distribution. A binomial distribution for the frequencies of families of size n in Table 7.1 can be fitted with expected counts

$$\mathrm{E}[\,X_{ni}\,] = f_n \binom{n}{i} p^i\,(1-p)^{n-i} \tag{7.2}$$

and is also given in (6.5).

The expected frequencies in (7.2) are the product of the binomial (n, p) probability distribution and f_n, the number of families of size n. If we estimate p in (7.2) by 60/203=.296, then the Pearson $\chi^2 = 312.3$ (15 df) indicates a poor fit for the IPF data in Table 7.1. An exact test of significance for the model of independence of disease occurrences summarized in Table 6.6 obtains a p-value of .00883 for this table. This lack of fit is indicative of dependence among individuals within the same family.

Our development in this chapter of models for disease clustering within families is based on the distribution of the sum of dependent Bernoulli random variables. The family frequency and binomial models given in (7.1) and (7.2) respectively, are useful in describing the counts in Table 7.1 under the null hypothesis model of homogeneous risk and independence of disease state among family members.

Let us introduce some notation. For each $n = 1, 2, \ldots,$ define

$$Y_n = Z_{n1} + \cdots + Z_{nn},$$

where the Z_{ni} are Bernoulli random variables for $i = 1, \ldots, n$.

The Z_{ni} are indicator variates of the disease status of each of the individuals in a family of size n ($n = 1, 2, \ldots$). In the remainder of the discussion, the first 'n' subscript will be omitted but understood on the Z_{ni}. Each Z_i equals one if the ith family member is a diseased case and Z_i is zero if this member is otherwise healthy. The random variable Y_n counts the number of diseased cases in the family of size n. In this chapter, we do not make the assumption that the Z_i are independent nor do we assume that they are identically distributed unless specifically stated.

Different models are developed in this chapter to describe possible alternative hypotheses of dependence among the Z_i. These models specify that the expected counts in each row of Table 7.1 are equal to f_n times the probability distribution of the sum Y_n of dependent Bernoulli random variables. That is,

$$\mathrm{E}[\, X_{ni} \,] = f_n \Pr[\, Y_n = i].$$

Johnson *et al.* (1992, pp 148–150) describe only a small number of models for the distribution of Y_n for dependent Z_i. Among these, Altham (1978) derives the model

$$\Pr[\, Y_n = i \,] \propto \binom{n}{i} p^i (1-p)^{n-i} \exp[-i(n-i)\theta] \qquad (7.3)$$

for parameters $\theta > 0$ and $0 < p < 1$.

The parameter $\theta < 0$ models a negative association and $\theta > 0$ indicates a positive association between the disease status of exchangeable family members $Z_1, \ldots, Z_n$. The binomial model (7.2) is obtained in (7.3) for $\theta = 0$. Properties of the Altham distribution is discussed in Section 8.2.

Section 7.2 develops a class of models for $\Pr[Y_n]$, for which the conditional distribution of family members' disease status is dependent on the data from previously assessed members. Section 7.2.1 provides general recurrence relations for probabilities and moments of these distributions. Section 7.2.2 describes a model based on the medical usage of the term 'family history.' Section 7.2.3 describes another useful model that has a very good fit to the IPF data of Table 7.1.

Other models for $\Pr[Y_n]$ with a finite number of exchangeable Z_i are described in Section 7.3. Exchangeability is a property that models equivalence of all family members. The important features of this property are discussed in that section. Section 7.4 compares all of the models developed in this chapter using several real data examples that are also examined in the previous chapter.

A different class of models for dependent counts is developed in Chapter 8 that is analogous to the functional form of the Altham model (7.3). These weighted models are less rigorous in their mathematical development but are intuitive and can easily be fit to data using standard software. Chapter 9 also models data on family units that include covariate values and applies these methods to the analysis of teratology experiments.

7.2 Conditional Models

Models for the distribution of the number of affected family members Y_n are developed in this section and assume that the Bernoulli indicators of individual disease status Z_i are dependent. Specifically, we assume that the conditional probability of disease in any one additional individual, given the status of other assessed members of the same family, is only a function of the number of those family members who are already known to be affected.

Symbolically, we can write this as

$$\Pr[\, Z_{n+1} = 1 \mid Z_1, \ldots, Z_n \,] = \Pr[\, Z_{n+1} = 1 \mid Z_1 + \cdots + Z_n \,]. \qquad (7.4)$$

The assumption in (7.4) is the basis for the models developed in Sections 7.2.1 through 7.2.4. We need to model the dependence of disease status in multiple individuals in the same family. Different expressions for the conditional probability in (7.4) are used to develop models for this dependence.

Model (7.4) has a useful interpretation when the sampling mechanism represents a sequential screening of family members. One family member may want to have a mammogram, for example, after a sister is diagnosed with breast cancer. Klaren *et al.* 2003 reports that women with a first degree relative diagnosed with ovarian cancer are more likely than the overall population to be screened for the BRCA1 and BRCA2 breast-cancer markers. We will not address whether the rate of screening is related to the perceived risk. Such biases are discussed by Miller (1993), for example. In this chapter, we develop methods that can be used to model the risk of cancer in one sister following its discovery in another.

7.2.1 General results for conditional models

For $i = 0, 1, \ldots, n$, denote the conditional probability

$$C_n(i) \;=\; \Pr[\, Z_{n+1} = 1 \mid Z_1 + \cdots + Z_n = i\,] \;=\; \Pr[\, Z_{n+1} = 1 \mid Y_n = i\,]$$

of disease in an additional individual, given the status of n previously assessed members of his or her family. We also define $C_0 = C_0(0) = \Pr[\, Z_1 = 1\,]$.

For general probabilities C_n, the indicators $\{Z_i\}$ are not identically distributed and hence not exchangeable. This point is illustrated at (7.7), below. Exchangeability is defined and discussed in Section 7.3.

If $C_n(i)$ is a constant probability (i.e., $C_n(i) = p$ for all n and i), then the Z_i are independent Bernoulli random variables and Y_n has a binomial (n, p) distribution.

In this section, we describe models for the distribution of Y_n

$$\Pr[\, Y_n = i\,] = \Pr[\, Z_1 + \cdots + Z_n \; = \; i\,]$$

for $i = 0, 1, \ldots, n$.

A useful recursive relation for $\Pr[Y_n]$ is

$$\begin{aligned}\Pr[\, Y_{n+1} = i + 1\,] &= \Pr[\, Z_{n+1} \; = 1 \mid Y_n = i\,] \; \Pr[\, Y_n = i\,] \\ &\quad + \Pr[\, Z_{n+1} \; = 0 \mid Y_n = i + 1\,] \; \Pr[\, Y_n = i + 1]. \qquad (7.5)\end{aligned}$$

Several probability models of Y_n developed in this section are based on this relation. Specific examples are given in Sections 7.2.2 through 7.2.4 of this chapter.

In settings in which C_n has a suitable form (as in Sections 7.2.3 and 7.2.4), it may be useful to apply (7.5) repeatedly to show

$$\Pr[\, Y_{n+1} = n + 1\,] = C_n(n) \Pr[\, Y_n = n\,] = \cdots = \prod_{i=0}^{n} C_i(i) \qquad (7.6)$$

and similarly,

$$\Pr[\, Y_{n+1} \; = 0\,] = \prod_{i=0}^{n} (1 - C_i(0)).$$

Expressions for (7.6) are also useful for describing models of sums of exchangeable $Z_1, \ldots, Z_n$. These are discussed in Section 7.3.

In situations (such as in Section 7.2.2) in which $C_n(i)$ is not a function of n, that is, $C_n(i) = C(i)$, $\Pr[Y_n = i]$ can be written as

$$\Pr[\, Y_n = i\,] = \left\{ \prod_{k=0}^{i-1} C(k) \right\} \left\{ \sum_{\boldsymbol{X}} \prod_{k=0}^{i} (1 - C(k))^{x_k} \right\},$$

where

$$\boldsymbol{X} = \boldsymbol{X}_n(i) = \{x_k = 0, 1, \ldots; \;\; k = 0, 1, \ldots, i; \;\; \sum_k x_k = n - i\}.$$

The marginal distribution of each Z_i $(i = 1, 2, \ldots)$ can be expressed as

$$\Pr[\, Z_i = 1\,] = \sum_{j=0}^{i-1} \Pr[\, Z_i = 1 \mid Y_{i-1} = j\,] \Pr[\, Y_{i-1} = j\,]. \qquad (7.7)$$

In (7.7), we see that in general, $\Pr[Z_i = 1]$ is not equal to $\Pr[Z_{i'} = 1]$ for $i \neq i'$. This demonstrates that the Bernoulli indicators $\{Z_i\}$ are not necessarily exchangeable.

The joint distribution of the Bernoulli indicators $\{Z_i\}$ does not have simple expressions in general. Two examples that illustrate this are

$$\Pr[\, Z_{i+1} = Z_i = 1\,] = \sum_{j=0}^{i-1} \Pr[\, Z_{i+1} = Z_i = 1 \mid Y_{i-1} = j\,]\ \Pr[\, Y_{i-1} = j\,]$$

and similarly,

$$\Pr[\, Z_{i+2} = Z_i = 1\,] = \sum_{j=0}^{i-1} \{C_{i+1}(j+2)\, C_i(j+1) \\ + C_{i+1}(j+1)\,[1 - C_i(j+1)]\}C_{i-1}(j)\ \Pr[Y_{i-1} = j].$$

Recursive expressions for the factorial moments of these conditional distributions can be derived from (7.5). For each $r = 1, 2, \ldots,$

$$\begin{aligned} \mathrm{E}[\, Y_{n+1}^{(r)}\,] &= \sum_{i=0}^{n+1} i^{(r)}\ \Pr[\, Y_{n+1} = i\,] \\ &= \sum_i i^{(r)}\,\{C_n(i-1)\ \Pr[\, Y_n = i-1\,] + (1 - C_n(i))\ \Pr[\, Y_n = i\,]\} \\ &= \mathrm{E}[\, Y_n^{(r)}\,] + \sum_i i^{(r)}\,\{\, C_n(i-1)\ \Pr[Y_n = i-1\,] \\ &\qquad - C_n(i)\ \Pr[\, Y_n = i\,]\}. \end{aligned}$$

This last summation can be rewritten giving

$$\mathrm{E}[\, Y_{n+1}^{(r)}\,] \;=\; \mathrm{E}[\, Y_n^{(r)}\,] + \sum_{i=0}^{n} [(i+1)^{(r)} - i^{(r)}]\, C_n(i)\ \Pr[\, Y_n = i\,].$$

Since

$$(i+1)^{(r)} - i^{(r)} = r\, i^{(r-1)},$$

we have

$$\mathrm{E}[\, Y_{n+1}^{(r)}\,] = \mathrm{E}[\, Y_n^{(r)}\,] + r \sum_i i^{(r-1)}\, C_n(i)\ \Pr[\, Y_n = i\,]. \tag{7.8}$$

In particular, the expected value of Y_n can be expressed using either (7.7) or (7.8) to show

$$\mathrm{E}[\, Y_{n+1}\,] \;=\; \mathrm{E}[\, Y_n\,] + \Pr[\, Z_{n+1} = 1\,] \;=\; \mathrm{E}[\, Y_n\,] + \sum_i C_n(i)\ \Pr[\, Y_n = i\,].$$

We can also use (7.8) to show that the variance of Y_n follows

$$\mathrm{Var}[\,Y_{n+1}\,] = \mathrm{Var}[\,Y_n\,] + \mathrm{Var}[\,Z_{n+1}\,] + 2\mathrm{Cov}\,[\,Y_n,\ Z_{n+1}\,],$$

where

$$\mathrm{Cov}\,[\,Y_n,\ Z_{n+1}\,] = \sum_i i\,C_n(i)\,\Pr[\,Y_n = i\,] \ - \ \mathrm{E}[\,Y_n\,]\,\mathrm{E}[\,Z_{n+1}\,].$$

The moment generating function M_n of Y_n is defined by

$$M_n(t) = \mathrm{E}\,[\,\exp\,(tY_n)\,]$$

and follows the recursive relation

$$M_{n+1}(t) = M_n(t) + \sum_i \mathrm{e}^{it}\,(\mathrm{e}^t - 1)\,C_n(i)\,\Pr[\,Y_n = i\,].$$

Sections 7.2.2 through 7.2.4 of this chapter examine specific examples of the general methods derived in this section.

7.2.2 Family history model

Specific models can be derived from the recursive relation given in (7.5). For the first of these models, suppose for probability parameters p and p' we specify the conditional probability C_n as

$$C_n(i) = \begin{cases} p' & \text{for } i = 0 \\ p & \text{for } i = 1, \ldots, n \end{cases} \tag{7.9}$$

In words, the conditional probability of one affected family member is p' if no other members are known to be affected. If there is already at least one known case in the family, then p is the conditional probability that an additional member is affected. If $p = p'$, then the Bernoulli counts Z_i are independent and their sum Y_n has a binomial (n, p) distribution.

For the model of a highly contagious disease such as influenza, $p' < p$. That is, once one child contracts the flu, the others are more likely to get it as well. In polio, however, exposure to the virus at an early age can have a preventative effect so we may have $p' > p$.

Model (7.9) is consistent with the medical usage labeling an individual as having a *family history* for the disease. Specifically, when a doctor asks a patient if he or she has a family history of some condition, this is another way of asking if there is at least one family member who has it.

The family history distribution of Y_n follows (7.5) and its mass function can be written as

$$\Pr[\, Y_n = i\,] = \begin{cases} (1-p')^n & \text{for } i = 0 \\ p'\, p^{i-1} \displaystyle\sum_{k=0}^{n-i} \binom{n-k-1}{i-1} (1-p')^k\, (1-p)^{n-i-k} & \\ & \text{for } i = 1, \ldots, n. \end{cases} \tag{7.10}$$

Intuitively, $(1-p')^n$ is the probability of no cases in a sample of n family members. For $i = 1, \ldots, n$, let k denote the number of healthy family members recorded before the first diseased case is recorded. We sum over all possible choices for k. The patients up to and including the first recorded case will occur with probability $p'(1-p')^k$. After the first case is recorded, there are $i-1$ additional cases and $n-i-k$ additional healthy individuals. These $i-1$ cases, after the first, need to be arranged into positions among the last $n-k-1$ family members examined. This explains the terms in the functional form of the probability $\Pr[Y_n = i]$ for $i = 1, \ldots, n$ in (7.10).

Examples of this distribution are plotted in Fig. 7.1 for parameter values $n = 10$ and $p' = .4$. The values of p in this figure vary from .2 to .8 by .1. The special case of $p = p'$ in this example corresponds to the binomial distribution with parameters $n = 10$ and $p = .4$. In this figure, the binomial distribution is plotted with a dashed line to distinguish it from the others. Overall, this figure demonstrates that the

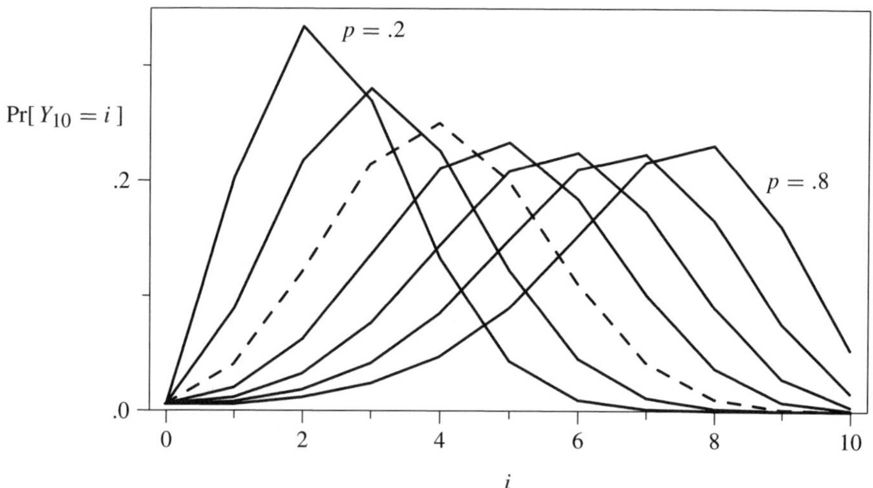

Figure 7.1 The family history distribution mass function (7.10) for $n = 10$ and $p' = .4$. Values of p range from .2 to .8 by .1. The distribution with dashed lines has $p = p' = .4$ and is also the binomial (10, .4) distribution.

Table 7.2 The expected frequencies for the IPF data under the two-parameter family history disease clustering model (7.10). ($\widehat{p}' = .24$; $\widehat{p} = .52$; $\chi^2 = 27.46$; 14 df; $p = .017$).

			Number of affected siblings i						
n	f_n	$\widehat{m}_n$	0	1	2	3	4	5	6
1	48	11.66	36.34	11.66					
2	23	12.73	13.18	6.90	2.91				
3	17	15.56	7.38	4.81	3.69	1.12			
4	7	9.21	2.30	1.68	1.76	1.01	.24		
6	5	10.99	.94	.77	1.10	1.12	.74	.283	.0469
Totals	100	60.16							

shape of the family history distribution (7.10) is not very different from that of the binomial distribution when p' is close in value to p.

The family history model (7.10) can be fitted to the IPF data of Table 7.1. The expected counts for this fitted model are given in Table 7.2. The maximum likelihood estimated parameter values are $\widehat{p}' = .24$ (SE $= .02$) and $\widehat{p} = .52$ (SE $=$ .07). These estimates of p and p' and their estimated standard errors were obtained using numerical methods to maximize the log likelihood and approximate its second derivative using finite differences. These estimates indicate a large difference in the risk of IPF between those individuals with and without affected siblings.

The fit of this model has $\chi^2 = 27.46$, with 14 df and p-value .017. While this is far from a good fit for the data, it does provide a large improvement over the binomial model (7.2) that has $\chi^2 = 312$, with 15 df. The source of the large value of $\chi^2 = 27.46$ for the fitted model in Table 7.2 is the single family with six members, all of whom have IPF. This one family is also the largest contributor to the χ^2 for the binomial model. In the case of the fitted family history model in Table 7.2, the expected number of families in this category is .0469 and the contribution this one family makes to the χ^2 is

$$(1 - .0469)^2/.0469 = 19.37,$$

more than 70% of the value 27.46 of the χ^2 statistic.

Notice that the fitted values in Table 7.2 do not correctly estimate the number of cases m in the original data. The estimated number of IPF cases $\widehat{m}$ is 60.16, or just slightly larger than the observed value of $m = 60$. The estimated value $\widehat{m}$ is obtained from the values in Table 7.2 as

$$\widehat{m} = \sum_n \widehat{m}_n,$$

where

$$\widehat{m}_n = \sum_{i=0}^{n} i \, \mathrm{E}[X_{ni} \mid \widehat{p}', \widehat{p}]$$

is the number of cases expected among the families of size n. (The m_n values do not have useful interpretations by themselves except for their use in the enumeration algorithm of Section 6.2.1.)

The values of m and $\widehat{m}$ are close but not equal in value. There is no reason that the maximum likelihood estimates of p and p' lead to estimates that equate m and $\widehat{m}$, as is the case with the binomial and hypergeometric models given in (7.2) and (7.1) respectively. The family history model has a useful interpretation for explaining disease clustering but may provide a bias in estimating the disease incidence rate. The separate concepts of clustering and incidence are addressed in Section 6.1.3. The issue of estimating incidence by equating m and $\widehat{m}$ is discussed in Section 8.6. A number of other models will be fitted to this data example and these are summarized in the remainder of this chapter.

Let us next describe other properties of the family history model and, specifically, derive expressions for the moments of this distribution. Moments of distribution (7.10) can be found as follows. For $r = 1, 2, \ldots$, the factorial polynomial is

$$Y^{(r)} = Y(Y-1)\cdots(Y-r+1).$$

In the family history distribution, it is convenient to omit the first term in this sequence. Specifically, we next obtain an expression for the expected value of

$$(Y_n - 1)^{(r)} = (Y_n - 1)(Y_n - 2)\cdots(Y_n - r).$$

For $r = 1, 2, \ldots$, these factorial moments of the family history distribution given in (7.10) satisfy

$$\begin{aligned}
\mathrm{E}[\,(Y_n-1)^{(r)}\,] &= (-1)^r r!\,\Pr[\,Y_n = 0\,] + \sum_{i=r+1}^{n} (i-1)^{(r)} \Pr[\,Y_n = i\,] \\
&= (-1)^r r!(1-p')^n + \sum_{i=r+1}^{n} (i-1)^{(r)} p' p^{i-1} \\
&\quad \times \sum_{k=0}^{n-i} \binom{n-k-1}{i-1} (1-p')^k (1-p)^{n-i-k}.
\end{aligned}$$

Write

$$(i-1)^{(r)} \binom{n-k-1}{i-1} = (n-k-1)^{(r)} \binom{n-k-r-1}{i-r-1}$$

and change the order of the two summation signs to show

$$\begin{aligned}
\mathrm{E}[\,(Y_n-1)^{(r)}\,] &= (-1)^r r!(1-p')^n \\
&\quad + p'/p \sum_{k=0}^{n-r-1} (n-k-1)^{(r)} (1-p')^k (1-p)^{n-k} \\
&\quad \times \sum_{i=r+1}^{n-k} \binom{n-k-r-1}{i-r-1} [p/(1-p)]^i.
\end{aligned}$$

The inner summation can be simplified as

$$\sum_{i=r+1}^{n-k} \binom{n-k-r-1}{i-r-1} [p/(1-p)]^i = p^{r+1}/(1-p)^{n-k}$$

so that

$$\mathrm{E}[\,(Y_n-1)^{(r)}\,] = (-1)^r r!(1-p')^n + p'\,p^r \sum_{k=0}^{n-r-1} (n-k-1)^{(r)}(1-p')^k. \tag{7.11}$$

Use (7.11) to show that the expected value of the family history distribution (7.10) is

$$\mathrm{E}[\,Y_n\,] = 1 + \mathrm{E}[\,(Y_n-1)^{(1)}\,] = np + (p'-p)/p'\,[1-(1-p')^n]$$

for every $n = 1, 2, \ldots$ and the variance is

$$\begin{aligned}\mathrm{Var}[\,Y_n\,] &= \mathrm{E}[\,(Y_n-1)^{(2)}\,] + 3\mathrm{E}[\,Y_n\,] - (\mathrm{E}[\,Y_n\,])^2 - 2 \\ &= np(1-p) + (p'-p)[(1+2np)p'(1-p')^n \\ &\quad - (p'-p)(1-p')^{2n} - p]/(p')^2.\end{aligned}$$

The expected value and variance of the family history distribution (7.10) both correspond to those of the binomial distribution when $p = p'$.

7.2.3 Incremental risk model

The family history distribution is based on the conditional probability given in (7.9) that the risk of disease is changed once there is at least one other case recorded in the family. Another useful model is one in which the conditional probability of disease $C_n(i)$ in an additionally assessed family member is a strictly monotone function of the known number of affected siblings i. In the *incremental risk model*,

$$C_n(i) = \exp(\alpha + i\beta)/[1 + \exp(\alpha + i\beta)] \tag{7.12}$$

specifies that the log odds of an individual having the disease is a linear function of the number of affected cases among the other family members.

This model has the intuitive interpretation that for $\beta > 0$, the more cases that are recorded in a family, the more likely that additional cases will be found. Bad news, if you will, increases the chances of being followed by even worse news. When $\beta = 0$, the binomial model is obtained in (7.12) with

$$p = \exp(\alpha)/[1 + \exp(\alpha)].$$

The probabilities $\Pr[Y_n = i]$ for the incremental risk model are difficult to describe in closed form but can be computed numerically using the recursive relation given in (7.5). As a graphical illustration of this distribution, Figs. 7.2 and 7.3 demonstrate the wide range of shapes that the incremental risk distribution can attain. Both of these figures model the distribution with $n = 10$. Fig. 7.2 varies

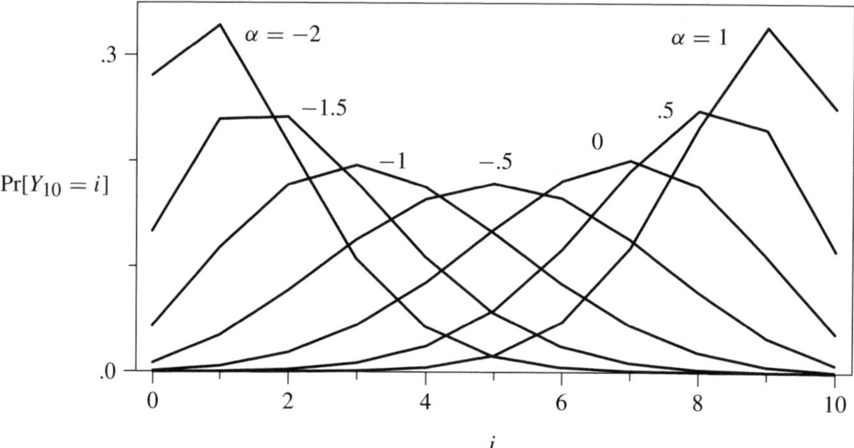

Figure 7.2 The incremental risk mass function for $\beta = .25$, $n = 10$, and values of α as given.

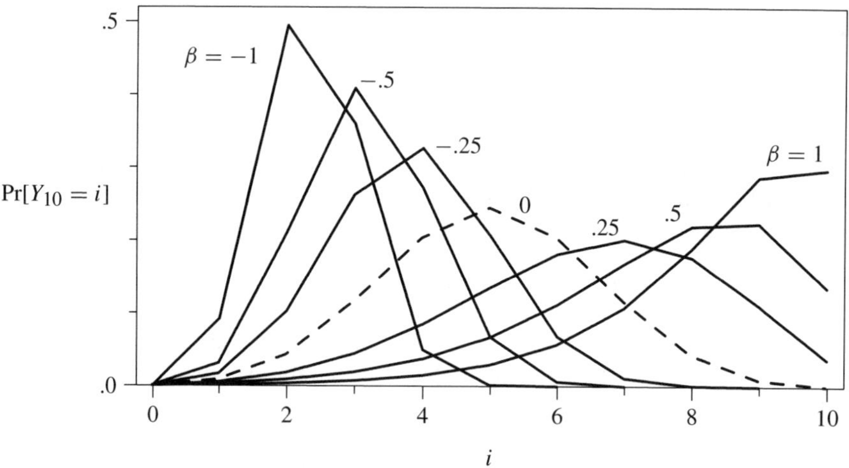

Figure 7.3 The incremental risk mass function for $n = 10$, $\alpha = 0$ and values of β as given. The distribution in dashed line for $\beta = 0$ is also the binomial with parameters $n = 10$ and $p = .5$.

values of α for a fixed value of $\beta = .25$. Similarly, Fig. 7.3 fixes $\alpha = 0$ and changes the values of β. The special case of $\alpha = \beta = 0$ in Fig. 7.3 is also the binomial distribution with parameters $n = 10$ and $p = .5$. This special case is highlighted with a dashed line.

Increasing either α or β moves the incremental risk distribution to the right. Intuitively, large values of α and/or β will increase the probability of more diseased cases. Another way to describe this is through the contour plot of the expected values of this distribution given in Fig. 7.4. The means increase with both α and β. These numerical properties are easy enough to demonstrate computationally but mathematical results are difficult to describe for this distribution.

The estimated parameter values for the IPF data are $\widehat{\alpha} = -1.15$ (SE = .11) and $\widehat{\beta} = .87$ (SE = .21). The expected frequencies are given in Table 7.3. This model has a very good fit to the IPF data with $\chi^2 = 9.17$; 14 df; $p = .82$. This fit is the best of all models we consider for this data example. Families of size $n = 6$ with all members affected have an expected frequency of .241. This one unusual family that contributed to the lack of fit in previous analyses is well explained by this model.

As we also see in the fitted family history distribution in Table 7.2, the estimated number of cases $\widehat{m} = 59.21$ in Table 7.3 does not correctly estimate the number of cases $m = 60$ in the original data. This issue is discussed in Section 8.6.

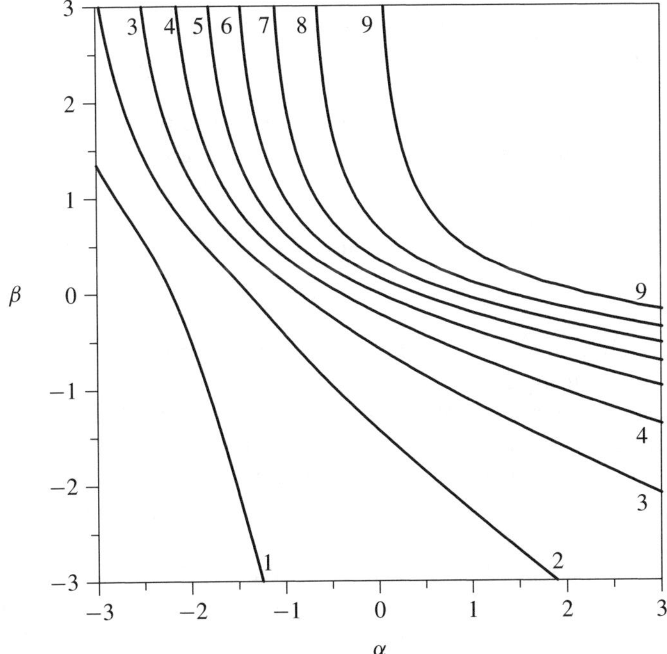

Figure 7.4 Contours of means for the incremental risk distribution for $n = 10$.

Table 7.3 The expected frequencies for the IPF data under the two-parameter incremental risk disease clustering model (7.12). The fitted estimates are $\widehat{\alpha} = -1.15$ (SE = .11) and $\widehat{\beta} = .87$ (SE = .21). ($\chi^2 = 9.17$; 14 df; $p = .82$).

			Number of affected siblings i						
n	f_n	$\widehat{m}_n$	0	1	2	3	4	5	6
1	48	11.57	36.43	11.57					
2	23	12.15	13.25	7.36	2.40				
3	17	14.83	7.43	5.45	2.98	1.14			
4	7	8.99	2.32	2.01	1.40	.880	.384		
6	5	11.66	.96	.993	.871	.773	.669	.498	.241
Totals	100	59.21							

7.2.4 The exchangeable, beta-binomial distribution

Neither the family history (7.9) nor the incremental risk (7.12) conditional probability models takes into account the size of the family n. Consider the conditional probability

$$C_n(i) = (i\alpha + p)/(n\alpha + 1) \tag{7.13}$$

with parameters $0 < p < 1$ and $\alpha \geq -p/I$, where I is the size of the largest family. The sign of α determines the sign of the correlation between the Z_i. The binomial model is obtained when $\alpha = 0$.

The conditional probability C_n in (7.13) is motivated by the form of a Bayesian estimator of a binomial parameter. The Bayes estimator is typically a weighted average of the prior mean (p) and the empirical fraction i/n. The function $C_n(i)$ in (7.13) also has this property.

Specifically, we can write the conditional probability C_n in (7.13) as

$$C_n(i) = \xi p \; + \; (1 - \xi)\,(i/n),$$

where the weight $\xi = (n\alpha + 1)^{-1}$ given to the fixed probability p becomes smaller as the family size n increases.

In words, small families do not provide much empirical data about the risk of their members. The estimated risk of disease for one individual in a small family is similar to that of the marginal population probability p. In larger families, the estimated risk for one unassessed individual is closer to the rate i/n among the other members of that family.

For the choice of C_n in (7.13), the joint distribution of $\{Z_1, \ldots, Z_n\}$ depends on their sum $Y_n = Z_1 + \cdots + Z_n$ but not on their individual values. The exchangeable indicators $\{Z_i\}$ for this model all have the same marginal Bernoulli (p) distribution. Their bivariate moments satisfy

$$\text{Cov}\,[\,Z_i,\; Z_{i'}\,] = \alpha p(1 - p)/(\alpha + 1)$$

for all $i \neq i'$ so that

$$\text{Corr}[\, Z_i,\; Z_{i'} \,] = \alpha/(\alpha + 1).$$

If we define $\prod_0^{-1} = 1$, then the probability mass function of Y_n can be written as

$$\Pr[\, Y_n = i \,] = \binom{n}{i} \prod_{r=0}^{i-1} (r\alpha + p) \prod_{s=0}^{n-i-1} (s\alpha + 1 - p) \Big/ \prod_{t=0}^{n-1} (t\alpha + 1) \qquad (7.14)$$

for $i = 0, 1, \ldots, n$.

If we restrict $\alpha > 0$, then we can write

$$\Pr[\, Y_n = i \,] = \binom{n}{i} \frac{\Gamma(i + p/\alpha)\, \Gamma[n - i + (1 - p)/\alpha]\, \Gamma(\alpha^{-1})}{\Gamma(p/\alpha)\, \Gamma[(1 - p)/\alpha]\, \Gamma(n + \alpha^{-1})}, \qquad (7.15)$$

which is the mass function of the beta-binomial distribution with parameters p/α and $(1 - p)/\alpha$.

This distribution is described at (1.21) in Section 1.7.1. More details and properties of the beta-binomial distribution (7.15) are available in (Johnson, *et al.* (1992) pp 239–42). This distribution often appears in the analysis of litter effects in teratology experiments. A recent example of these applications and extensions of the beta-binomial distribution are given in (Moore, Park, and Smith (2001)). Additional examples, references, and methods are discussed in Chapter 9. The more general expression for the mass function in (7.14) allows for mutual negative correlation among the Bernoulli indicators Z_i. The property of modeling negative correlations may have limited application with the examples described here and elsewhere.

The moments of Y_n in (7.15) satisfy

$$\text{E}[\, Y_n \,] = np$$

and

$$\text{Var}[\, Y_n \,] = np(1 - p)[1 + (n - 1)\alpha/(\alpha + 1)].$$

This variance is larger than that of the corresponding binomial distribution for $\alpha > 0$.

The fitted maximum likelihood estimates of the IPF data under the beta-binomial model are given in Table 7.4. The estimated $\widehat{p} = .282$ (SE = .03) is comparable to the corresponding maximum likelihood estimate (.296) for the binomial model. The fitted $\widehat{\alpha} = .270$ (SE = .10) estimates a slight positive correlation of

$$\widehat{\alpha}/(\widehat{\alpha} + 1) = .212$$

between the exchangeable disease indicators $\{Z_i\}$.

The fit is adequate ($\chi^2 = 17.43$, 14 df, $p = .23$). The largest contribution to the χ^2 statistic is the single family of size $n = 6$, all of whose members exhibit IPF. The estimated expected number of such families is .090 in Table 7.4, contributing to more than half of the value of the χ^2 statistic. This single family has also been shown to be the source of poor fit in other models of this chapter and in the previous chapter.

Table 7.4 The expected frequencies for the IPF data with the beta-binomial model (7.15). The fitted estimates are $\widehat{p} = .28$ (SE = .03) and $\widehat{\alpha} = .27$ (SE = .10). ($\chi^2 = 17.43$; 14 df; $p = .23$).

			Number of affected siblings i						
n	f_n	$\widehat{m}_n$	0	1	2	3	4	5	6
1	48	13.54	34.46	13.54					
2	23	12.98	12.84	7.33	2.82				
3	17	14.39	7.75	5.22	2.91	1.11			
4	7	7.90	2.70	1.99	1.31	.728	.277		
6	5	8.47	1.46	1.20	.920	.660	.430	.237	.090
Totals	100	57.28							

7.2.5 Application to IPF example

Through the material described so far in this chapter, we have fitted the family history, incremental risk, and beta-binomial models to the IPF data. The expected frequencies, estimated parameters, and measures of goodness of fit are provided in each case. Before we describe other models of sums of dependent Bernoulli random variables for this data, let us demonstrate that each of these fitted models also allows us to obtain an estimate of properties of the indicators Z_i and their sum Y_n.

Specifically, Table 7.5 provides the fitted means and standard deviations for the number of IPF cases Y_n in families of each size $n = 1, \ldots, 6$. The empirical column refers to the original data. The Altham distribution is given in (7.3) and described in greater detail in Section 8.2. The fitted parameter values for the Altham model are given in Table 7.9.

The marginal distribution of each Bernoulli indicator can then be found from the mean of the fitted expectation of Y_n according to

$$\text{fitted}\,\Pr[\,Z_n = 1\,] = (\text{fitted}\mathrm{E}\,[\,Y_n\,])/n$$

for $n = 1, \ldots, 6$.

These estimates of the distributions of the Bernoulli indicators Z_n are given in Table 7.6 for the IPF data. In the case of the binomial and beta-binomial distributions, the expectations of Y_n follow the relation

$$\mathrm{E}\,[\,Y_n\,] = n\mathrm{E}\,[\,Y_1\,],$$

for every $n = 1, 2, \ldots$, so the fitted probabilities $\Pr[Z_n = 1]$ are constant in these columns of Table 7.6.

The Altham distribution is also the sum of exchangeable Bernoulli random variables but its expected value does not follow this relation in general. The expected value of the Altham distribution is discussed in Section 8.2.

Table 7.5 Estimated means and standard deviations of the number of IPF cases Y_n.

Family size n	Distribution model					
	Empirical	Binomial	Altham	FH	Beta-binomial	IR
Means						
1	.25	.30	.33	.24	.28	.24
2	.39	.59	.63	.55	.56	.53
3	1.12	.89	.89	.91	.84	.89
4	.71	1.18	1.10	1.31	1.12	1.29
5	—	1.48	1.24	1.74	1.41	1.78
6	3.00	1.77	1.32	2.19	1.69	2.34
Standard deviations						
1	.43	.46	.47	.43	.45	.43
2	.57	.65	.69	.71	.70	.68
3	.96	.79	.87	.95	.93	.93
4	.70	.91	1.04	1.17	1.15	1.21
5	—	1.02	1.18	1.36	1.37	1.46
6	2.00	1.12	1.30	1.53	1.58	1.79

Table 7.6 Estimated marginal probability $\Pr[Z_n = 1]$ of IPF.

	Distribution model				
n	Binomial	Altham	FH	Beta-binomial	IR
1	.296	.334	.242	.281	.242
2	.296	.317	.361	.281	.346
3	.296	.297	.400	.281	.414
4	.296	.274	.430	.281	.488
5	.296	.249	.452	.281	.565
6	.296	.219	.469	.281	.638

7.3 Exchangeable Models

Exchangeability is a property that generalizes identically distributed random variables. The definition of exchangeable is that all subsets of the random variables of the same size have the same distribution. Specifically, the random variables $Z_1, \ldots, Z_n$ are *exchangeable* if

$$\Pr[\, Z_1 = z_1, \ \ldots\ , Z_k = z_k \,] = \Pr[\, Z_{i_1} = z_1, \ \ldots\ , Z_{i_k} = z_k \,]$$

for any indices $\{i_1, \ldots , i_k\}$, a subset of $\{1, \ldots , n\}$ and all $k = 1, 2, \ldots , n$.

Exchangeability is a way of saying that individuals and all subsets are equivalent and can be substituted for all other individuals and subsets of the same size. Independent and identically distributed random variables are exchangeable. Exchangeable also means identically marginally distributed and usually is meant as dependent. This dependence is often a mutual positive correlation between all possible pairs, triples, and so on. Negative correlations are possible but tend to be restrictive, as we see in this section, particularly when the family size is large. In the limit, exchangeable infinite sized populations cannot be mutually negatively correlated.

There are several methods for describing the sum

$$Y_n = Z_1 + \cdots + Z_n$$

of exchangeable Bernoulli random variables $Z_1, \ldots, Z_n$.

The general principle of de Finetti is that if the Z_i are exchangeable and sampled from an infinitely large population, then the distribution of Y_n is expressible as

$$\Pr[\, Y_n = i \,] = \binom{n}{i} \int_0^1 p^i \,(1-p)^{n-i}\, \mathrm{d}F(p) \tag{7.16}$$

for some distribution F defined on 0–1.

The idea behind this expression is that a value of the p parameter is sampled from the distribution F and then a binomial distribution is sampled using this choice of p. In an infinite population, the exchangeable random variables must be positively correlated. Similarly, expression (7.16) only models positively correlated Bernoulli indicators Z_i. This model includes the specific examples of the beta-binomial distribution described in Section 7.2.4, for which F represents the beta distribution.

The Altham distribution discussed in Section 8.2 allows for mutual negative correlation among the Bernoulli indicators Z_i. Consequently, the Altham model is not expressible in the form (7.16). More generally, this section describes methods for developing new distributions to model the sum Y_n of exchangeable Bernoulli random variables.

The sampling mechanism that is modeled by exchangeability is different from that of the conditional models described in Section 7.2. In conditional models, we consider sampling one family member at a time and model the conditional risk of disease in the next screened member, given the information from previously measured family members. Models for exchangeability, on the other hand, are best used to describe a process where all family members are screened at the same time.

Specifically, the IPF frequencies (Table 6.1) and the childhood cancer example (Table 6.2) lend themselves to interpretation using conditional models. In both of these examples, the disease status of one or more individuals brought the family to the attention of epidemiologists, who then examined the remaining family members. These two examples are consistent with the conditional sampling methods described in Section 7.2.

In contrast, the infant mortality data in Table 6.3 and the incidence of *T. cruzi* (Table 6.4) represent random samples of whole families or entire households, all of whose members were examined at the same time. These latter two examples lend themselves to an examination using exchangeable methods.

In this section, we develop models for sums of exchangeable Bernoulli random variables using a method developed by Bowman and George 1995; George and Bowman 1995; and George and Kodell 1996. These authors derive the relationship

$$\Pr[\, Y_n = i \,] \quad = \quad \binom{n}{i} \sum_{k=0}^{n-i} (-1)^k \binom{n-i}{k} \lambda_{i+k}, \tag{7.17}$$

where $\lambda_0 = 1$ and

$$\lambda_k = \Pr[\, Y_k = k \,] = \Pr[\, Z_1 = \cdots = Z_k = 1 \,]$$

for $k = 1, 2, \ldots$.

Every λ_k in (7.17) is the probability that all individuals are affected in a family of size k. We also note that

$$\lambda_1 = \mathrm{E}[\, Z_i \,]$$

for $i = 1, 2, \ldots, n$ defines the marginal distribution of any one individual's disease risk.

Expression (7.17) is central to the development of discrete distributions developed in this section. A key feature leading to the development of the distribution in (7.17) is the exchangeable property of the disease status Z_i of the individual family members. The proof of this important expression is given in the Appendix of Section 7.5.

Exchangeability includes independence as a special case. If we set $\lambda_k = p^k$ for probability p and every $k = 1, 2, \ldots$, then (7.17) simplifies to the binomial (n, p) distribution mass function. The binomial distribution represents independence among the Bernoulli indicators $\{Z_1, \ldots, Z_n\}$. Of course, modeling dependence is of greatest interest to us.

We can describe dependence between the Bernoulli indicators Z_i and Z_j (for $i \neq j$) in terms of their odds ratio

$$\psi = \frac{\Pr[\, Z_i = 1;\ Z_j = 1 \,]\ \Pr[\, Z_i = 0;\ Z_j = 0 \,]}{\Pr[\, Z_i = 1;\ Z_j = 0 \,]\ \Pr[\, Z_i = 0;\ Z_j = 1 \,]}.$$

The Bernoulli indicators random variables are exchangeable so the value of ψ does not depend on i and j. If we use the exchangeability property, we can write

$$\begin{aligned}\Pr[\, Z_i = 1;\ Z_j = 1 \,] &= \Pr[\, Z_1 = 1;\ Z_2 = 1 \,]\\ &= \Pr[\, Y_2 = 2 \,]\\ &= \lambda_2.\end{aligned}$$

Similarly, we have

$$\begin{aligned}\Pr[\, Z_i = 0;\; Z_j = 0\,] &= \Pr[\, Y_2 = 0\,]\\ &= \lambda_2 - 2\lambda_3 + \lambda_4\end{aligned}$$

and

$$\begin{aligned}\Pr[\, Z_i = 1;\; Z_j = 0\,] &= \Pr[\, Z_i = 0;\; Z_j = 1\,]\\ &= \Pr[\, Y_2 = 1\,]/2\\ &= \lambda_2 - \lambda_3,\end{aligned}$$

using exchangeability and (7.17) in both cases.

This allows us to express the odds ratio

$$\psi = \lambda_2(\lambda_2 - 2\lambda_3 + \lambda_4)/(\lambda_2 - \lambda_3)^2$$

between any pair of exchangeable Bernoulli indicators Z_i and Z_j.

George and Bowman (1995) describe multivariate moments of the indicators $\{Z_1, \ldots, Z_k\}$ and demonstrate the relationship between these moments and the λ_k.

Define the kth order correlation ρ_k by

$$\rho_k = \mathrm{E}\,[\,(Z_1 - \lambda_1)\cdots(Z_k - \lambda_1)\,]\;/\;\mathrm{Var}\,[\,Z_1\,]^{k/2}$$

and $\lambda_1 = \mathrm{E}\,[\,Z_k\,]$ for $k = 1, 2, \ldots$.

Then

$$\rho_k = \sum_{j=0}^{k} (-\lambda_1)^{k-j} \binom{k}{j} \lambda_k \;\Big/\; [\lambda_1(1-\lambda_1)]^{k/2}\,.$$

This last relation shows that the joint moments of the exchangeable Bernoulli random variables $\{Z_i\}$ also determine the distribution of their sum. Bowman and George (1995) demonstrate how the higher order correlations ρ_k can be estimated from family data such as discussed in this chapter. They argue that a virtue of this approach over the more commonly used generalized estimating equations (GEE) is that the latter only models means and covariances. Their approach allows for models that include higher order interactions between the Bernoulli indicators.

In (7.17), there is also a connection to the conditional models of Section 7.2. Let us write

$$\lambda_k = \prod_{j=1}^{k} C_j(j)$$

for conditional probabilities

$$C_j(j) = \Pr[\, Y_j = j \mid Y_{j-1} = j - 1\,],$$

using the notation for the conditional probability developed in Section 7.2.1.

Similarly, we have

$$C_n(n) = \lambda_n/\lambda_{n-1}.$$

These expressions for λ_k are used in Section 7.3.2 to extend the incremental risk model to sums of exchangeable Bernoulli indicators.

In closed form, we can also express (7.17) as

$$\begin{aligned}\Pr[\,Y_n = i\,] = \binom{n}{i}&[C_1(1)\cdots C_i(i)]\\ &\times\left[1-\frac{(n-i)C_{i+1}(i+1)}{1}\left[1-\frac{(n-i-1)C_{i+2}(i+2)}{2}\right.\right.\\ &\left.\left.\cdots\left[1-\frac{2C_{n-1}(n-1)}{n-i-1}\left[1-\frac{C_n(n)}{n-i}\right]\right]\cdots\right]\right].\end{aligned}$$

This demonstrates the connection between the conditional and the exchangeable models (7.17) of $\Pr[Y_n]$. The conditional models also have this extension to an exchangeable form and examples are given in this section.

It should be noted that (7.17) is sufficient to generate the distribution of a sum of exchangeable Bernoulli random variables. Expression (7.17) is not necessary, however. That is, there are distributions of sums of exchangeable Bernoulli's that do not follow (7.17). This claim can be illustrated with two examples.

For the first of these two examples, consider the beta-binomial distribution described in Section 7.2.4. This distribution, with mass function at (7.15), describes the behavior of the sum of exchangeable Bernoulli random variables. In this model, with parameters p and α we have

$$\begin{aligned}\lambda_k(\beta\text{–binomial}) &= \Pr[\,Y_k = k\,]\\ &= \frac{\Gamma(k+p/\alpha)\,\Gamma(\alpha^{-1})}{\Gamma(p/\alpha)\,\Gamma(k+\alpha^{-1})},\end{aligned}$$

using expression (7.15).

If we use these values of λ_k, then (7.17) will reproduce (7.15). That is, the beta-binomial distribution is a member of distributions generated by (7.17).

For a second example in which (7.17) fails to reproduce the same distribution, consider the Altham model with mass function given in (7.3). In the Altham model, with parameters p and θ, we have

$$\lambda_k(\text{Altham}) = p^k \Bigg/ \sum_{j=0}^{k}\binom{k}{j}\,p^j\,(1-p)^{k-j}\exp\{-\theta j(k-j)\}\,.$$

To show that these values of λ_k used in (7.17) do not reproduce the Altham distribution, consider a single numerical example. In Fig. 7.5, we plot the Altham distribution mass function with parameters $n = 10$, $p = .4$ and $\alpha = .2$ connected with dotted lines. Figure 7.5 also plots the mass function generated by (7.17) using

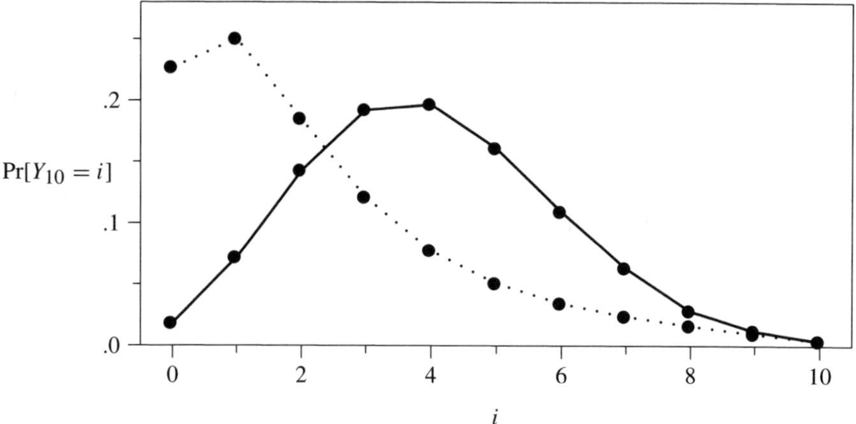

Figure 7.5 Altham mass function (7.3) in dots with parameters $n = 10$, $p = .4$ and $\alpha = .2$ and the exchangeable distribution (solid line) generated using this model of $\lambda_k = \Pr[Y_k = k]$ in (7.17).

the values of λ_k from this Altham distribution with the same parameter values. This plot clearly describes two very different distributions.

These two examples demonstrate that (7.17) is sufficient to generate distributions of sums of exchangeable Bernoulli random variables but it is not necessary that every such sum obey (7.17). Nevertheless, expression (7.17) is very helpful in generating useful models. The proof of this important expression is given in Section 7.5.

Overall, exchangeability is a good idea in principle but two problems arise in practice. The first of these is the restrictive parameter space necessary for (7.17) to describe valid probability distributions in the presence of mutual negative correlations. Expression (7.17) might not produce a valid probability distribution if we try to fit strong mutual negative correlations among the exchangeable disease indicators $\{Z_i\}$.

That is, (7.17) may not represent a valid probability distribution for arbitrary choices of $\{\lambda_k\}$. There are restrictions on the values of the λ's and these cannot be arbitrarily assigned values. Specific examples follow that illustrate these restrictions on the parameters. In the following narrative, we describe exchangeable analogies to the family history and incremental risk models described in Section 7.2. Both of those models are defined for all parameter values. Once we require that the Bernoulli indicators be exchangeable, then difficult restrictions on the parameters are also imposed.

The second problem with requiring exchangeability is that sums of exchangeable Bernoulli random variables often result in bimodal distributions when their correlations are strong. If there is a strong positive mutual correlation among the exchangeable indicators $\{Z_i\}$, then they are likely to all have the same value, resulting in large probability masses at $Y_n = 0$ and $Y_n = n$. Bimodal distributions do not pose a problem mathematically (*cf.* Fig. 2.3), but they do not often have an intuitive appeal in applied work. Despite this lack of appeal, Chapter 2 contains examples in which bimodal models are used in order to describe long-tailed datasets.

7.3.1 Exchangeable family history

Let us begin with the family history conditional probability from (7.9) in Section 7.2.2. The probability of the first case is p' and the probability of subsequent cases is p. Then

$$\lambda_k = \Pr[\, Z_1 = \cdots = Z_k = 1\,] = p' p^{k-1}$$

for $k = 1, 2, \ldots$ and $\lambda_0 = 1$.

We can use these values of λ_k in (7.17) to extend the family history model to a model of sums of exchangeable Bernoulli random variables. In closed form, the *exchangeable family history distribution* has mass function

$$\Pr[\, Y_n = i\,] = \begin{cases} 1 - p'[1 - (1-p)^n]/p & \text{for } i = 0 \\ \binom{n}{i} p' p^{i-1} (1-p)^{n-i} & \text{for } i = 1, \ldots, n. \end{cases} \tag{7.18}$$

The family history distribution given in (7.10) identifies one family member as the "first case" and labels others as "subsequent cases." There is also a distinction made between those healthy persons recorded before and those after the first disease case. The binomial coefficient in (7.10) reflects these distinctions. The names of the first and subsequent cases are in contrast to the exchangeable property of individuals described by (7.18). The similarity of (7.18) to the binomial distribution for $i = 1, \ldots, n$ shows that all i cases are considered exchangeable. The binomial coefficient $\binom{n}{i}$ in (7.18) does not distinguish between the different types of cases or the order in which they appeared. Similarly, all $n - i$ nondiseased, otherwise healthy family members are exchangeable and no distinction is made between those assessed before or after the first diseased case.

The probability generating function for this distribution is

$$\begin{aligned} G_n(t) &= \sum_i t^i \Pr[\, Y_n = i\,] \\ &= 1 - p'[1 - (1 - p + tp)^n]/p. \end{aligned}$$

The range of parameters p' and p are determined so that $\Pr[Y_n]$ is a valid probability. Specifically, we need to have

$$0 \le \Pr[\, Y_n = 0\,] \le 1.$$

This puts the restriction

$$0 \le p' \le p/[1 - (1-p)^n]$$

on the p' parameter in (7.18).

The range of p' as a function of p is plotted in Fig. 7.7 for various values of n. Parameter values along the dotted line have $p = p'$ and correspond to the binomial distribution. Values of $p' < p$ below the dotted line in this figure result in positive correlations among the Bernoulli disease indicators $\{Z_i\}$.

The exchangeable family history distribution with mass function at (7.18) is always valid if $p' \leq p$. The exchangeable indicators $\{Z_i\}$ are negatively correlated for parameter values located between the dotted line and the upper bound in Fig 7.7. Specifically, cases are negatively correlated when

$$p \leq p' \leq p/[\,1 - (1 - p)^n\,].$$

Figure7.7 illustrates that the larger the family size n, the more restrictive the parameter space is for models of mutual negative correlation.

The factorial moments of the exchangeable family history distribution are

$$\mathrm{E}[\,Y_n^{(r)}\,] = n^{(r)} p'\, p^{r-1}$$

for $r = 1, 2, \ldots$.

Specifically, the expected value is

$$\mathrm{E}[\,Y_n\,] = np'$$

and the variance is

$$\mathrm{Var}[\,Y_n\,] = np'[\,n(p - p') + 1 - p\,].$$

This variance is larger than the corresponding binomial variance when $p' < p$, or when the Z_i are mutually positively correlated. Conversely, if $p' > p$, then the Z_i are negatively correlated and the variance of Y_n is smaller than that of the corresponding binomial distribution.

The third central moment is

$$\mathrm{E}[\,(Y_n - np')^3\,] = np'\{\,n(p - p')\,[\,n(p - 2p') + 3(1 - p)\,] \\ + (1 - p)(1 - 2p)\,\}.$$

These three moments agree with those of the binomial distribution when $p' = p$. Every Bernoulli indicator has expected value

$$\mathrm{E}[\,Z_i\,] = \mathrm{E}[\,Y_n\,]/n = p'.$$

In this exchangeable distribution, any one indicator Z_i behaves marginally as Bernoulli (p') in the absence of knowledge of other family members. The disease risk for one randomly chosen individual is the same as that of the first case in any family.

The bivariate moments of indicators $\{Z_i\}$ for exchangeable family members are

$$\mathrm{Cov}[\,Z_i;\ Z_{i'}\,] = p'(p - p')$$

and

$$\text{Corr}[\,Z_i;\; Z_{i'}\,] = (p - p')/(1 - p')$$

for all $i \neq i'$.

These covariances are positive for $p' < p$. Intuitively, a second diseased case is more likely once the first is found so disease status is positively correlated.

Mutual negative covariances between the exchangeable Z_i occur when p' is greater than p and smaller than the valid upper range plotted in Fig. 7.7.

Negative correlations among family members appear because recording the first case lowers the risk of a second when $p' > p$. As the family size n increases, models with mutual negative correlations between members are restricted to narrower parameter ranges.

The range of the correlation between the Bernoulli distributed indicators is

$$-(n-1)^{-1} \leq \text{Corr}[\,Z_i;\; Z_{i'}\,] \leq 1.$$

The upper limit of the correlation occurs when $p = 1$ for any value of probability p'. The lower limit of the correlation is attained as p approaches zero and $p' = 1/n$. These limits occur when the parameters p and p' take values along the left edge of Fig. 7.7.

Figure 7.6 demonstrates that the exchangeable family history distribution often has more than one mode. Extreme positive correlation results in distributions in which all family members are either diseased or disease-free. The distributions

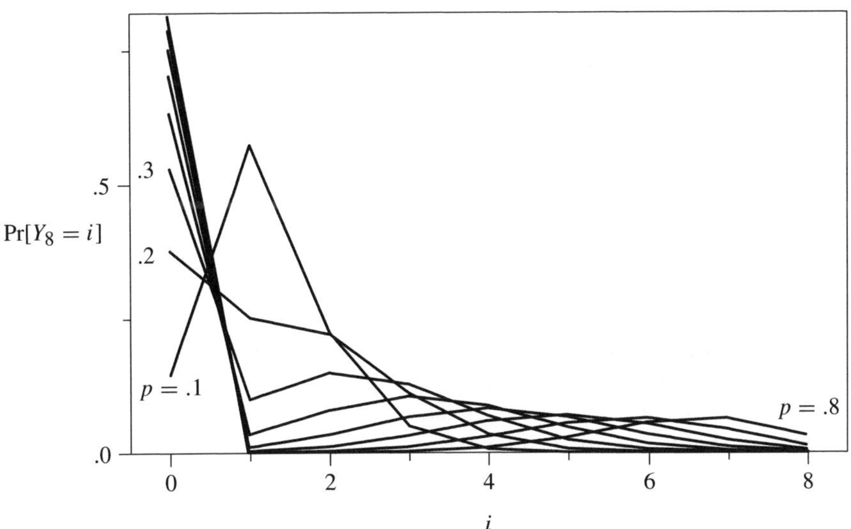

Figure 7.6 Exchangeable family history distribution mass function given in (7.18) with $n = 8$, $p' = .15$ and values of p between .1 and .8. All of these distributions have expected value $np' = 1.2$.

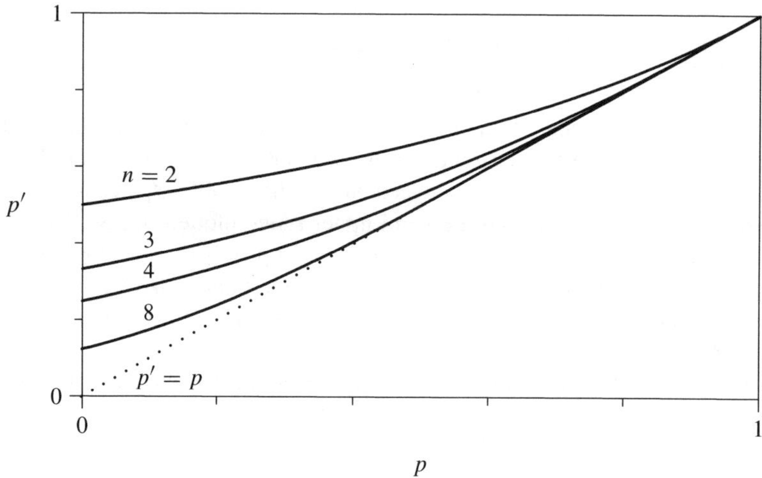

Figure 7.7 Upper limits of p' for the exchangeable family history distribution and $n = 2, 3, 4$, and 8. The dotted line is $p' = p$, corresponding to the binomial distribution.

in Fig. 7.6 all have the same expected value. This can only be achieved if the distribution has a large probability at zero and also in the upper tail. Bimodal distributions generally occur when p is much larger than p'. More specific details are described next.

A local mode at $Y_n = 0$ occurs in (7.18), when

$$\Pr[\, Y_n = 0\,] \geq \Pr[\, Y_n = 1\,]$$

or equivalently, when

$$p' \leq p/[1 - (1-p)^n + np(1-p)^{n-1}].$$

These bounds are plotted in Fig. 7.8. Every set of parameter values below these bounds results in a distribution with a local mode at $Y_n = 0$. Although these bounds on p' are not linear, they almost coincide with the dashed line $p' = p$ when n is large. As a general rule, a local mode at $Y_n = 0$ occurs when $p' < p$ or when the Bernoulli indicators are positively correlated.

Another mode in the distribution of Y_n occurs at the closest integer to

$$\tilde{i} = (n+1)p - 1.$$

The fitted expected counts for the IPF data are given in Table 7.7. The maximum likelihood estimates for the two parameters of the exchangeable family history distribution are $\widehat{p'} = .287$ (SE = .023) and $\widehat{p} = .411$ (SE = .039). The fit with $\chi^2 = 66.67$, 14 df is much better than that of the original binomial distribution

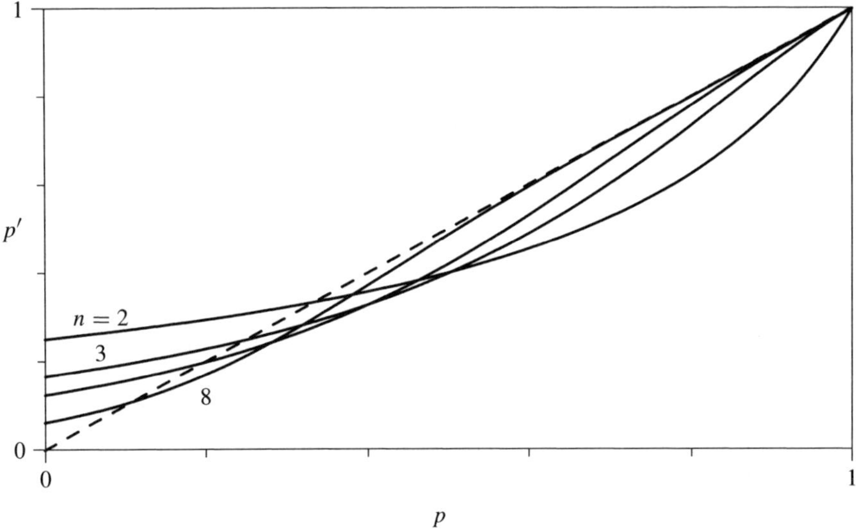

Figure 7.8 The EFH distribution has a local mode at $Y_n = 0$ with parameter values below these lines for $n = 2, 3, 4$, and 8. If the parameter values are below the dashed line, then $Y_n = 0$ is also the global mode.

Table 7.7 The expected frequencies for the IPF data under the two-parameter exchangeable family history disease clustering model (7.12). The fitted estimates are $\widehat{p}' = .287$ (SE = .023) and $\widehat{p} = .411$ (SE = .039). ($\chi^2 = 66.67$; 14 df; $p < 10^{-4}$).

			Number of affected siblings i						
n	f_n	$\widehat{m}_n$	0	1	2	3	4	5	6
1	48	13.76	34.24	13.76					
2	23	13.18	12.53	7.76	2.71				
3	17	14.62	7.57	5.07	3.54	.823			
4	7	8.02	2.71	1.64	1.72	.799	.139		
6	5	8.60	1.66	.609	1.06	.989	.518	.145	.0168
Totals	100	58.17							

but not as good as that obtained by other models we propose for this data. Almost all of this value of the χ^2 statistic is attributable to the single family of size six with all affected members and an expected frequency of .0168.

The expected counts in families of size four and six in Table 7.7 exhibit a bimodal shape. The expected counts in families of sizes four and six have a global mode at zero cases but also exhibit a local mode at two cases. As with the conditional models, the number of cases m in the original data is not correctly estimated.

7.3.2 Exchangeable incremental risk model

The incremental risk distribution is described in Section 7.2.3. The extension of the incremental risk model to describe sums of exchangeable Bernoulli indicator random variables is examined here. As with the incremental risk distribution, closed form mathematical results are also difficult to achieve for its extension to exchangeability.

In the incremental risk model, the conditional probability of one additional case, given by (7.12), is a monotonic function of the number of cases already known in the same family. The expression for this conditional probability can be extended to a model for exchangeable family members as we see next.

Expression (7.17) can be used after writing

$$\lambda_k = \Pr[\, Y_k = k\,] = \prod_{j=1}^{k} \exp(\alpha + j\beta)/[1 + \exp(\alpha + j\beta) \qquad (7.19)$$

for $k = 1, 2, \ldots$ and $\lambda_0 = 1$.

The marginal distribution of disease status in any one family member is Bernoulli with parameter

$$\mathrm{E}[\, Z_i\,] = \lambda_1 = \mathrm{e}^{\alpha}/(1 + \mathrm{e}^{\alpha}).$$

The expected value of the exchangeable incremental risk random variate Y_n is

$$\mathrm{E}[\, Y_n\,] = n\lambda_1 = n\mathrm{e}^{\alpha}/(1 + \mathrm{e}^{\alpha}).$$

The resulting distribution of Y_{10} given by (7.17) is plotted in Fig. 7.9 for $\beta =$ .25 and a range of values of α. These are the same parameter values as in Fig. 7.2. Large values of the α parameter can result in bimodal distributions as seen in this figure. Fig. 7.10 illustrates examples of this distribution when we vary the β parameter.

Not every set of parameter values of α and β result in a valid probability distribution. There are combinations of values of parameters α and β in λ_k that result in negative values in expression (7.17). The valid parameter regions are plotted in Fig. 7.11. The invalid regions are generally for positive values of α and negative values of β. In this invalid region, there would be a probability greater than 1/2 of a first disease case and subsequent cases would be less likely to occur. This setting is indicative of negative correlations among the exchangeable family disease indicators $\{Z_i\}$ and are not useful to us.

Extremely large values of β are also invalid. These regions are not plotted in Fig. 7.11. When $n = 10$, values of β greater than approximately 3.5 do not have valid distributions. Smaller values of n have higher upper limits for the β parameter. Such extreme values of β indicate large differences in the risk between

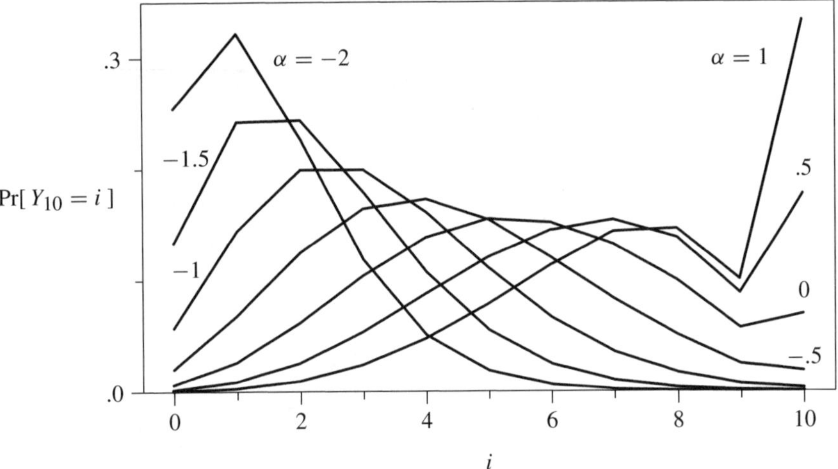

Figure 7.9 Exchangeable incremental risk distribution mass function for $\beta = .25$, $n = 10$ and values of α given.

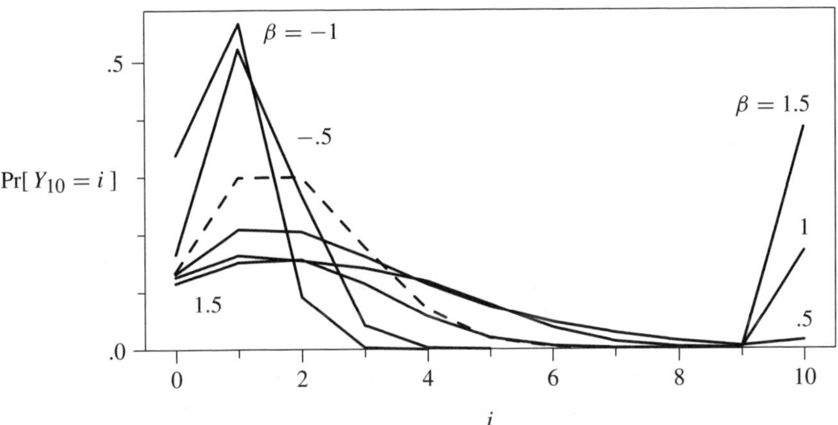

Figure 7.10 Exchangeable incremental risk mass function for $\alpha = -1.5$ and values of β given. The dashed line for $\beta = 0$ is also the binomial(10, .182) mass function. All of these distributions have the same expected value.

the first and subsequent disease cases. Such parameter values are unlikely to appear in practice.

The fitted expected frequencies for the IPF data are given in Table 7.8. The maximum likelihood parameter estimates are $\widehat{\alpha} = -.95$ (SE = .13) and $\widehat{\beta} = .72$ (SE = .17). The fitted expected values for the families of size $n = 6$ exhibit modes

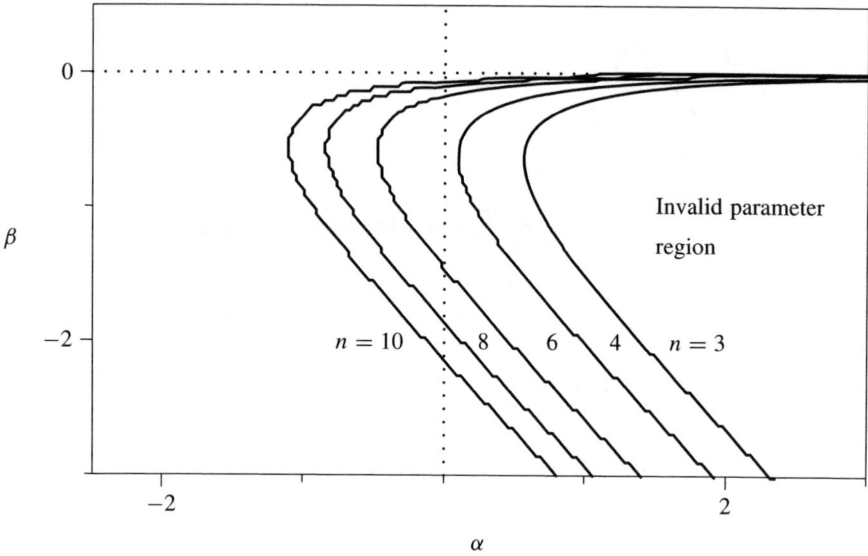

Figure 7.11 Valid parameter regions of the exchangeable incremental risk distribution for values of n given.

Table 7.8 The expected frequencies for the IPF data under the two-parameter exchangeable incremental risk clustering model (7.19). The fitted estimates are $\widehat{\alpha} = -.95$ (SE = .13) and $\widehat{\beta} = .72$ (SE = .17). ($\chi^2 = 10.69$; 14 df; $p = .7$).

			Number of affected siblings i						
n	f_n	$\widehat{m}_n$	0	1	2	3	4	5	6
1	48	13.43	34.56	13.43					
2	23	12.88	12.97	7.17	2.85				
3	17	14.28	7.74	5.55	2.41	1.31			
4	7	7.84	2.63	2.22	1.24	.497	.413		
6	5	8.40	1.35	1.40	.991	.607	.309	.104	.240
Totals	100	56.83							

at one and six cases. The latter mode makes a large contribution to the good fit of the one family that was the source of lack of fit in other models. The overall fit of the model is excellent: $\chi^2 = 10.7$; 14 df; $p = .7$.

The positive estimated value of β indicates the increasing risk of IPF for individuals with more affected siblings. A positive value of β is also estimated in the exchangeable risk model fitted to the IPF data in Table 7.3.

7.4 Applications

The models fit to the IPF data in this chapter are summarized in Table 7.9. The Altham model is given in (7.3). This model is listed here for completeness but is described more fully in Section 8.2 in the following chapter. The beta-binomial is both a conditional model and an exchangeable model so it could be listed under either category in Table 7.9.

All the fitted conditional and exchangeable models in this table have 14 df. The description of degrees of freedom becomes less meaningful when we discuss sparse tables in Chapter 9.

Table 7.9 Deviance, chi-squared goodness of fit, and fitted parameters for the IPF/COPD data and all models described in this chapter. The 2Λ statistics are likelihood ratio tests compared to the binomial model and behave as 1 df chi-squared.

Model and (eq'n. #)	Parameter estimates: Point	Parameter estimates: S.E.	χ^2	Deviance	2Λ
Homogeneous risk models					
Hypergeometric (7.1)			373.23	23.15	
Binomial (7.2)	$\widehat{p}=.30$	.03	312.30	22.55	
Conditional models					
Family history (7.10)	$\widehat{p}' = .24$ $\widehat{p} = .52$	.02 .07	27.46	14.73	7.82
Incremental risk (7.12)	$\widehat{\alpha} = -1.15$ $\widehat{\beta} = .87$	.11 .21	9.13	10.93	11.62
Exchangeable models					
Beta-binomial (7.15)	$\widehat{p} = .28$ $\widehat{\alpha} = .27$	.03 .10	17.43	13.73	8.83
Altham (7.3)	$\widehat{p} = .33$ $\widehat{\theta} = .23$	.04 .12	49.43	18.99	3.56
Exchangeable family history (7.18)	$\widehat{p}' = .29$ $\widehat{p} = .41$	.02 .04	66.67	16.75	5.80
Exchangeable incremental risk (7.19)	$\widehat{\alpha} = -.94$ $\widehat{\beta} = .72$	.13 .17	10.69	11.84	10.71

The two best fitting models, as judged by the chi-squared statistic, are those associated with the incremental risk models. These two models summarize the data well, especially the single outlying family of size six with all members affected. Both the conditional and exchangeable incremental risk models have the smallest values of this goodness-of-fit statistic of all the fitted models in Table 7.9. This appears to indicate that IPF is not merely a disease that clusters within families but that the risk to one individual is directly related to the number of affected siblings.

Another application of the methods given in this chapter is the household incidence of *T. cruzi* given in Table 6.4. The summary statistics are presented in Table 7.10.

The chi-squared and deviance statistics are provided but the concept of degrees of freedom is not meaningful in this example. All families of size six or greater contain only one household, for example, so the usual definition of degrees of freedom does not apply.

Table 7.10 Summary statistics for the *T. cruzi* data.

Model and (eq'n. #)	Parameter estimates: Point	S.E.	χ^2	Deviance	2Λ
Homogeneous risk models					
Hypergeometric (7.1)			250.48	51.43	
Binomial (7.2)	$\widehat{p} = .35$	.04	217.31	50.28	
Conditional models					
Family history (7.10)	$\widehat{p}' = .26$ $\widehat{p} = .54$	.03 .07	94.33	45.10	5.27
Incremental risk (7.12)	$\widehat{\alpha} = -1.05$ $\widehat{\beta} = .73$	.13 .17	67.40	40.11	10.17
Exchangeable models					
Beta-binomial (7.15)	$\widehat{p} = .36$ $\widehat{\alpha} = .31$	.04 .10	42.98	36.95	13.33
Altham (7.3)	$\widehat{p} = .42$ $\widehat{\theta} = .80$	.02 .03	45.66	37.83	12.46
Exchangeable family history (7.18)	$\widehat{p}' = .35$ $\widehat{p} = .40$	.02 .03	161.67	48.56	1.73
Exchangeable incremental risk (7.19)	$\widehat{\alpha} = -.61$ $\widehat{\beta} = .58$	.15 .13	39.27	35.82	14.46

The difference of the deviances of nested models should behave as chi-squared even if the individual deviances do not behave as chi-squared. The precise conditions are described by Haberman (1977). This result allows us to test the statistical significance of parameters in a model but does not help in our assessment of overall goodness of fit.

Let us consider the exchangeable incremental risk model for the *T. cruzi* data. In Table 7.10, this model has the smallest chi-squared and deviance statistics of all models considered. All of these models consist of one parameter more than the binomial, null hypothesis model of no disease clustering. We do not fully understand the underlying distribution of the chi-squared or deviances so we cannot assign a p-value to the goodness of fit.

The expected frequencies for this fitted model are given in Table 7.11. There are a large number of observed frequencies equal to one and these are identified with a '*' mark in this table. Many of these occur where there is only one household of that size.

We cannot provide a p-value for the goodness of fit but can examine the chi-squared residuals to this model, and these are plotted in Fig. 7.12. The horizontal axis is the log of expected frequency and the vertical axis is the chi-squared residual. The diameters of the bubbles correspond to the sizes of the various households.

The apparent pattern of these residuals is emphasized by dotted lines linking all residuals corresponding to observed frequencies of zero and one. The residuals corresponding to zero observed frequencies are all negative and small in magnitude. The observed frequencies equal to one tend to be larger than expected and

Table 7.11 The expected frequencies for the *T. cruzi* data under the two-parameter exchangeable incremental risk clustering model (7.19). The fitted estimates are $\widehat{\alpha} = -.61$ (SE = .15) and $\widehat{\beta} = .58$ (SE = .13). The locations of single observed frequencies are identified with a '*.'

			Number of affected siblings i					
n	f_n	$\widehat{m}_n$	0	1	2	3	4	5+
1	1	.35	.65*	.35				
2	8	5.65	3.74	2.87	1.39			
3	13	13.77	4.58	4.50	2.49	1.43		
4	5	7.06	1.37	1.57	.54	.42		
5	5	8.83	1.09	1.40*	1.13	.71*	.32	.35*
6	4	8.48	.71	1.00	.88*	.63	.38*	.41
7	1	2.47	.15	.22*	.21	.16	.11	.15
8	1	2.83	.12	.20	.20	.16*	.12	.20
9	1	3.18	.10	.17*	.19	.16	.13	.25
13	1	4.59	.05	.11	.14*	.14	.13	.43
Totals	40	57.22						

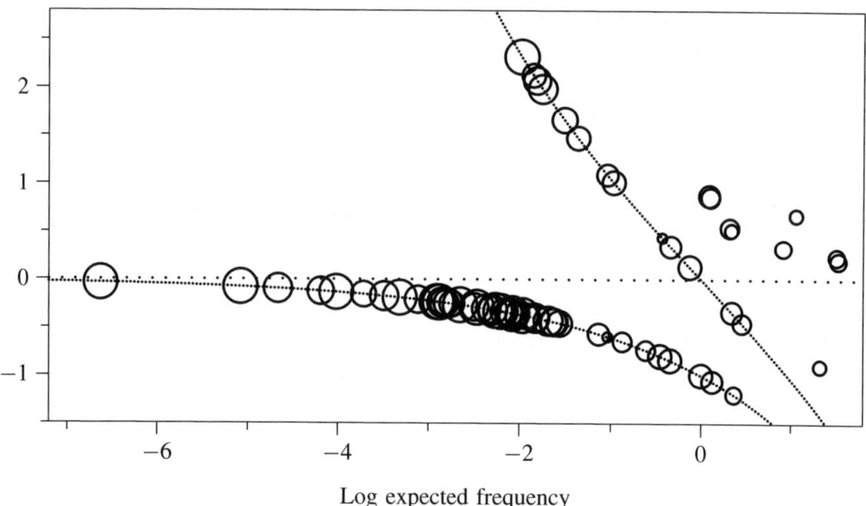

Figure 7.12 Chi-squared residuals for exchangeable incremental risk model of *T. cruzi* data. The dotted lines locate chi-squared residuals corresponding to observed frequencies of either zero (bottom) or one (top).

positive, especially for the largest sized households. This is not surprising because all households of size six or more represent single frequencies.

7.5 Appendix: Proof of Exchangeable Distribution

In this section, we present a proof of expression (7.17) for the distribution of the sum of exchangeable Bernoulli random variables.

For $r = 1, 2, \ldots, n$, let $\{Z_r\}$ denote a set of n exchangeable Bernoulli random variables. Recall that exchangeable means that

$$\Pr[\, Z_1 = z_1,\ Z_2 = z_2,\ \ldots\ , Z_n = z_n \,] = \Pr[\, Z_{\pi(1)} = z_1,\ Z_{\pi(2)} = z_2,\ \ldots\ , Z_{\pi(n)} = z_n \,]$$

for every set of permutations $\pi(1), \ldots, \pi(n)$ of the integers $1, \ldots, n$ and every integer $n = 1, 2, \ldots$.

Define

$$\lambda_n = \Pr[\, Z_1 = 1,\ Z_2 = 1,\ \ldots\ , Z_n = 1 \,]$$

for each $n = 1, 2, \ldots$ and $\lambda_0 = 1$.

For each $n = 1, 2, \ldots,$ define

$$Y_n = Z_1 + \cdots + Z_n.$$

The aim of this section is to prove that (7.17) expresses the probability $\Pr[Y_n = r]$ in terms of the λ's. Specifically, we want to prove

$$\Pr[\,Y_n = r\,] = \binom{n}{r} \sum_{k=0}^{n-r} (-1)^k \binom{n-r}{k} \lambda_{r+k}.$$

Begin by writing

$$\lambda_r = \Pr[\,\mathcal{A}\,]$$

for $r = 0, 1, \ldots, n$, where $\mathcal{A} = \mathcal{A}(r)$ is the event

$$\mathcal{A} = \{\,Z_1 = 1,\;Z_2 = 1,\;\ldots,Z_r = 1\,\}.$$

We can write this probability of r exchangeable random variables as a marginal probability imbedded within a larger set of $n(\geq r)$ Bernoulli variates:

$$\lambda_r = \sum_{z_{r+1}=0}^{1} \sum_{z_{r+2}=0}^{1} \cdots \sum_{z_n=0}^{1} \Pr[\,\mathcal{A} \cap \{\,Z_{r+1} = z_{r+1},\;Z_{r+2} = z_{r+2},\;\ldots,Z_n = z_n\,\}\,]. \tag{7.20}$$

This summation is over all possible outcomes among the $\{Z_{r+1}, \ldots, Z_n\}$ random variables. Consider partitioning the universe of all events summed in (7.20) into the following sets:

$$\begin{aligned}
\mathcal{B} &= \{\,Z_{r+1} = 0,\;\ldots,Z_n = 0\,\}\\
\mathcal{C}_1 &= \{\,Z_{r+1} = 1\,\}\\
\mathcal{C}_2 &= \{\,Z_{r+2} = 1\,\}\\
&\;\;\vdots\\
\mathcal{C}_{n-r} &= \{\,Z_n = 1\,\}.
\end{aligned}$$

The sets $\mathcal{B}, \mathcal{C}_1, \ldots, \mathcal{C}_{n-r}$ overlap but also partition the universe of all possible events among the $\{Z_{r+1}, \ldots, Z_n\}$ in the sense that

$$\Pr[\,\mathcal{B} \cup \mathcal{C}_1 \cup \mathcal{C}_2 \cup \cdots \cup \mathcal{C}_{n-r}\,] = 1.$$

The set $\mathcal{B}$ is incompatible with each of $\mathcal{C}_1, \ldots, \mathcal{C}_{n-r}$, so

$$\Pr[\,\mathcal{B} \cup \mathcal{C}_1 \cup \mathcal{C}_2 \cup \cdots \cup \mathcal{C}_{n-r}\,] = \Pr[\,\mathcal{B}\,] + \Pr[\,\mathcal{C}_1 \cup \mathcal{C}_2 \cup \cdots \cup \mathcal{C}_{n-r}\,].$$

The *inclusion–exclusion principle* (see, for example, Stuart and Ord, 1987, p. 276) allows us to write

$$\begin{aligned}
&\Pr[\,\mathcal{C}_1 \cup \mathcal{C}_2 \cup \cdots \cup \mathcal{C}_{n-r}\,]\\
&\quad= \sum_{i=1}^{n-r} \Pr[\,\mathcal{C}_i\,] - \sum_{i<j}^{n-r} \Pr[\,\mathcal{C}_i \cap \mathcal{C}_j\,] + \sum_{i<j<k}^{n-r} \Pr[\,\mathcal{C}_i \cap \mathcal{C}_j \cap \mathcal{C}_k\,]\\
&\qquad \cdots (-1)^{n-r+1} \Pr[\,\mathcal{C}_1 \cap \mathcal{C}_2 \cap \cdots \cap \mathcal{C}_{n-r}\,]
\end{aligned} \tag{7.21}$$

If we return to (7.20), we can write

$$\begin{aligned}\lambda_r &= \Pr[\,\mathcal{A}\,]\\ &= \Pr[\,\mathcal{A}\cap(\mathcal{B}\cup\mathcal{C}_1\cup\cdots\cup\mathcal{C}_{n-r})\,].\end{aligned}$$

Since $\mathcal{B}$ is incompatible with each of the $\mathcal{C}_i$'s, we have

$$\lambda_r = \Pr[\,\mathcal{A}\cap\mathcal{B}\,] + \Pr[\,\mathcal{A}\cap(\mathcal{C}_1\cup\mathcal{C}_2\ldots\cup\mathcal{C}_{n-r})\,].$$

The inclusion–exclusion rule (7.21) allows us to write

$$\begin{aligned}\lambda_r = \Pr[\,\mathcal{A}\cap\mathcal{B}\,] + \sum_{i=1}^{n-r}\Pr[\,\mathcal{A}\cap\mathcal{C}_i\,] - \sum_{i<j}^{n-r}\Pr[\,\mathcal{A}\cap(\mathcal{C}_i\cap\mathcal{C}_j)\,]\\ \cdots(-1)^{n-r+1}\Pr[\,\mathcal{A}\cap(\mathcal{C}_1\cap\mathcal{C}_2\cap\cdots\cap\mathcal{C}_{n-r})\,].\end{aligned} \tag{7.22}$$

The set $\mathcal{A}\cap\mathcal{B}$ is r 1's followed by $n-r$ 0's in $Z_1,\ldots,Z_n$ so $\mathcal{A}\cap\mathcal{B}$ is only one possible realization in the set of events that comprise $\{Y_n = r\}$. We use the exchangeability of $Z_1,\ldots,Z_n$ to write

$$\Pr[\,Y_n = r\,] = \binom{n}{r}\Pr[\,\mathcal{A}\cap\mathcal{B}\,].$$

Similarly, use the exchangeability of $Z_1,\ldots,Z_n$, giving

$$\Pr[\,\mathcal{A}\cap\mathcal{C}_i\,] = \lambda_{r+1}$$

for each $i = 1, 2, \ldots, n-r$,

$$\Pr[\,\mathcal{A}\cap(\mathcal{C}_i\cap\mathcal{C}_j)\,] = \lambda_{r+2}$$

for $i < j$, and so on up to

$$\Pr[\,\mathcal{A}\cap(\mathcal{C}_1\cap\mathcal{C}_2\cap\cdots\cap\mathcal{C}_{n-r})\,] = \lambda_n.$$

This allows us to write (7.22) as

$$\begin{aligned}\lambda_r = \Pr[\,Y_n = r\,]\Big/\binom{n}{r} + \binom{n-r}{1}\lambda_{r+1}\\ - \binom{n-r}{2}\lambda_{r+2} + \cdots + (-1)^{n-r+1}\lambda_n\end{aligned}$$

so that

$$\Pr[\,Y_n = r\,] = \binom{n}{r}\sum_{k=0}^{n}(-1)^k\binom{n-r}{k}\lambda_{r+k}$$

for $r = 0, 1, \ldots, n$, completing the proof of (7.17).

8

Weighted Binomial Distributions and Disease Clusters

The methods of this chapter are developed in a spirit very different from those described in Chapter 7. The derivations in this chapter are based more on intuition and less on mathematical formality. The good features of the methods described here are their intuitive appeal and the relative ease with which these models can be fit using standard linear model software.

The weighted binomial models described here are discussed more generally by Johnson *et al.* (1992, Section 12.4), including the references contained therein. Our discussion is limited to those weighted models that provide good descriptions of the family data we examine here.

8.1 Weighted Models and Clustering

The development of a weighted model for disease clustering depends on what we mean by the word 'clustering.' Intuitively, clustering means that we expect to see large numbers of cases appearing in the same families. An example of this is the family of size six in the IPF frequency data (Table 7.1) with all members affected. Such a family is very unlikely to occur under the null hypothesis model of homogeneous risk. Under a suitable alternative hypothesis of disease clustering, the expected numbers of such families with large numbers of cases should be much greater than anticipated by the binomial, nonclustering model (7.2).

However, this statement represents only a portion of the complete story.

Discrete Distributions Daniel Zelterman
 ISBN: 0-470-86888-0 (PPC)

Recall that the X_{ni} are the number of families of size n with i disease cases. The number of diseased cases m is constrained by

$$\sum_{ni} i \, X_{ni} = m, \tag{8.1}$$

also given in (6.2).

A model for clustering cannot simply increase the frequencies of the families with large numbers of affected individuals without also increasing the expected number of cases in the sample. A model for clustering cannot just move the expected counts for data in Table 7.1 to the right within each row. This naïve process would also increase the estimated number of cases in the whole data set. Clearly then, the cases to be clustered have to come from somewhere else.

Clustering in this type of data means that we expect to see more families with large numbers of diseased cases and at the same time we should also observe fewer families of the same size with few cases. The cases to be clustered need to come from families with small numbers of cases. In other words, under disease clustering we would expect to see a greater frequency than expected for families with a large number of disease cases and additionally, to make up for these many cases in the same family, there will also be a corresponding decrease in the number of families with few cases. There might also be an increase in the number of families with no cases in order to provide further cases to be clustered.

Clustering means that more families than would be expected by chance will have a large number of cases. But in addition, these cases must come from elsewhere. We would then see a greater frequency of families with zero cases and fewer families with only one case. Intuitively then, we are looking for models with both tails lengthened and the center flattened relative to the binomial distribution.

Mathematically then, this definition of clustering leads us to consider models of the form

$$\mathrm{E}[\, X_{ni} \,] = f_n \, \Pr[\, Y_n = i \,], \tag{8.2}$$

where

$$\Pr[\, Y_n = i \,] = w_n(i) \binom{n}{i} p^i \, (1-p)^{n-i} \tag{8.3}$$

for positive valued weights $w_n(i)$. The f_n are the number of families of size n.

The weights $w(i)$ are 'U-shaped' or convex in i, and serve to increase the frequencies of families with large number of cases as well as the number of families with no disease cases, all relative to the numbers expected by the binomial distribution. These weights also decrease the frequency of families with a small number of cases.

The weights $w_n(i)$ are normalized for each value of n so that the weighted distribution at (8.3) is a valid distribution and sums to one. Specifically, the weights

$w(i)$ are also functions of n and p such that

$$\sum_{i=0}^{n} w(i) \binom{n}{i} p^i (1-p)^{n-i} = 1 \tag{8.4}$$

for each value of $n = 0, 1, \ldots$ and $0 < p < 1$.

One example of this type of weighted model is described in Section 6.2.2, in which the sample exhibits a length bias. In such a sample, the linear weight function is

$$w_{\mathrm{L}}(i) \;\propto\; i.$$

That is, families with $i = 2$ affected members are twice as likely to be sampled as families with only $i = 1$ affected member. This weight is used by Patil and Rao (1978) to model length or ascertainment bias in samples. This ascertainment bias does not alter the basic shape of the underlying distribution, only its parameters, as explained in Proposition 6.2.1. Specifically, the linear weight function w_{L} used in (8.3) results in another binomial distribution. The function w_{L} is not useful for modeling clustering because it is not strictly convex in i.

Before we go on with specific examples, let us describe the method of model fitting in SAS. A model of the form described in (8.2) and (8.3) for $w \equiv 1$ is a special case of the binomial model for this data, namely

$$\mathrm{E}[\,X_{ni}\,] = f_n \binom{n}{i} p^i (1-p)^{n-i}, \tag{8.5}$$

also described at (6.5).

Models of the form (8.2) and (8.3) can be fit using standard software after we express them as log-linear models. The binomial model in (8.5) can be expressed as the log-linear model

$$\log \mathrm{E}[\,X_{ni}\,] = \log[f_n\, n!(1-p)^n] - \log[i!(n-i)!] + i\, \log[p/(1-p)]. \tag{8.6}$$

The first term in (8.6) acts as an intercept. This first term involves parameters but is not a function of i. The second term $-\log[i!(n-i)!]$ is a function of i but does not involve any parameters to be estimated. Such a term is called the *offset* in SAS. It is included in the model with no estimated regression coefficient. The offset may be a function of i but not unknown parameters. Log-linear models containing an offset are called *flats* by Haberman (1974, Chapter 9).

The last term in (8.6) is a linear regression slope on i. The slope parameter is the log odds $\log[p/(1-p)]$. Additional log-linear models of this form are described in the following sections of this chapter. The maximum likelihood parameter and frequency estimates are obtained in SAS by specifying that the frequencies $\{X_{ni}\}$ behave as independent Poisson random variables with expected values that follow this log-linear model.

It is not necessary to use log-linear models to fit Poisson or binomial distributions, of course. Writing the binomial model in (8.6), however, is the first step in allowing us to generalize to weighted models, as we show next.

8.2 The Altham Distribution

This model was developed by Patricia M.E. Altham. The Altham (1978) distribution of a sum of n exchangeable Bernoulli random variables is

$$\Pr[\, Y_n = i\,] \;\propto\; \binom{n}{i} p^i\,(1-p)^{n-i}\,\exp[\,-\theta i(n-i)] \tag{8.7}$$

for $i = 0, 1, \ldots, n$ and parameters $0 \le p \le 1$ and all real θ.

This distribution is an example of a weighted binomial model of the form (8.2). In the Altham model, we have

$$w_{\mathrm{A}}(i) \;\propto\; \exp[\,-\theta i(n-i)] \tag{8.8}$$

for real parameter θ.

The constant of proportionality is determined so that the probabilities in (8.7) sum to one over $i = 0, 1, \ldots, n$ and for each $n = 1, 2, \ldots$ according to the constraint in (8.4). The special case of $\theta = 0$ reduces $w_{\mathrm{A}} = 1$, corresponding to the binomial (n, p) distribution for all probabilities $0 < p < 1$.

The Altham mass function in (8.7) is proportional to w_{A} times the binomial probability distribution. The specific case of $\theta > 0$ in the Altham model is of the greatest interest to us. Values of $\theta > 0$ in the Altham model (8.7) correspond to our intuition of how the frequencies of clustered cases should occur. (The maximum likelihood estimate of θ is .23 for the IPF data, for example.) A graph of $w_{\mathrm{A}}(i)$ in (8.8) is convex in i for $\theta > 0$. Relative to the binomial distribution, the Altham model with $\theta > 0$ exhibits less frequent families with few cases and more frequent families with many or no cases. The Altham distribution is also flattened in the middle of its range, relative to the binomial distribution, in order to assure that it sums to one.

As a graphical illustration, consider the Altham distribution with parameters $n = 10$ and $p = .3$ plotted on a log scale in Fig. 8.1. The values of θ range from -0.1 to 0.5 by 0.05. The flattening of the Altham model relative to the binomial distribution is illustrated for values of $0.05 \le \theta \le 0.5$. The binomial distribution with $n = 10$ and $p = .3$ is the special case of this Altham distribution for $\theta = 0$. This binomial distribution is plotted in dashed lines to contrast it with the other Altham distributions. All of the Altham distributions flatten the center of the binomial distribution and lengthen both of its tails when $\theta > 0$. Larger values of θ exaggerate this effect. Values of θ greater than 0.35 in this figure start to become bimodal.

Values of $\theta < 0$ corresponding to mutual negative correlations among family members have the opposite effect but are not of interest to us. Two of these distributions are plotted in Fig. 8.1. These distributions have shorter tails than the binomial model with the same value of the p parameter.

Let $\{Z_i, i = 1, 2, \ldots\}$ denote exchangeable Bernoulli indicators of disease status among family members and set

$$Y_n = Z_1 + \cdots + Z_n.$$

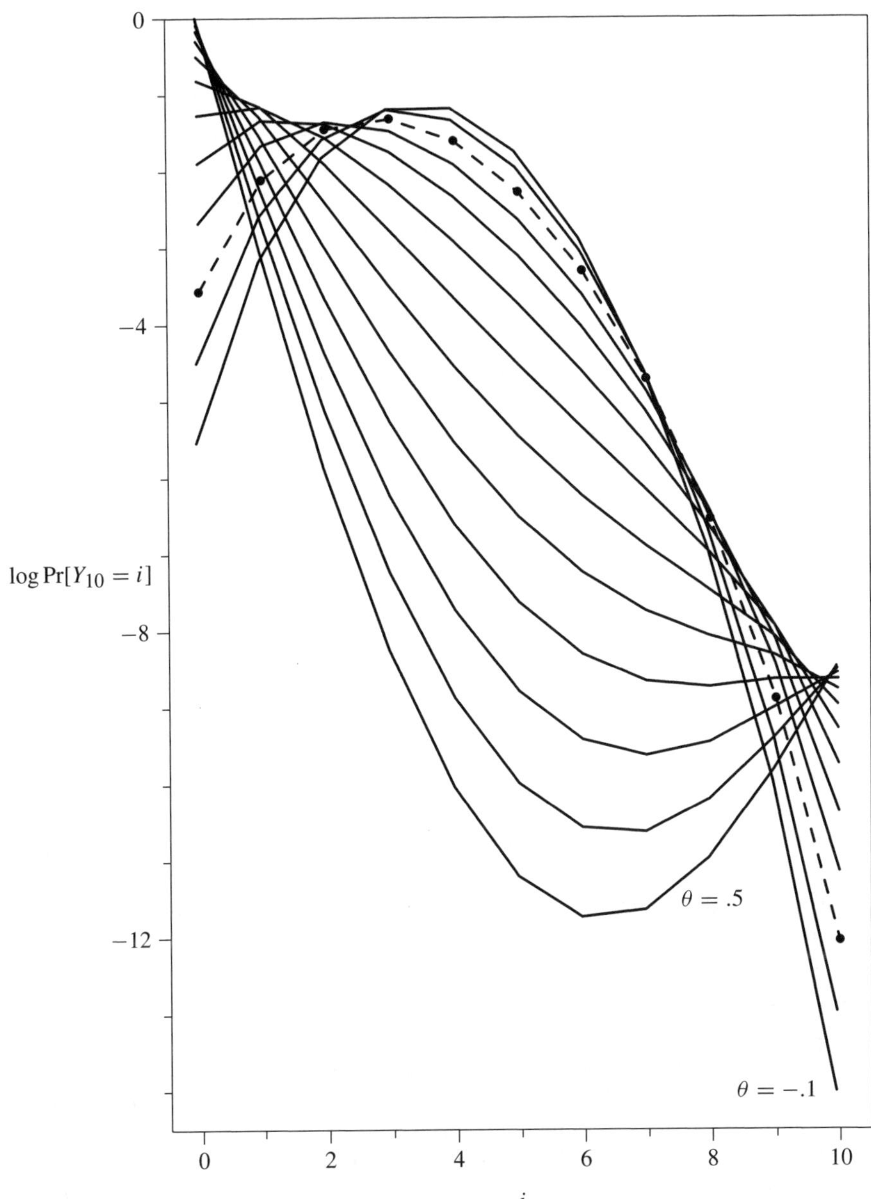

Figure 8.1 The Altham distribution mass function (8.7) plotted on a log scale for $n = 10$, $p = .3$ and values of θ from -0.1 to 0.5 by 0.05. The unweighted ($\theta = 0$) distribution in dashed lines is also the binomial (10, .3).

Let us demonstrate a connection between the parameter θ in the Altham distribution and the log-odds ratio

$$\phi = \log \left\{ \frac{\Pr[\, Z_1 = 1,\ Z_2 = 1\,]\ \Pr[\, Z_1 = 0,\ Z_2 = 0\,]}{\Pr[\, Z_1 = 1,\ Z_2 = 0\,]\ \Pr[\, Z_1 = 0,\ Z_2 = 1\,]} \right\}.$$

Since Z_1 and Z_2 are exchangeable, we have

$$\begin{aligned} \Pr[\, Z_1 = 1,\ Z_2 = 1\,] &= \Pr[\, Y_2 = 2\,] \\ &= p^2 / K_{\mathrm{A}}, \end{aligned}$$

where K_{A} is the normalizing constant

$$K_{\mathrm{A}} = p^2 + 2p(1-p)\mathrm{e}^{-\theta} + (1-p)^2$$

for $n = 2$ in the Altham distribution (8.7).

Similarly we have

$$\begin{aligned} \Pr[\, Z_1 = 0,\ Z_2 = 0\,] &= \Pr[\, Y_2 = 0\,] \\ &= (1-p)^2 / K_{\mathrm{A}} \end{aligned}$$

and

$$\begin{aligned} \Pr[\, Z_1 = 1,\ Z_2 = 0\,] &= \Pr[\, Z_1 = 0,\ Z_2 = 1\,] \\ &= \Pr[\, Y_2 = 1\,]/2 \\ &= p(1-p)\mathrm{e}^{-\theta} / K_{\mathrm{A}} \end{aligned}$$

so that $\phi = 2\theta$.

From this derivation we see that larger values of θ are associated with stronger positive correlations among the disease indicators. As θ becomes larger, the correlation between the exchangeable Bernoulli random variables increases. At a certain point these correlations become so strong that most of the Bernoulli indicators Z_i have the same value and the sum of these Bernoulli's becomes bimodal, as seen in Fig. 8.1. Bimodal distributions of sums of exchangeable random variables are also described in Section 7.3.

In the limit, when θ becomes very large, all of the Bernoulli indicators have the same value and the Altham distribution becomes a pair of point masses at zero or n with probabilities $1 - p$ and p respectively.

The expected values of the Altham distribution with $n = 10$ are plotted in Fig. 8.2 against θ. These expected values were all calculated numerically and generally do not have closed form mathematical expressions. The plotted lines in this figure correspond to values of p from .05 to .95 by .05 from the bottom to the top. Altham (1978) points out that the expected value of this distribution is an increasing function of p, as is clearly the case in this figure. The symmetry of the p parameter shows that

$$\mathrm{E}[\, Y_n \mid p\,] = n - \mathrm{E}[\, Y_n \mid 1-p\,].$$

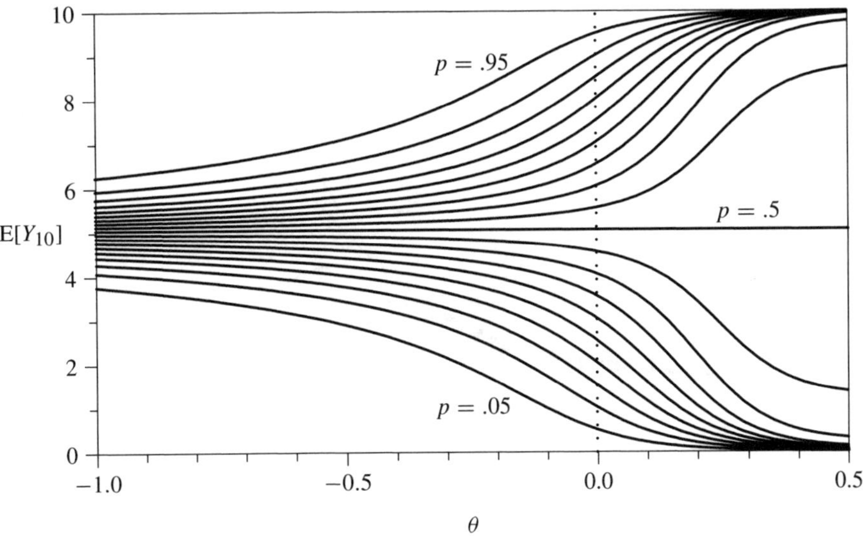

Figure 8.2 Expected value of the Altham distribution for $n = 10$ and values of p from .05 to .95 by .05. The dotted line at $\theta = 0$ corresponds to the binomial distribution.

At the right side of Fig. 8.2, the exchangeable Bernoulli indicators have a strong mutually positive correlation. Such indicators are likely to all have the same value.

At the left side of Fig. 8.2, large negative values of θ correspond to strong mutual negative correlations between the exchangeable Bernoulli indicators. This is achieved when exactly half of the indicators are 0 and 1. In this case, the expected value of Y_n is close to $n/2$ regardless of the value of p.

The standard deviation of the distribution (8.7) is plotted in Fig. 8.3 with values of $p = .05$ to .95 by .05. The symmetry of p shows

$$\text{Var}[\,Y_n \mid p\,] = \text{Var}[\,Y_n \mid 1 - p\,],$$

as is also the case with the binomial distribution.

At the left extreme edge of Fig. 8.2, the Altham distribution has expected value $n/2$ for all p and at the left edge of Fig. 8.3, we see that all of the variances become small. Large negative values of θ result in distributions with small variances. This can be explained as follows. When θ is a large negative, then there is a high probability that exactly half of the strongly negatively correlated indicators Z_i have the value one and exactly half are equal to zero regardless of the value of the p parameter. Such extreme negative correlations among the Bernoulli indicators are unlikely to be useful in practice.

When $p = 1/2$ and θ is a large positive, then the positively correlated Bernoulli indicators are either all 0 or 1 with equal probability. In this case Y_n will equal 0 or n with equal probability and the variance of Y_n will achieve the value of $n^2/4$.

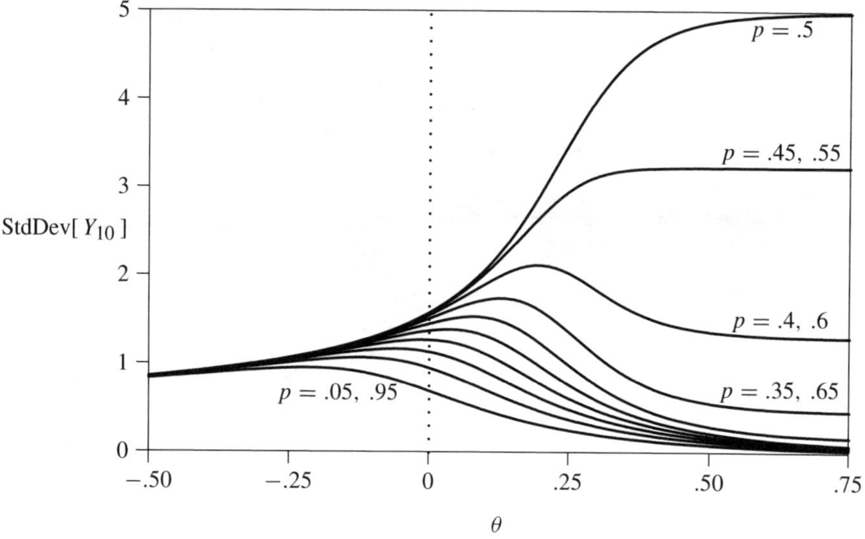

Figure 8.3 Standard deviation of the Altham distribution with $n = 10$. The dotted line at $\theta = 0$ is also the binomial distribution.

Table 8.1 Fitted expected frequencies for the IPF data using the Altham clustering model (8.7). The fitted parameter values are: $\widehat{\theta} = 0.23$ (SE = .12) and $\widehat{p} = .33$ (SE = 0.04). ($\chi^2 = 49.4$, 14 df, $p < 10^{-5}$).

			Affected siblings i						
n	f_n	$\widehat{m}_n$	0	1	2	3	4	5	6
1	48	16.01	31.99	16.01					
2	23	14.57	11.25	8.93	2.82				
3	17	15.15	6.68	6.32	3.16	.838			
4	7	7.68	2.41	2.41	1.43	.603	.151		
6	5	6.58	1.63	1.54	.960	.508	.241	.0965	.0256
Totals	100	60							

The large standard deviation approaching 5 appears at the top of Fig. 8.3. Extreme positive and negative values of θ are of limited use to us.

The fitted expected values of the Altham distribution for the IPF data are given in Table 8.1. The maximum likelihood estimates of $\widehat{\theta} = 0.23$ and $\widehat{p} = .33$ are obtained in SAS using the program given in Section 8.9. The goodness of fit is less than adequate ($\chi^2 = 49.4$, 14 df, $p < 10^{-5}$) but represents a great 1 df improvement over the fit for the unweighted binomial model ($\chi^2 = 312$, 15 df) given in (6.5).

Most of the value of the χ^2 for the Altham-fitted model in Table 8.1 can be traced to the single family of size six with members exhibiting IPF. This single category has an expected count of 0.0256. This single family contributes approximately 1/.0256 or more than 39 to the χ^2 statistic. This single extreme family has already been identified in several analyses of this data. We discuss this example again several times in this chapter.

Unlike the models described in Chapter 7, notice that the Altham model correctly estimates the number of cases in the data so that $\widehat{m} = m$ in Table 8.1. The issue of unbiased estimates of the number of cases is described in Section 8.6.

In order to fit the Altham model in SAS, let us next describe it as a log-linear model. Within the nth row of the triangular shaped family frequency data, the expected counts are f_n times the Altham distribution probability mass function.

Following (8.2) and (8.3), the Altham model is

$$\mathrm{E}[\, X_{ni} \mid w_\mathrm{A}\,] = f_n \exp[\,-\theta i(n-i)\,] \binom{n}{i} p^i\,(1-p)^{n-i}/K_\mathrm{A}$$

for normalizing constant

$$K_\mathrm{A} = \sum_{j=0}^{n} \exp[\,-\theta j(n-j)\,] \binom{n}{j}\, p^j\,(1-p)^{n-j}.$$

The normalizing constant K_A is a function of θ, p and n but not i. The number of families of size n is denoted by f_n. The frequencies X_{ni} are the number of families of size n with i affected members. The log-linear model for the frequencies X_{ni} can be written as

$$\begin{aligned}\log \mathrm{E}[\, X_{ni} \mid w_\mathrm{A}\,] = \log[\, f_n\,(1-p)^n n!/K_\mathrm{A}\,] \;-\; \log[\, i!(n-i)!\,]\\ +\, i\{\log[\, p/(1-p)\,] - n\theta\} + i^2\theta.\end{aligned} \tag{8.9}$$

The first term here is a function of unknown parameters (but not i) and acts as an intercept. The second $-\log[i!(n-i)!]$ term does not involve any estimated parameters. This term is the offset in SAS. The offset in the Altham log-linear model (8.9) is the same as the offset for the binomial model given in (8.6).

Implicit in writing the log-linear model for the Altham distribution in the form (8.9) is that i is the observed value of the random variable Y_n in (8.3). That is,

$$\mathrm{E}[\, X_{ni}\,] = f_n \;\Pr[\, Y_n = i\,].$$

The intercept in (8.9) is not a function of i. The offset term may depend on i but not on any parameters to be estimated. The log-linear model expressed in (8.9) demonstrates that the Altham model can be fit as a log-linear regression on i and i^2 with frequencies X_{ni}.

A drawback to writing the Altham model in the form (8.9) is that most computer packages will not be able to separately estimate parameters p and θ, nor will these packages provide separate variance estimates.

A better parameterization of the model (8.9) is

$$\begin{aligned} \mathrm{E}[\, X_{ni} \mid w_{\mathrm{A}}\,] = \log[\, f_n(1-p)^n n!/K_{\mathrm{A}}\,] - \log[\, i!(n-i)!\,] \\ + i \log[\, p/(1-p)\,] - i(n-i)\theta. \end{aligned}$$

Written in this form, most packages will provide separate maximum likelihood estimates $\widehat{\theta}$ of θ and an estimate of the log odds

$$\widehat{l} = \log[\, \widehat{p}/(1-\widehat{p})\,]$$

as the fitted coefficient for regression on i.

We can then write

$$\widehat{p} = \exp(\widehat{l})/(1+\exp(\widehat{l}))$$

to obtain the maximum likelihood estimate $\widehat{p}$ from $\widehat{l}$.

Given the software estimate of the variance of $\widehat{l}$, we can use the delta-method to approximate

$$\begin{aligned} \mathrm{Var}[\,\widehat{p}\,] &\approx (\partial\widehat{p}/\partial\widehat{l}\,)^2 \mathrm{Var}[\,\widehat{l}\,] \\ &= [\,\widehat{p}(1-\widehat{p})\,]^2 \mathrm{Var}[\,\widehat{l}\,] \end{aligned}$$

or

$$\mathrm{SE}[\,\widehat{p}\,] \approx \widehat{p}(1-\widehat{p})\,\mathrm{SE}[\,\widehat{l}\,]$$

in order to obtain a variance estimate of $\widehat{p}$ from the software. This is the method used to estimate the SE of $\widehat{p}$ in this section and the following.

This completes the discussion of the Altham distribution in the context of weighted distributions (8.2). We next provide an application of this model using the mortality data of Brazilian children given in Table 6.3. Following that example, we propose two additional choices for the weights $w(i)$ that modify the basic model provided by the binomial distribution towards the definition of clustering proposed in this chapter.

8.3 Application to Childhood Mortality Data

The set of models described here is motivated by the pattern of outlying frequencies displayed in Table 6.9 for the Brazilian childhood mortality data. Table 6.9 is copied here as Table 8.2 for convenience. This data is also examined in Section 6.3.3. The extremely poor fit of the binomial model ($\chi^2 = 2300$, 35 df) suggests that there is considerable modeling needed to explain this data. The models considered are based on the Altham distribution just described in the previous section.

Table 8.2 Unusually large frequencies in the Brazilian family data are given by + and counts much smaller than expected are denoted with a −.

			Number of affected siblings i							
n	f_n	m_n	0	1	2	3	4	5	6	7+
1	267	12	255	12−						
2	285	48	239	44−	2					
3	202	80	143	41	15	3				
4	110	54	69	30	9	2	0			
5	104	103	43	34	15	9+	3+	0		
6	50	67	15	18	8	5	3+	0	1+	
7	21	38	4	4	7	4	2+	0	0	0
8	12	28	1	2	4	3	1	1+	0	0
Totals	2946	430								

Table 8.2 demonstrates a striking pattern of extreme positive and negative residuals. Frequencies of multiple childhood deaths in the same family are much larger than expected in several large families. Conversely, many small families have mortality frequencies that are much lower than expected. This suggests that the binomial p parameter varies with the size of the family in this data. In other words, the incidence of deaths appears to be directly related to the family size. Smaller families experienced fewer deaths than expected and larger families had many more.

The θ parameter in the Altham distribution can be used to model the clustering of cases within families, relative to the binomial distribution. We might also ask if the pattern of clustering, as measured by θ, also varies with family size. The separate concepts of incidence rate and clustering are described in Section 6.1.3. The Altham model is a good choice for illustrating these separate concepts because there are two different parameters to describe these. The p parameter measures incidence and θ models the amount of clustering.

As in the models of Chapter 6, the expected frequency of X_{ni} is the number f_n of families of size n times a binomial distribution

$$\mathrm{E}[\,X_{ni}\,] = f_n \binom{n}{i} p^i\,(1-p)^{n-i}, \tag{8.10}$$

under the null hypothesis that mortality affected all children independent of their siblings and family size.

The pattern of extreme residuals in Table 8.2 suggests that the binomial p parameter is not constant throughout the data set. In particular, the pattern of large positive and negative outliers in Table 8.2 suggests that p is increasing with the family size n. A popular method for modeling the binomial p parameter is through the use of logistic regression. In this example, we need to regress p on the family size and we will use the logit model to accomplish this.

Specifically, let us set

$$\text{logit}(p) = \log[p/(1-p)] = \alpha + n\beta$$

or

$$p = p_n = \exp(\alpha + n\beta)/[1 + \exp(\alpha + n\beta)]$$

in (8.10).

Then we can write

$$\log \text{E}[\,X_{ni}\,] = \log\{\, f_n\, n!/[1 + \exp(\alpha + n\beta]^n\} - \log[i!(n-i)!] + i\alpha + ni\beta. \tag{8.11}$$

This is the form of the log-linear model discussed in this chapter beginning with (8.6) and including (8.9).

The first term

$$\log\{\, f_n\, n!/[1 + \exp(\alpha + n\beta]^n\}$$

in (8.11) acts as an intercept. There is a separate intercept for every family size n.

The second term

$$-\log[i!(n-i)!]$$

in (8.11) is the same offset as for the binomial and Altham log-linear models given in (8.6) and (8.9), respectively. Finally, there are coefficients α and β for regressing on the variables i and ni respectively.

We could also simplify the expression (8.11) and use an abbreviated notation

$$\log \text{E}[\,X_{ni}\,] = \text{intercept}(n) + \text{offset}(i) + i\alpha + ni\beta.$$

Including the θ term of the Altham distribution gives us

$$\text{E}[\,X_{ni}\,] \propto f_n \binom{n}{i} [1 + \exp(\alpha + n\beta)]^{-n} [\exp(\alpha + n\beta)]^i \exp[\,-\theta i(n-i)\,]$$

and the corresponding log-linear model,

$$\log \text{E}[\,X_{ni}\,] = \text{intercept}(n) + \text{offset}(i) + i\alpha + ni\beta - i(n-i)\theta. \tag{8.12}$$

The intercept contains the normalizing constant K_{A} that is different for different choices of n, α and β but K_{A} is not a function of i. This log-linear model contains an intercept, an offset and regression slopes on i, ni and $i(n-i)$. Equivalently, we could also regress on i, ni, and i^2 but as pointed out at the end of the preceding section, the present model formulation offers computational advantages when using standard software. As with the binomial and Altham models, the offset here is equal to $-\log[i!(n-i)!]$.

We also found it useful for models of the mortality data to include a quadratic term in the logit of p. That is,

$$\text{logit}(p_n) = \log[p/(1-p)] = \alpha + n\beta + n^2\gamma.$$

The corresponding log-linear model with a quadratic logit and Altham parameter is then

$$\log \text{E}[\,X_{ni}\,] = \text{intercept}(n) + \text{offset}(i) + i\alpha + ni\beta + n^2 i\gamma - i(n-i)\theta.$$

This demonstrates how the p parameter can be described in a log-linear model identifying varying childhood mortality rates across different family sizes. We can also model how the degree of clustering changes with family size. Let us ask if the mortality patterns in larger families behave less as expected by the binomial distribution than the pattern seen in smaller families. Is the mortality status of family members more or less correlated depending on the size of the family? Let us next show how to model changing values of θ with the family size.

Begin by writing

$$\theta = \theta_n = \xi + n\psi \tag{8.13}$$

for parameters ξ and ψ to be estimated.

Positive values of ψ indicate a greater positive dependence among the Bernoulli indicators of childhood mortality status within larger sized families. Values of θ near zero are indicative of independence of mortality status.

The largest model we consider for this data contains a logit (p) that is quadratic in family size n and an Altham parameter θ that is linear in n. This model is given by

$$\begin{aligned} \text{E}[\,X_{ni}\,] \propto f_n \binom{n}{i} [1 + \exp(\alpha + n\beta + n^2\gamma)]^{-n} \\ \times [\exp(\alpha + n\beta + n^2\gamma)]^i \ \exp\{-(\xi + n\psi)[\,i(n-i)\,]\} \end{aligned}$$

or

$$\begin{aligned} \log \text{E}[\,X_{ni}\,] = \text{intercept}(n) + \text{offset}(i) \\ + i\alpha + ni\beta + n^2 i\gamma - i(n-i)\xi - ni(n-i)\psi. \end{aligned} \tag{8.14}$$

Log-linear regression on $-i(n-i)$ here is the term for fitting a single Altham θ parameter in the model. The regression on $-ni(n-i)$ allows us to model change in the Altham θ parameter with family size.

All of these combinations of log-linear models are summarized in Table 8.3. The p parameters are expressed as either constant, linear or quadratic logistic models of the family size n with parameters α, β, and γ respectively. There are also three different models of mutual dependence among family members

Table 8.3 Deviance of log-linear models for the Brazilian children data.

	Binomial $\theta = 0$		Altham model with a single θ		Models (8.13) and (8.14) with $\theta = \xi + n\psi$	
Logit p	Dev	df	Dev	df	Dev	df
Constant	152.10	35	144.30	34	106.73	33
Linear	59.70	34	38.98	33	38.44	32
Quadratic	56.86	33	29.91	32	21.45	31

through the weight function. The choice of weight function fits a binomial ($\xi = \psi = 0$) distribution, the Altham model (8.9) with a single value of θ, and the Altham model (8.14) in which $\theta = \theta_n$ varies linearly with the family size according to (8.13).

Every combination of models is fitted to this data and these are summarized in Table 8.3. Every row in Table 8.3 represents an addition of one parameter to the previous row. Every row in this table summarizes a different logistic model for the p parameter. Similarly, the pairs of columns of this table represent the addition of one parameter to the column on their left. The binomial model does not include the Altham θ parameter. The Altham columns add a single θ parameter for the whole data set. The last pair of columns summarizes models that estimate ξ and ψ, allowing the Altham θ parameter to vary across family sizes according to (8.13). All of these models can be fit using the SAS program in Section 8.9.

Two models in adjacent rows or columns in this table are nested and differ by one parameter. The differences of the deviances of these nested models represent 1 df chi-squared tests and almost all identify a large improvement over the simpler model. The sparse nature of the original data suggests that the chi-squared approximation may not be valid. Haberman (1978) provides conditions for the differences of deviances to behave as chi-squared. His general conclusion is that the difference of the deviances of two nested models may often behave as chi-squared even though the individual deviances do not. This topic of the chi-squared approximation to the behavior of the deviance is also discussed in Section 6.3.

The largest of the models summarized in Table 8.3 represents a very good fit: $\chi^2 = 20.89$, 31 df, $p = .91$. This model (8.14) offers a huge improvement over the simple binomial model with the addition of only four parameters. Summary statistics of the fitted parameters for this model are given in Table 8.4. The residuals of this model are plotted in Fig. 8.5. All of the chi-squared residuals are smaller than 2 in absolute magnitude.

Fitted parameter values for p and θ are plotted in Fig. 8.4 against the family size n. In the smallest sized families, children in one-child families have an estimated mortality rate of under 7%. This mortality rate increases with family size and appears to level off at about 30% among the largest families in this data.

Table 8.4 Parameter estimates in model (8.14) for the Brazilian children.

Parameter	Estimate	Std Err	Wald Chi-squared	p-value
Logit(p) intercept i	−3.52	.27	169.21	< .0001
Linear logit ni	.87	.14	36.36	< .0001
Quadratic logit n^2i	−.067	.018	14.35	.0002
θ_n intercept ξ $-i(n-i)$	.623	.15	17.08	< .0001
θ_n slope ψ $-ni(n-i)$	−.0727	.027	7.55	.0060

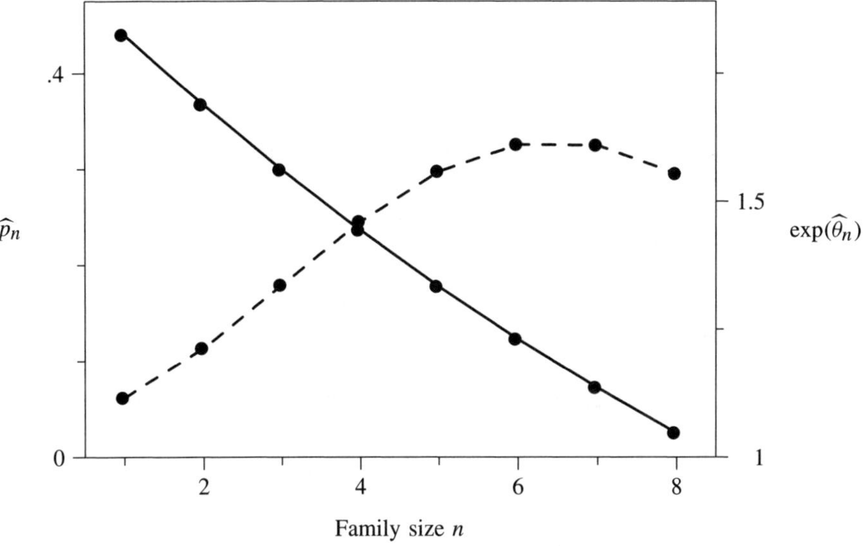

Figure 8.4 Estimated $\widehat{p}$ parameters for the Brazilian children (dashes, left scale) and Altham $\widehat{\theta}$ parameter (solid line, right scale) fitted to model (8.14). The mortality rate p increases and then levels off with family size but family members' mortality becomes more independent of others as θ approaches zero.

The θ parameter decreases with family size. Smallest families have an estimated θ of 0.62 and these parameters decrease to almost zero with the largest sized families. Values of the estimated θ are plotted on an exponential scale in order to encourage their interpretation as odds. In this figure, there is an estimated high positive dependence among members of small families. Members of larger families tend to have independent mortality status.

To summarize this analysis of the childhood mortality data, small families have the lowest mortality rate. This rate increases with family size up to about

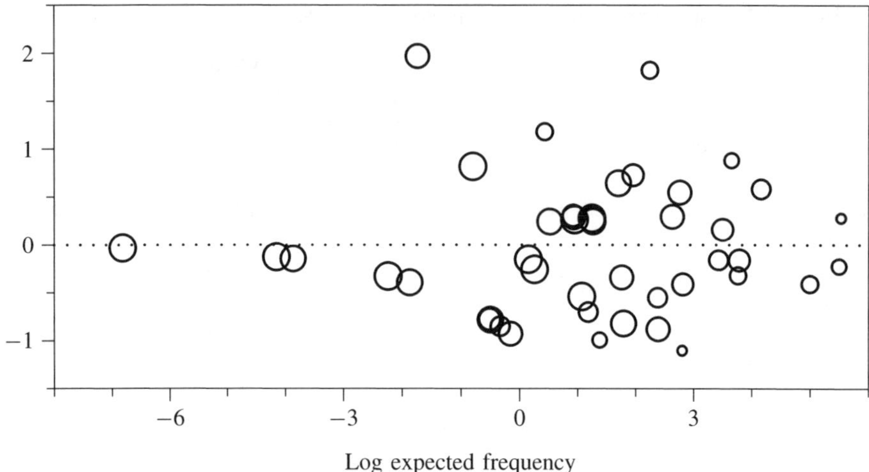

Figure 8.5 Residual bubble plot for Brazilian children with frequencies in Table 8.2. Bubble areas are proportional to the family size. The log-linear Altham model (8.14) contains quadratic logit parameters for p parameter.

five children, then appears to level off or even drop slightly. The fitted Altham model shows a high degree of positive dependence in the survival among children in smaller families. As family sizes increase, the patterns of mortality appear to follow a binomial model with independence in survival among the children.

These two parameters of the Altham model can be used in this fashion to separately estimate incidence and clustering, as described in Section 6.1.3. We next demonstrate other possible weight functions and their corresponding log-linear models.

8.4 A Log-linear Weighted Distribution

A useful one parameter example of a weight function w is

$$w_1(i) \propto i!\,\mathrm{e}^{-i\beta}, \tag{8.15}$$

where the parameter β is to be estimated.

All values of β in this model provide the proper convex 'U' shape necessary to conform to the definition of clustering used in this chapter. The constant of proportionality in (8.15) is determined by the constraint given by (8.4) and is given below, at (8.19). The constant of proportionality depends on n, β, and p but not i.

Unlike the Altham model, the binomial distribution is not a special case of the w_1 weighted distribution. There is no value of β in (8.15) that gives us $w_1 = 1$, corresponding to the binomial distribution. The binomial distribution is not nested within the w_1 weighted distribution so we cannot use a likelihood ratio test to compare these two models.

The w_1 weighted binomial distribution of Y_n is a right-truncated Poisson distribution that is reversed, left to right. To demonstrate this, let us write

$$w_1(i)\binom{n}{i}\, p^i(1-p)^{n-i} \;\propto\; (n!p^n \mathrm{e}^{-n\beta})\,\lambda^{n-i}/(n-i)! \qquad (8.16)$$

for

$$\lambda = \mathrm{e}^{\beta}\,(1-p)/p \qquad (8.17)$$

and $i = 0, 1, \ldots, n$.

The constant of proportionality and normalizing constant in (8.16) depends on n and parameters (p, β) but not the number of affected siblings i. This term plays the role of the intercept in the log-linear model, as we will see at (8.20) below. The only terms in (8.16) involving i, the number of affected siblings in a family of size n, are

$$\lambda^{n-i}/(n-i)!.$$

If we ignore the normalizing constant in (8.16), we see that the number of *unaffected* siblings $n - Y_n$ follows a truncated Poisson distribution defined on $0, \ldots, n$. The number of unaffected family members is represented by $n - i$, where i is the number of affected cases out of the n total members of the family.

Examples of the distribution resulting from the choice of w_1 in (8.3) are plotted on a log scale in Fig. 8.6 for $n = 10$, $p = .3$, and values of λ specified. This figure includes the binomial (10, .3) distribution for comparison. This binomial reference distribution is also plotted in Fig. 8.1 for the Altham distribution. In both figures, the binomial distribution is plotted using dashed lines to make it stand out in comparison. When we compare these two figures, note how the w_1 distribution greatly increases both tails, but especially the upper tail, and generally flattens the center. This distortion of the binomial distribution is even more extreme in Fig. 8.6 than the examples plotted for the Altham distribution in Fig. 8.1.

The Altham distribution can be bimodal, as we see in Fig. 8.1. The Poisson distribution is unimodal, as well as its truncated and reversed versions. The w_1 weighted binomial distribution will never have two separated local modes.

The w_1 model is log-linear in its parameter λ, and can be fitted by the SAS program of Section 8.9. Let us describe how the w_1 weighted model is fitted using this software by describing it as a log-linear model.

The expected value of the family frequency X_{ni} under the w_1 weighted model can be written as

$$\mathrm{E}[\,X_{ni} \mid w_1\,] = f_n\,\lambda^{n-i}/[(n-i)!\,K_1], \qquad (8.18)$$

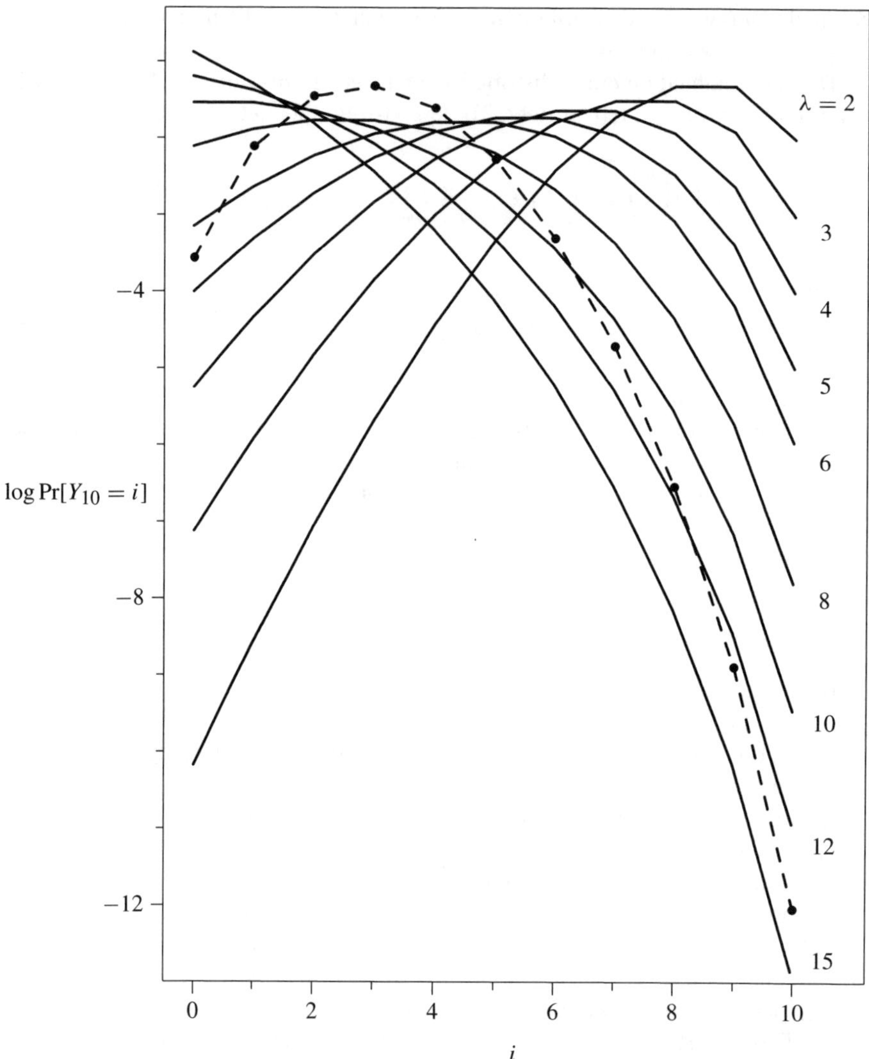

Figure 8.6 The w_1 distribution plotted on a log scale for $n = 10$ and values of λ as given. The unweighted binomial (10, .3) distribution is plotted in dashed lines for comparison with Fig. 8.1 but is not a member of the w_1 family.

where the normalizing constant is

$$K_1 = \sum_{j=0}^{n} \lambda^j / j! \tag{8.19}$$

and λ is given in (8.17).

Table 8.5 Fitted expected frequencies for the IPF data using the w_1 weighted model (8.15). The fitted parameter value is $\widehat{\lambda} = 3.62$ with SE = .35 ($\chi^2 = 12.86$, 15 df; $p = .61$).

			Number of affected siblings i						
n	f_n	$\widehat{m}_n$	0	1	2	3	4	5	6
1	48	10.38	37.62	10.38					
2	23	11.56	13.49	7.45	2.06				
3	17	14.95	7.05	5.84	3.22	.890			
4	7	9.57	1.91	2.11	1.75	.965	.266		
6	5	13.53	.453	.751	1.04	1.14	.948	.523	.144
Totals	100	60							

The normalizing constant K_1 is a function of n and λ. This denominator is determined by (8.4) so that w_1 times the binomial mass function is a valid distribution and sums to one. We can then write

$$\log \mathrm{E}[\, X_{ni} \mid w_1 \,] = \log[f_n \, \lambda^n / K_1] - \log[(n-i)!] - i \log(\lambda) \, . \tag{8.20}$$

The first term in (8.20) is a function of n and λ and acts as an intercept in this log-linear model. The intercept is not a function of i. The second $-\log[(n-i)!]$ term does not involve any estimated parameters. This second term is the offset. This offset is different from that of the binomial and Altham models.

The final term in (8.20) contains a regression slope to be estimated. The parameter for the regression slope on i is $-\log(\lambda)$.

This completes the description of the w_1 weighted model (8.20) as a log-linear model. The model has been reparameterized so that the two parameters to be estimated are an intercept and a slope on i.

The w_1 weighted model has a greatly improved fit over the binomial model (8.6) for the IPF data. The expected frequencies for this data are given in Table 8.5. The goodness of fit is excellent: $\chi^2 = 12.9$, 15 df, $p = .6$. The estimated value of λ is 3.62 with an estimated standard error of 0.35. The K_1 constant of proportionality in (8.15) can be found from the intercept in this log-linear model, but this is generally of limited interest to us.

Finally we note that the w_1 weighted model correctly estimates the number of disease cases in Table 8.5. That is, the estimate of $\widehat{m}$ of m is equal to the observed value 60. This point is discussed again in Section 8.6 in more generality.

8.5 Quadratic Weighted Distributions

Another useful model for $w(i)$ in (8.2) is

$$w_2(i) \;\propto\; \exp(i\beta_1 + i^2\beta_2) \tag{8.21}$$

with two parameters, β_1 and β_2.

When $\beta_2 \geq 0$, the w_2 weight function also has a convex shape and provides a meaningful mathematical representation corresponding to our definition of disease clustering. This two-parameter model for disease clustering is

$$\mathrm{E}[\, X_{ni} \mid w_2\,] \;=\; f_n \exp(i\beta_1 + i^2\beta_2) \binom{n}{i} p^i (1-p)^{n-i} / K_2. \tag{8.22}$$

The normalizing constant K_2 corresponding to w_2 is

$$K_2 = \sum_j \exp(j\beta_1 + j^2\beta_2) \binom{n}{j} p^j (1-p)^{n-j}.$$

This normalizing constant is a function of n, β_1, β_2, and p but not i. The log-linear model used in fitting (8.22) with the w_2 weighted distribution is given by

$$\log \mathrm{E}[\, X_{ni} \mid w_2\,] = \mathrm{intercept}(n) - \log[i!(n-i)!]$$
$$+\, i\,[\beta_1 \log(p/(1-p))] + i^2\beta_2. \tag{8.23}$$

This model is also fitted in SAS with the program given in Section 8.9. The model (8.23) is a log-linear regression on i and i^2. The offset term in the log-linear model $-\log[i!(n-i)!]$ is a function of i but does not depend on any parameter to be estimated. The offset term in (8.23) is the same as the offset for both the Altham model in (8.9) and the binomial model at (8.6).

Written as the log-linear model in (8.23), it is clear that the β_1 and p parameters are confounded and cannot be estimated separately. The parameter that is linear in i will be denoted by

$$\eta = \exp(\beta_1)\, p/(1-p) \tag{8.24}$$

for the w_2 weighted model.

Similarly, it is sufficient to consider weights

$$w_2'(i) \;\propto\; \exp(i^2\beta)$$

in (8.21) in order to achieve the same model as in (8.22) and (8.23).

The parameters for the w_2' model are β and η given in (8.24). The fitted values for the w_2' model with the IPF data are given in Table 8.6 and the residuals are plotted in Fig. 8.7.

A more general weighted model of the form

$$w_3(i) \;\propto\; \exp(\beta\, i^{\phi}) \tag{8.25}$$

is also possible but the corresponding model (8.2) and (8.3) is not log-linear in the parameter ϕ and cannot be fitted using standard software unless ϕ is specified.

The fitted expected frequencies of the w_2 model for the IPF data are given in Table 8.6. The overall fit as measured by ($\chi^2 = 9.69$, 14 df, $p = .78$) is one of the best of any model we consider for this data. This measure of fit is just behind that of the incremental risk model described in Section 7.2.3.

Table 8.6 Fitted expected frequencies w_2 for the IPF data using the disease clustering model (8.22). The fitted parameter values are: $\widehat{\eta} = -1.53$ (SE = 0.24) and $\widehat{\beta} = .26$ (SE = 0.06) $\chi^2 = 9.69$, 14 df, $p = .78$.

			Number of affected siblings i						
n	f_n	$\widehat{m}_n$	0	1	2	3	4	5	6
1	48	10.50	37.50	10.50					
2	23	11.18	13.61	7.61	1.78				
3	17	14.08	7.28	6.11	2.86	.747			
4	7	9.05	2.03	2.27	1.59	.832	.273		
6	5	15.20	.433	.727	.850	.888	.872	.764	.467
Totals	100	60							

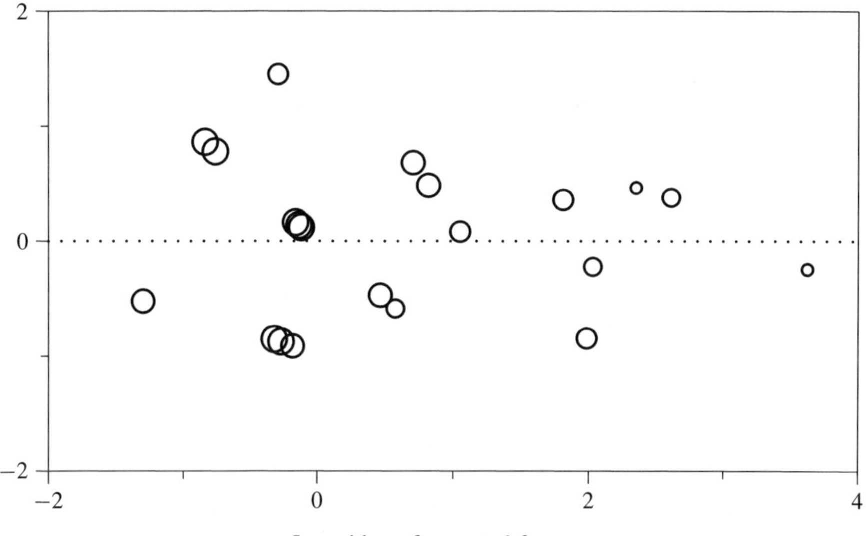

Figure 8.7 Bubble plot of chi-squared residuals for the IPF/COPD data plotted against log-fitted value. The w_2 weighted distribution model (8.22) is fitted and the expected counts are given in Table 8.6.

The fitted means of model (8.22) are given in Table 8.6 for the IPF/COPD data. The chi-squared residuals of this fitted clustering model are given in the bubble plot of Fig. 8.7. The areas of the bubbles are proportional to the sizes of the families that make up each residual. There were few large-sized families in the observed data and these had correspondingly smaller estimated frequencies.

The horizontal axis in Fig. 8.7 is the logarithm of the fitted expected value. Almost half of the fitted means are smaller than one. Taking logs of the expected counts spreads these values out and makes this plot easier to see. The largest absolute residual is less than 1.5 and all others are less than 1 in magnitude. This is indicative of a very good fit for the model (8.22).

8.6 Weighted Distributions in General

Let us develop some properties of weighted distributions of the form (8.2), in general terms. The form of the log-linear models described so far in this chapter is

$$\log \mathrm{E}[\, X_{ni} \,] = \text{intercept}(n) + \text{offset}(i) + i\theta_1, \tag{8.26}$$

corresponding to the binomial model given in (8.6) and the w_1 weighted distribution given in (8.20).

We also have models with a quadratic term

$$\log \mathrm{E}[\, X_{ni} \,] = \text{intercept}(n) + \text{offset}(i) + i\theta_1 + i^2\theta_2,$$

as in the Altham in (8.9) and the w_2 weighted distribution in (8.23).

These log-linear models all contain a term that is linear in the number i of affected family members. The intercept can be a function of unknown parameters and n but does not depend on i. The intercept is specified in the computer program as a separate indicator variable for each n-sized family. If there is a separate intercept for each n, then there is no need to include f_n in the program. This point is demonstrated below in Lemma 8.6.1. The models in Chapter 7 are generally not log-linear in their parameters and not expressible in the form (8.26).

The offset can contain functions of i but not parameters to be estimated. Useful choices of the offset include

$$-\log[\, i!(n-1)!\,]$$

as in the binomial, w_2, and Altham log-linear models, and

$$-\log[\,(n-i)!\,]$$

as in the w_1 weighted distribution at (8.20).

Additional terms could also be added to these models that are linear in their parameters. Such additional terms could include $i^2\theta_2$ as in the Altham model for example, or more generally be of the form

$$f_3(i)\,\theta_3 + f_4(i)\,\theta_4 + \cdots .$$

The functions $f_3,\ f_4 \ldots$ depend on i but not other parameters. The models in Section 8.3 include examples where $f_3,\ f_4, \ldots$ are polynomials in i and n.

The parameters $\theta_2,\ \theta_3, \ldots$ are said to be linear in i even though the functions of i are not themselves linear. The weighted binomial distribution of Kocherlakota and Kocherlakota (1990), for example, uses $w(i) \propto i^{\psi}$ and is also of this form with $f_3 = \log(i)$. The w_3 weight function given in (8.25) is not expressible in this form if the parameter ϕ is to be estimated.

Log-linear models containing an offset term are referred to as *flats* by Haberman (1974, Chapter 9). In terms of the space spanned by varying the parameters of the log-linear model, a model containing an offset is not a linear space, but rather an *affine* linear space. An affine space is a linear space that might not contain the origin. Instead, an affine linear space is a plane that is located at a fixed offset from the origin, hence the name used by SAS. All of what we know about log-linear models also holds true for affine models as well.

Specifically, in this section we use the *Birch criteria* for estimating parameters in log-linear models. Briefly, the Birch criteria for log-linear models (Birch 1963; Zelterman 1999, p 115–8) asserts that maximum likelihood estimates for parameters of log-linear models for Poisson data are determined by equating sufficient sums of data with the corresponding sums taken over the expected counts. Although Birch (1963) is only concerned with a single specific setting, these conditions hold more generally and continue to be referred to as the Birch criteria.

We next use the Birch criteria to explain a situation encountered in Chapter 7. Specific examples appear in Tables 7.2, 7.3 and 7.4. In each of these tables, the estimated number of affected cases $\widehat{m}$ is not equal to the observed value, m. Specifically, the observed number of cases

$$m = \sum_{n} \sum_{i=0}^{n} i\, X_{ni}$$

and the estimated number of cases

$$\widehat{m} = \sum_{n} \sum_{i} i\, \mathrm{E}[\, X_{ni} \mid \text{fitted parameters}\,] \tag{8.27}$$

are not generally equal for the models of Chapter 7.

The models of Chapter 7 are not log-linear in their parameters so the Birch criteria are not applicable to them. On the other hand, fitted values for the weighted distributions given in Tables 8.1, 8.5 and 8.6 all exhibit equality of the number of diseased cases m in the observed data and its estimate $\widehat{m}$.

The following lemma shows that the number of cases m and the family size frequencies $\boldsymbol{f} = \{f_n\}$ need not be specified in the computer program for fitting log-linear models of weighted binomial distributions for family frequency data. In many of these models, estimates of $\boldsymbol{f}$ and m are equal to their observed values.

Lemma 8.6.1 *If the affine log-linear model contains a separate intercept for each value of n, then the fitted number of families of size n is equal to the observed value f_n. If the affine log-linear model contains a linear term in i, then the estimated number of cases $\widehat{m}$ is equal to the observed value m.*

Proof. Sufficient statistics for parameters in the log-linear model are

$$\sum_n \sum_i^n X_{ni} \log \mathrm{E}[\, X_{ni}\,]$$

$$= \sum_{ni} X_{ni}[\text{intercept}(n) + \text{offset}(i) + i\theta_1 + \text{other terms}] \tag{8.28}$$

for independent Poisson distributed counts X_{ni}.

For the weighted distributions considered here, the number of families of size n

$$f_n = \sum_i X_{ni}$$

and the total sample size

$$N = \sum_n \sum_i X_{ni}$$

are sufficient statistics corresponding to the intercepts. As a consequence of the Birch criteria, the sum over all fitted expected values of the weighted log-linear models provide unbiased estimates of the total sample size N and the individual f_n.

The offset does not contain any unknown parameters. Similarly, the term

$$\sum_{ni} X_{ni} \,\text{offset}(i)$$

in (8.28) is not a sufficient statistic corresponding to any parameters to be estimated.

Finally, the linear term in (8.28)

$$\sum_{ni} i\, X_{ni} = m$$

corresponding to θ_1, is equal to m, the number of affected cases in the sample.

The proof is completed by noting that m is a sufficient marginal sum in log-linear models with a linear term in i. The Birch criteria asserts that the corresponding sum over maximum likelihood fitted expected values $\widehat{m}$ given in (8.27) is equal to the observed value m. ■

The Birch conditions are not specific to Poisson distributed data and apply to log-linear models of other distributions as well (*cf.* Waller and Zelterman, 1997).

Let us next identify another interpretation of the weight functions w. Specifically, the weights $w(i)$ can be interpreted as odds ratios relative to the binomial model and the frequency of families with zero disease cases.

Let $\mathrm{E}_0[X_{ni}]$ denote expectation with respect to the binomial model (8.5) of homogeneous risk among all family members. Similarly, let $\mathrm{E}_w[X_{ni}]$ denote

Table 8.7 Weight ratios $w(i)/w(0)$ for the Altham, w_1, and w_2 models fitted to the IPF frequency data in families of size $n = 6$.

	Number of affected siblings i						
Model	0	1	2	3	4	5	6
Altham (8.8)	1	.375	.223	.211	.318	.759	2.87
w_1 (8.15)	1	.658	.866	1.71	4.50	14.8	58.4
w_2 (8.21)	1	.667	.744	1.39	4.34	22.6	198.

expectation with respect to the general weighted distribution model (8.2) and (8.3). The weights $w(i)$ satisfy

$$w(i)/w(0) = \frac{\mathrm{E}_w [\, X_{ni} \,] \, \mathrm{E}_0 [\, X_{n0} \,]}{\mathrm{E}_w [\, X_{n0} \,] \, \mathrm{E}_0 [\, X_{ni} \,]}. \tag{8.29}$$

Intuitivcly we can speak of the weights $w(i)$ as the relative risk of i affected family members relative to the binomial model for $i = 1, 2, \ldots$. Table 8.7 illustrates this relative risk and demonstrates the convex 'U' shape of the $w(i)$ for fitted models of the form (8.2) in the IPF data. The weights are for the Altham w_1 and w_2 functions described here. In all three cases, relative to the number of families with no affected siblings, these models anticipate fewer families with 1 or 2 cases than are expected by the binomial model. Relatively many more families with 4 or more cases are expected for the w_1 and w_2 weighted distributions.

The fitted weights w_A of the Altham distribution are less extreme in their effects, as seen in Table 8.7. The effects of the Altham distribution are to increase the relative number of families with all six members with IPF. This effect of the Altham distribution is more subtle than the effects of the w_1 and w_2 weighted distributions. This coincides with our definition of clustering used in this chapter. Table 8.7 demonstrates the convex 'U'-shape required for the $w(i)$ weights in (8.2).

8.7 Family History Log-linear Model

The family history distribution described in Section 7.2.2 and exchangeable family history distribution in Section 7.3.1 each have analogies to the weighted binomial distributions described in this chapter. Once one family member has been identified as a diseased case, then the risk for the remaining members is changed under these two different family history distributions. In this section, we develop a weighted binomial model that has the same interpretation.

The exchangeable family history distribution with mass function given in (7.18) is

$$\Pr[\, Y_n = i \,] = \begin{cases} 1 - p'[1 - (1-p)^n]/p & \text{for } i = 0 \\ \binom{n}{i} p' \, p^{i-1} (1-p)^{n-i} & \text{for } i = 1, \ldots, n. \end{cases} \tag{8.30}$$

This distribution has a clear analogy to the binomial distribution. For $i = 1, \ldots, n$, we see that the mass function is the same as that for the binomial (n, p) multiplied by the weight p'/p. The probability of zero events is whatever is left over in order to make the mass function sum to one over i.

The analogous weight function w_{FH} for use in (8.3) takes the form

$$w_{FH}(i) = \begin{cases} \exp(\theta')/K_{FH} & \text{for } i = 0 \\ \exp(\theta)/K_{FH} & \text{for } i = 1, \ldots, n \end{cases} \tag{8.31}$$

In other words, there is a different weight once one case has been recorded in the family. There is a clear analogy with these sets of weights to the conditional probabilities given in (7.9).

The normalizing constant in (8.4)

$$K_{FH} = \exp(\theta')(1-p)^n + \exp(\theta)[1-(1-p)^n]$$

assures that the probabilities in this weighted distribution sum to unity.

Written as a log-linear model, we have

$$\log \mathrm{E}[\, X_{ni} \,] = \text{intercept}(n) - \log[\, i!(n-i)!\,] + \alpha i + \beta \mathrm{I}(i = 0),$$

where the indicator I(i = 0) is equal to one if $i = 0$ and zero otherwise. The offset $-\log[i!(n-i)!]$ is the same as for the binomial and Altham distributions. The parameter α is equal to the logit of p.

The fitted values for the IPF data are given in Table 8.8. The model correctly estimates the number of cases m, as described in the previous section. The fit is not particularly good for this model: $\chi^2 = 48.86$, 14 df, $p < 10^{-5}$.

Notice how the number of families with zero cases is also correctly estimated in Table 8.8, as well as the number of cases m in the entire sample. Another application of the Birch criteria described in Section 8.6 can be used to demonstrate that this fitted model retains the number of families with zero cases that appear in the observed data. The proof of this equality would closely follow that of Lemma 8.6.1. This property would make model (8.30) useful for a sample in which cases are very rare, and a large number of families have no cases at all.

8.8 Summary Measures and IPF Example

All of the weighted log-linear models described in this chapter were fitted to the COPD/IPF data. The fitted parameters and measures of goodness of fit for all of these models are summarized in Table 8.9.

The binomial and hypergeometric models have huge values of χ^2 because of the single family of size six with all members exhibiting IPF. Both of these models anticipate a small frequency of such families but one appeared in the data, greatly contributing to the value of the test statistics.

Table 8.8 Fitted expected frequencies for the family history log-linear model and the IPF data. $\chi^2 = 48.86$, 14 df, $p < 10^{-5}$. Note how the estimated number of cases and number of families with no cases is the same as those in the original data.

			Number of affected siblings i						
n	f_n	$\widehat{m}_n$	0	1	2	3	4	5	6
1	48	10.26	37.74	10.26					
2	23	12.30	13.25	7.20	2.55				
3	17	15.99	6.72	5.48	3.88	.916			
4	7	9.76	1.80	1.96	2.08	.982	.174		
6	5	11.68	.49	.804	1.42	1.34	.712	.202	.0238
Total	100	60	60						

All of the models summarized in Table 8.9 provide a large improvement over the binomial model in terms of the differences of their deviances. These differences are given in the column headed by 2Λ. The best fitting of all 1 df additions to the binomial model is that of the w_2 quadratic model described in Section 8.5.

Another model with a very good fit is the Altham model in which the logit of p is linear over the family size n. That is,

$$\text{logit}(p) = \alpha + \beta n.$$

The corresponding log-linear model is given in (8.12). This model also exhibits a good fit to the data. The two fitted Altham models in Table 8.9 demonstrate a positive association among family members because of the positive values of the estimated $\widehat{\theta}$ in both cases.

8.9 SAS Program for Clustered Family Data

All of the weighted distributions described in this chapter can be fit using standard log-linear model-fitting procedures in SAS. One of the features of the weighted models described in this chapter is that they can easily be fit using standard software. The software given here uses the SAS GENMOD procedure, which fits log-linear models and provides maximum likelihood estimates for the parameters.

The data is initially expressed as a rectangle with the upper triangle filled in with dots, which is the way SAS expresses missing values. This is the most convenient way for us to see the triangular shape of the raw data. In subsequent steps, the triangle shape is unraveled producing a long file with one frequency on each line.

Each line in the long version of the data also includes the indexes n and i to identify the frequency, as well as marginal sums such as f_n and m. The `estim`

Table 8.9 Deviance, chi-squared and parameter estimates for the weighted log-linear models described in this chapter fitted to the IPF data. The 2Λ compares nested hypotheses with the binomial model and are all 1 df chi-squared except as noted.

Model and (Eq'n #)	Parameter estimates Point	SE	χ^2	Deviance	2Λ
Hypergeometric			373.23	23.15	
Binomial	$\widehat{p} = .30$	.03	312.30	22.55	
Altham	$\widehat{p} = .33$	.04	49.43	18.99	3.56
	$\widehat{\theta} = .23$	.12			
Altham with	$\widehat{\theta} = .32$	.11	7.46	9.81	12.74*
logit(p) linear	$\widehat{\alpha} = -1.39$	.29			
in family size	$\widehat{\beta} = .23$	.07			
w_1	$\log \widehat{\lambda} = 1.29$	.14	12.86	12.01	—
w_2	$\widehat{\eta} = -1.53$	.24	8.69	10.35	12.20
	$\widehat{\beta_2} = .26$	.06			
Family history	$\widehat{\alpha} = -.35$	.24	48.86	16.28	6.27
log-linear model	$\beta = .96$	.38			

* This deviance difference has 2 df.

macro verifies that the sum of expected number of cases $\widehat{m}$ is equal to the observed number of cases m.

```
options linesize=75 center pagesize=59 nodate nonumber;
/*
   Family clusters in GENMOD: IPF Models from Chapter 8
*/

%let outfile=0;
%macro estim(fileno);
title3 'Find the number of cases from estimated counts';
data em&fileno;
  array mn(&max) mn1-mn&max;
  set plus&fileno;
  mn(n)=i*pred;
  estm=i*pred;
run;
proc means data=em&fileno sum;
  var mn1-mn&max estm;
run;
%mend estim;
```

```
/*  Macro to retain fitted, expected values */

%macro outp(fileno);
  ods output obstats = fit&fileno; /* retain obstats data */
  ods exclude listing obstats;/* omit the obstats listing */
run;

data plus&fileno; /* add log-predicted values to the data */
  merge long fit&fileno;
  logpred=log(pred);                   /* log-fitted value */
run;

proc print data=plus&fileno noobs;
  var n i pred;
run;
%mend outp;

%macro e0(fileno);
title3 'The estimated number of families with zero cases';
data ez&outfile;
  array m0(&max) m01-m0&max;
  set plus&outfile;
  estm=0;
  do k=1 to &max;
     m0(k)=0;
  end;
  if (i = 0) then m0(n)=pred;
  if (i = 0) then estm=pred;
run;
proc means data=ez&outfile sum;
  var m01-m0&max estm;
run;
title3 ' ';
%mend e0;

title1 'IPF Data:  Models of Chapter 8'; /* Program begins*/
title2 'Raw triangular data';
%let max=6;                /* Specify: maximum family size */
data raw;
  input n xn0-xn&max;      /* family frequencies of size n */
  array xn(0:&max) xn0-xn&max;    /* each row is an array */
  fn=0;          /* initialize number of families of size n */
  mn=0;                       /* initialize number of cases */
  do i=0 to n;          /* loop over the families of size n */
     if xn(i)=. then xn(i)=0; /* fill in zeros if missing */
     mn=mn+i*xn(i);          /* accumulate number of cases */
     fn=fn+xn(i);         /* accumulate number of families */
```

```
  end;
  nfn=n*fn;   /* number of siblings in families of size n */
  label
     n= 'family size'
     fn='# of families of size n' ;
  datalines;
      1  36  12   .   .   .   .   .
      2  15   7   1   .   .   .   .
      3   5   7   3   2   .   .   .
      4   3   3   1   0   0   .   .
      6   1   0   1   1   1   0   1
run;

proc print data=raw noobs;    /* echo the triangular data */
  var n fn xn0-xn&max;
run;

proc means noprint sum data=raw;    /* Find marginal sums */
  var nfn mn;                      /* n=sum of ns; m=sum of mi */
  output out=sum1 sum=nn m; /* dataset with marginal sums */
run;

data full;   /* Build a full table with the marginal sums */
  if _N_=1 then set sum1;/* merge the marginal sums . . . */
  set raw;                         /* . . . with the raw data */
  label
     m = 'affected individuals'
     nn = 'total number of siblings' ;
  drop mn nfn _TYPE_ _FREQ_;
run;

title2 'Full trianglular data with marginal summary values';
proc print noobs data=full;
  var n fn xn0-xn&max nn m;
run;

/*  Build list version of the data with binomial and
 hypergeometric expected values under the null hypothesis */

data long;
  set full;      /* begin with triangle and marginal sums */
  array xn(0:&max) xn0-xn&max;          /* Xij frequencies */
  array in(0:&max) in0-in&max;  /* family size indicators */
  do k=0 to &max;
     in(k)=0;        /* initialize family size indicators */
  end;
  in(n)=1;              /* indication of this family's size */
            /* constant term in hypergeometric log-means */
```

```
  lhypcon=lgamma(m+1)+lgamma(nn-m+1)-lgamma(nn+1)
     + lgamma(nn-n+1)+lgamma(n+1);
  phat=m/nn;   /* proportion with disease: Binomial p-hat */
  do i=0 to n;            /* loop over families of size n */
     lbin=lgamma(n+1)-lgamma(i+1)-lgamma(n-i+1);
     lbin=lbin+i*log(phat)+(n-i)*log(1-phat);
     bin=exp(lbin)*fn;        /* Binomial expected counts */
           /* Expected counts under the conditional model */
     lhyp=lhypcon-lgamma(i+1)-lgamma(n-i+1)-lgamma(m-i+1)
        -lgamma(nn-m-n+i+1); /* Hyper'c log-probabilities */
     hyp=exp(lhyp)*fn;  /* Hypergeometric expected counts */
     freq=xn(i);          /* individual family frequency */
     lop=i;                   /* log-odds of p parameter */
     linear=n*i;         /* linear logit p in family size */
     alo=-lgamma(i+1)-lgamma(n-i+1);      /* Altham offset */
     theta=-(n-i)*i;            /* theta in Altham model */
     output;     /* switch from triangular to list format */
  end;
  label
     n='family size'
     i='number of affected sibs'
     freq='frequency Xni'
     bin='binomial H0 expectation'
     hyp='hypergeometric H0 expectation'
     lbin='log binomial H0 probability'
     lhyp='log hypergeometric probability'
     lop='log-odds of p'
     linear='linear logit of p'
     alo = 'PME Altham model offset'
     theta = 'Altham theta' ;
run;

title2 'Expected values with no clustering null hypothesis';
proc print data=long noobs;
  var n i freq bin hyp;
run;

/* Use GENMOD to obtain goodness of fit statistics  */

title2 'Hypergeometric null hypothesis model';
%let outfile=%eval(&outfile+1);
proc genmod data=long;
  model freq = in2-in&max
        / dist=Poisson offset=lhyp obstats;
  %outp(&outfile);
run;
%estim(&outfile);
```

```
title2 'Binomial null hypothesis model';
%let outfile=%eval(&outfile+1);
proc genmod data=long;
  model freq = in2-in&max
        / dist=Poisson offset=lbin obstats;
  %outp(&outfile);
run;
%estim(&outfile);

title2 'P.M.E. Altham''s exchangeable model for clustering';
%let outfile=%eval(&outfile+1);
proc genmod data=long;                 /* fit Altham model */
  model freq = theta lop in2-in&max
      / dist=Poisson offset=alo obstats;
  %outp(&outfile);
run;
%estim(&outfile);

title2 'Altham model with linear logit(p) in family size';
%let outfile=%eval(&outfile+1);
proc genmod data=long;                 /* fit Altham model */
  model freq = theta lop linear in2-in&max
      / dist=Poisson offset=alo obstats;
  %outp(&outfile);
run;
%estim(&outfile);

    /*    Fit weighted alternative clustering models    */

data weighted;    /* build offset variables for w1 and w2 */
  set long;
  w1offset=-lgamma(n-i+1);                         /* w1 offset */
  loglambda=n-i;   /* neg. truncated Poisson w1 parameter */
  w2offset=-lgamma(i+1)-lgamma(n-i+1);       /* w2 offset */
  eta=i;
  beta2=i*i;          /* quadratic regression coefficient */
  label
     loglambda='Poisson parameter'
     beta2 = 'i-squared';
run;

title2 'Negative truncated Poisson w1 clustering model';
%let outfile=%eval(&outfile+1);
proc genmod data=weighted;
  model freq = loglambda in2-in&max
        / dist=Poisson offset=w1offset obstats;
  %outp(&outfile);
run;
```

```
%estim(&outfile);

title2 'Binomial weighted w2 clustering model';
%let outfile=%eval(&outfile+1);
proc genmod data=weighted;
  model freq = eta beta2 in2-in&max
     / dist=Poisson offset=w2offset obstats;
  %outp(&outfile);
run;
%estim(&outfile);

title2 'Family history weighted log-linear model';
data efh;
  set long;
  efhoff=-lgamma(i+1)-lgamma(n-i+1);
  lop=i-1;
  zeroin=0;
  if i EQ 0 then zeroin=1;
run;

%let outfile=%eval(&outfile+1);
proc genmod data=efh;
  model freq=  lop zeroin in2-in&max
     / dist=Poisson offset=efhoff obstats;
  %outp(&outfile);
run;
%estim(&outfile);
%e0(&outfile);
```

9

Applications to Teratology Experiments

A common experiment used to determine the teratological properties of substances is to expose pregnant laboratory animals to teratogenic agents, usually at one of various levels of exposure, and record the outcomes in terms of birth defects in the resulting litter. Experiments of this type often provide the most important link between industrial or environmental exposure and any resulting health outcome.

9.1 Introduction

The study of teratology refers to the measurement of birth defects. The word teratology derives from the Greek word for monster. It has long been known that exposure to radiation or certain drugs will induce birth defects in unborn humans and laboratory animals. A developing fetus or any other rapidly dividing cells are very susceptible to genetic and developmental damage. Much of the treatment for cancer, for example, seeks to exploit this property.

A distinct advantage to those working with this type of data stems from the laboratory nature of the experiment. The data represents a complete census of all exposed individuals and the level of exposure is known with certainty. All individual members of the litter are recorded, including those that did not exhibit the outcome of interest. These properties of the data are in contrast to the examples of Section 6.1.1, in which the data may represent a sample obtained through a biased mechanism.

The evaluation of human exposure level through environmental contact continues to remain a difficult task. There are examples where exposure can easily be estimated. For example, many health-care workers wear a badge containing a piece

Discrete Distributions Daniel Zelterman
 ISBN: 0-470-86888-0 (PPC)

of unexposed photographic film. After a period of time, the film is developed and its density or 'fog' is a measure of the worker's radiation exposure.

The experiments described here carefully measured the amount of exposure. The laboratory animals involved are often inbred over many generations, producing individuals with very little genetic variation. Even so, the examples described in this chapter tend to exhibit a much larger variability than what would be expected from commonly used statistical models such as the binomial or Poisson distributions.

A variety of outcomes may be of interest and these are modeled in the search to uncover a possible dose effect. Fertilized eggs might be reabsorbed or later result in delivery of a dead fetus. Litter sizes may be affected by the suspected teratogen in terms of the number of these stillborn pups. Malformations of surviving or dead fetuses may take the form of those easily identifiable (visceral) and those, such as skeletal, that may require dissection in order to record their presence. An example of the form this data takes appears in Table 9.1. This example is discussed at length in Section 9.2. Two other similar examples are explored in this chapter.

We can use the methods developed in the previous two chapters to model the incidence of these outcomes as well as their clustering or dependence within the individual litters. The incidence of birth defects is different from the clustering or correlation of defects in members of the same litter or family. These two characteristics of incidence and dependence in the data often need to be modeled separately. See Section 6.1.3 for a comparison of these two different issues. The degree of correlation of outcomes between members of the same litter often results in extra-binomial variation. Many statisticians choose to model this overdispersion using the beta-binomial distribution. This distribution is also discussed in Section 7.2.4.

In every example introduced in Section 6.1.1, we conditioned on the family size and frequency. In this chapter, we also examine litter size in relation to the dose of teratogen used.

The models used in this chapter are direct applications of the methods developed in Chapters 7 and 8 so there is little new methodology developed here. We will need, however, to describe a type of residual different from what we have used up to this point. The frequency X_{ni} denotes the number of families or litters of size n with i affected members. The expected frequency is

$$\mathrm{E}[\, X_{ni}\,] = f_n \ \Pr[\, Y_n = i\,],$$

where f_n is the number of litters of size n and Y_n is a random variable modeling the sum of n possibly dependent Bernoulli random variables. The individual Bernoulli indicators describe the outcome status of each of the n members of the litter.

The corresponding chi-squared residual we have been using up to this point is

$$\text{chi-squared residual} = (x_{ni} - \mathrm{E}[\, X_{ni}\,]) \,/ \sqrt{\mathrm{E}[\, X_{ni}\,]}.$$

This residual is defined in terms of the observed frequency x_{ni} of the outcomes. The observed value of X_{ni} is denoted by x_{ni}.

When the litters are large, many of the frequencies X_{ni} tend to have small expectations. Most of the observed frequencies x_{ni} are zero and few are two or

Table 9.1 Dominant lethal assay data. Frequency f_n of implant size n and numbers of fetal deaths m_n for offspring of male mice exposed to different doses of radiation. Source: Lüning *et al.* (1966); Rai and Van Ryzin (1985).

Dose	Implants			Number of dead fetuses i							
in R	n	f_n	m_n	0	1	2	3	4	5	6	7
0	5	71	60	30	27	9	5				
	6	156	95	86	51	14	4	1*			
	7	224	163	111	73	31	8	1*			
	8	150	104	79	44	23	3		1*		
	9	70	48	32	29	8	1				
	10	12	9	5	5	2					
Subtotal		683	479								
300	5	121	172	27	41	32	17	4			
	6	170	284	28	47	59	28	6	1	1*	
	7	186	310	31	61	54	20^a	19^b	1		
	8	99	183	12	32	24	22	8	1		
	9	24	51	1	6	9	6	1	1		
	10	4	4	1	2	1					
Subtotal		604	1004								
600	5	160	335	16	32	48	49	15			
	6	153	361	7	35	45	37	20	9		
	7	120	322	5	22	27	36	17	9	3	1
	8	45	142	1	4	12	11	8	7		2
	9	7	24			2	2	2		1	
	10	1	7								1^c
Subtotal		486	1191								
Totals		1773	2674								

Notes: Table 9.4 shows that frequency a is much smaller than expected and b is much larger. Observation c is identified as an outlier in Fig. 9.1 but not in Fig. 9.2. The four litters marked with *s are identified as outliers in Fig. 9.2.

more in some of the examples explored in this chapter. In such cases, we find it useful to describe the *response residuals* in terms of the numbers of affected individuals in each litter rather than the frequencies of these litters. The response residuals are defined in terms of the Y_n as

$$\text{response residual} = (y_n - \mathrm{E}[\,Y_n\,]) \,/ \sqrt{\mathrm{Var}[\,Y_n\,]},$$

where y_n is the observed number of affected pups in a litter of size n.

The observed value of Y_n for a given litter of size n is denoted by y_n. As is the case with the chi-squared residuals, the definition of response residuals depends on the choice of model for $\Pr[Y_n]$.

If an observed frequency x_{ni} is zero, then there are no litters of size n with i affected individuals and there is no corresponding response residual. If the observed frequency x_{ni} is larger than one, then there will be that multiple of response residuals.

The use of the chi-squared statistic by itself may be misleading when there are a huge number of degrees of freedom, but many of the observed frequencies are equal to zero. For example, if the experiment contains a single litter of size 10 animals, then this one observation will contribute nine or ten degrees of freedom but only one response residual. Similarly, the single frequency $X_{10,i} = 1$ may appear as a large outlier because almost all possible outcomes have rather small probabilities $\Pr[Y_{10} = i]$ of occurring. That is, $X_{10,i} = 1$ may be judged as an outlier for almost all values of $i = 0, 1, \ldots, 10$. Consequently, we will try to assess goodness of fit in terms of graphical displays and identification of specific outliers in addition to the use of the chi-squared test statistic.

These two types of residuals are plotted in order to assess model fit in the examples of this chapter. When the data are sparse and the observed frequencies x_{ni} are small, then these two types of plots are probably the best manner for use in judging goodness of fit for the various models and identifying outlying litters. In Section 9.2, for example, we see that observations identified as outliers using one type of residual may not be remarkable when we use the other type of residual.

9.2 Dominant Lethal Assay

In the most general case of the dominant lethal assay, males are exposed to the suspected mutagen or else kept separately to be used as control subjects. Each of these male laboratory animals is subsequently mated with one or more females and the resulting litters are examined for any of a number of abnormal fetal outcomes. Notice then, it is the males who are exposed and not the pregnant females, as is most often the case in teratology studies. A more detailed discussion of the more general experiment and some fundamental mathematical models are described by Haseman and Soares (1976).

In the experiment examined in this section, male mice were exposed to either 300 or 600 rads(R) of radiation. There was also a third unexposed control group. Following exposure to extreme levels of radiation, the mice might live up to three weeks but not much longer because of damage to their bone marrow and immune systems. Within seven days of radiation exposure, each of the male mice in this experiment were mated with one female. The outcome of interest is the number of dead fetuses out of the total number of implants.

Lüning *et al.* (1966) describe the experiment in detail and present the original data. More recent analyses of their data are given by Rai and Van Ryzin (1985) and by Moore, Park, and Smith (2001). Both of these two latter references examined these data using the beta-binomial distribution to model the within-litter correlation and binomial extra-variation. Rai and Van Ryzin (1985) also describe methods for extrapolating the response rate at low radiation-dose exposures.

Table 9.1 summarizes the frequencies of litter sizes and the number of dead fetuses at each radiation exposure level. Lüning *et al.* (1966) omitted a small number of litters of size 11 or more and those of size four or fewer. These litters are also omitted here. Rai and Van Ryzin chose to omit another litter as well in their analyses. This litter is pointed out in our examination of the data and is labelled as '*c*' in Table 9.1.

Table 9.2 contains a number of simple summary measures for these data. There is a monotone decrease in the implant size from over seven for the unexposed control mice and successively smaller average sizes in each of those resulting from irradiated males. In this table, we also see that higher levels of male radiation exposure result in more deaths per litter. The estimates of the death rates are 0.100, 0.253, and 0.398 per implant in each of the exposure levels, so there is a definite trend towards a higher rate of deaths associated with higher rates of exposure. Table 9.4 lists the most extreme chi-squared frequency residual outliers after fitting three separate binomial models for death rate in each group.

We fit Altham model with separate p and θ for each exposure dose. This model is identified by '†' in Table 9.3. The most extreme residuals of this model also appear in Table 9.4. The same extreme chi-squared frequency residuals under the binomial model are also those that are extreme under this Altham model.

A number of other models from Chapter 8 are fit to this data and are summarized in Table 9.3. The Altham model with separate p parameters and a single θ for all exposure levels shows a large statistically significant improvement over the three separate binomial models in terms of the difference of the respective deviances.

The improvement from one θ to three in the Altham model is statistically significant: $\chi^2 = 7.16$, 2 df, $p = .028$. Three fitted Altham θ parameters are 0.138

Table 9.2 Simple summary statistics for the dominant lethal assay data.

	Radiation dose			
	0	300R	600R	Overall
# of implants	4809	3975	2991	11,775
# of litters	683	604	486	1773
# deaths	479	1004	1191	2674
Average implant size	7.04	6.58	6.15	6.64
Death rate per implant	.100	.253	.398	.227
Death rate per litter	.70	1.66	2.45	1.51

Table 9.3 Summary statistics for fitted models to dominant lethal assay. The subscripts 0, 3, and 6 refer to the control, 300R and 600R exposure levels, respectively.

Model	Estimated Point	Estimated SE	Deviance	Pearson χ^2	df
Hypergeometric			136.87	203.87	132
Binomial	$\widehat{p}_0 = .100$	.004	136.48	202.50	132
	$\widehat{p}_3 = .253$	.007			
	$\widehat{p}_6 = .398$	.009			
Altham	$\widehat{p}_0$=.135	.009	108.33	118.85	131
One θ	$\widehat{p}_3$=.291	.010			
	$\widehat{p}_6$=.416	.010			
	$\widehat{\theta} = .071$	.013			
Altham †	$\widehat{p}_0$=.177	.023	101.17	107.78	129
Separate	$\widehat{p}_3$=.284	.014			
θ's at each	$\widehat{p}_6$=.411	.010			
radiation	$\widehat{\theta}_0 = .138$	.027			
level	$\widehat{\theta}_3 = .058$	.020			
	$\widehat{\theta}_6 = .050$	.021			
w_1 Poisson	$\log \widehat{\lambda}_0 = -.355$	.046	156.22	218.766	132
	$\log \widehat{\lambda}_3 = .514$	.032			
	$\log \widehat{\lambda}_6 = .934$	.031			
w_2	$\log \widehat{\eta}_0 = -2.27$	.06	132.28	168.76	131
One β	$\log \widehat{\eta}_3 = -1.20$	.06			
for all	$\log \widehat{\eta}_6 = -.56$	.08			
levels	$\log \widehat{\beta} = .028$	.014			
w_2	$\log \widehat{\eta}_0 = -2.38$	.10	129.88	160.96	129
Separate β's	$\log \widehat{\eta}_3 = -1.12$	.10			
for each	$\log \widehat{\eta}_6 = -.58$	.11			
radiation	$\log \widehat{\beta}_0 = .078$	.038			
level	$\log \widehat{\beta}_3 = .009$	.023			
	$\log \widehat{\beta}_6 = .032$	.019			

Notes: The chi-squared residuals of the model indicated by '†' are plotted in Fig. 9.1. The most extreme outliers for the binomial and Altham † models are given in Table 9.4. The response residuals for this model are plotted in Fig. 9.2.

(SE = 0.03), 0.059 (0.02), and 0.050 (0.02), showing a trend towards independence of fetal deaths at higher doses of radiation exposure. Recall that independence corresponds to the binomial distribution with $\theta = 0$ in the Altham model. This pattern of an improving fit of the binomial model with increasing exposure levels will be noted again below in the further analysis of this data.

The two w_2 weighted models with one β overall and separate β's for each dose do not fit this data particularly well. The weighted w_1 model of Section 8.4 can be modified to fit a Poisson distribution to $\Pr[Y]$ if we use an offset variable $-\log(i!)$ instead of $\log(i!)$. The fit of this model is given but it is not a particularly good fit relative to others available to us and summarized in Table 9.3.

The most extreme chi-squared residuals for frequencies x_{ni} are identified in Table 9.4 for both the binomial and Altham models. Outliers that are identified under one model are generally also identified as outliers under the other model as well. The two largest positive chi-squared residuals are in the unexposed group, litter size five, with three deaths. A frequency of $X_{5,3} = 5$ was observed but the expected frequencies are 0.56 under the binomial and 1.64 under the Altham models.

The second most extreme residual occurs in the 600-R exposure, litter size ten, with seven deaths. In this frequency, we observe one litter but only 0.05 are expected under both binomial and Altham models. This single litter is omitted in the analysis of Rai and Van Ryzin (1985) but is included here. This litter corresponds to the extreme outlier appearing at the top of Fig. 9.1. This single frequency is identified as c in Tables 9.1 and 9.4.

Curiously, there is also a large negative residual under both the binomial and Altham models. This frequency occurs in dose 300 R, litter size seven with three deaths. We observe 20 but expect 32.7 under binomial and 31.4 under Altham. It is possible that some of the 19 litters sized seven with four deaths in the 300-R

Table 9.4 Extreme outlying frequencies x_{ni} and their chi-squared frequency residuals in the dominant lethal assay. The fitted models are three binomial experiments and the Altham † model in Table 9.3 with a separate θ for each exposure level.

				Binomial		Altham	
Dose	n	i	x_{ni}	Fitted	Residual	Fitted	Residual
0	5	3	5	.569	5.88	1.64	2.62
600R	10	7	1^c	.042	4.70	.049	4.28
300R	6	6	1*	.044	4.55	.126	2.46
0	8	5	1*	.060	3.83	.244	1.53
600R	8	7	2	.344	2.82	.575	1.88
300R	7	4	19^b	11.06	2.39	12.48	1.85
600R	5	3	49	36.59	2.05	36.23	2.12
300R	7	3	20^a	32.74	−2.23	31.40	−2.03

Notes: Observations a and b appear in adjacent columns of Table 9.1. Observation c is identified in Figs. 9.1 and 9.2. The *ed observations are also identified in Table 9.1 and in Fig. 9.2.

group were misclassified from this adjacent category. These two frequencies are labelled as a and b in Table 9.1.

The bubble plot of chi-squared residuals for the Altham '†' model with a separate p and θ for each exposure level is given in Fig. 9.1. The diameters of the bubbles are proportional to the sizes of the litters rather than the areas, which have used up to this point. The difference between litters of size five and ten would differ in diameter by a factor of $\sqrt{2}$ if we used area, and the distinction of different litter sizes in this figure would be too subtle to detect.

The response residuals of the three exposure groups are plotted in Fig. 9.2 after fitting the Altham '†' model with separate p and θ for each exposure group.

The exposure category in Fig. 9.2 has been jittered slightly to aid in visualizing the pattern of residuals. Jittering is the addition of a small amount of random noise to the exposure level category. There is one point plotted in Fig. 9.2 for every litter so if $x_{ni} = 2$, then there are two residuals at the same value along the $y-$axis but jittered along their $x-$axis. Multiple litter sizes with the same number of affected pups result in horizontal bands when jittered.

Three litters in the unexposed control group experienced a large number of deaths beyond 3.5 standard deviations from the mean. The 300-R group only exhibited one such extreme litter and the 600-R group had none. These four litters are identified by *s in this figure. These four litters are plotted as dark circles in Fig. 9.1. All of these litters occur with frequency one and are found along the corresponding dotted line in this figure.

One of these *ed observations is the 300-R litter with all six affected littermates. This litter is an outlier under both criteria of frequency as well as response. One of the *ed litters identified as a large positive outlier in Fig. 9.2 exhibits a small negative residual in Fig. 9.1.

The pattern of improving fit to the binomial model with increasing exposure was noted earlier when we described the fit of three separate Altham distributions to this data. The Altham model indicates a tendency of independence of deaths within the same litter at increasing levels of the male's exposure to radiation. We also see fewer extreme outliers with higher exposure levels in Fig. 9.2.

The outlier labelled as c in Tables 9.1 and 9.4 is identified by a circle in Fig. 9.2. In this figure, it is not all remarkable. Similarly, only one of the three *ed outliers in this figure is identified as outstanding in Fig. 9.1.

The chi-squared residuals examined in Fig. 9.1 and Table 9.4 tell one story about the fit and reveal certain outliers. The plot of the response residuals in Fig. 9.2 provides a very different description of the data. In fitting models to data of this type, we need to examine both of these types of residual plots in order to properly judge fit and identify different kinds of outliers.

9.3 Shell Toxicology Experiment

This example examines an experiment in which 84 pregnant, banded Dutch rabbits were exposed to one of four doses of a toxic chemical agent and then the resulting

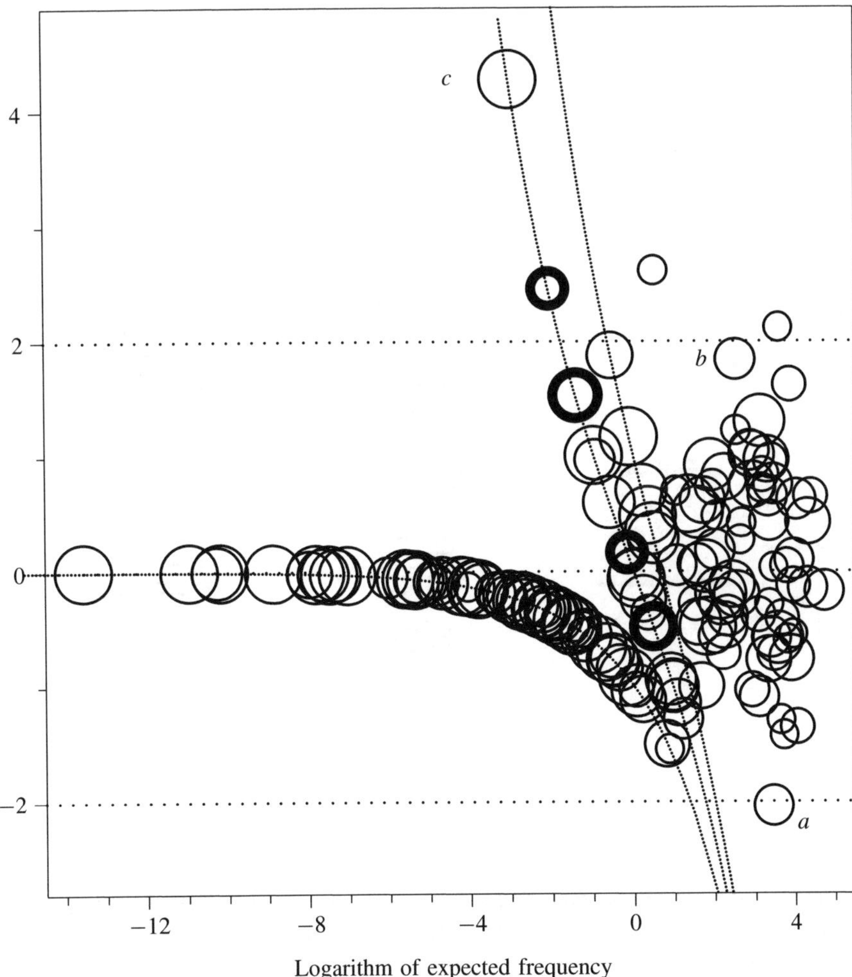

Figure 9.1 Bubble plot of chi-squared residuals for dominant lethal assay data and Altham model with separate p and θ parameters fitted to each exposure level. Bubble diameters (not areas) are in proportional to litter size. Observed frequencies x_{ni} of zero, one, and two are connected with dotted lines, from lower left to the upper right. The extreme outlier identified by c is for the single $x_{10,7} = 1$ litter at 600 R. This litter, identified in Tables 9.1 and 9.4, is also identified by Rai and Van Ryzin (1985). The outliers a and b are also identified. The four *ed outliers in Fig. 9.2 are depicted by bold circles along the line for frequencies equal to one.

litters were examined for birth defects. The data for this study was observed at the Shell Toxicology Laboratories in the U.K. The data represents a complete census and contains information on all individuals and litters, including those with no birth defects. There were four levels of exposure that are described as Low, Medium

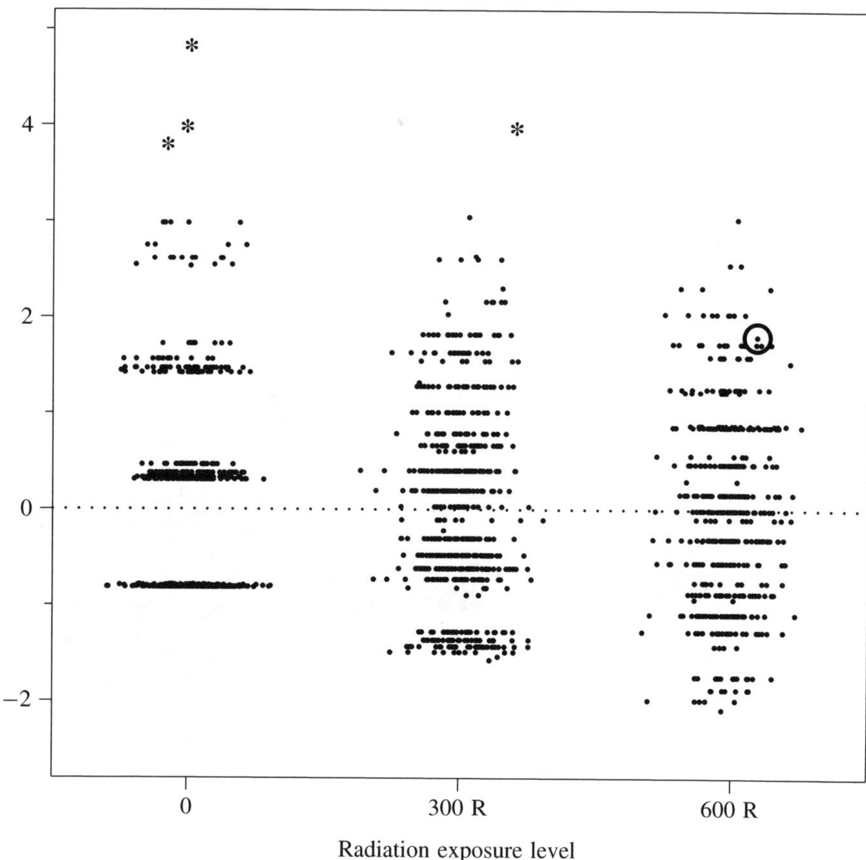

Figure 9.2 Response residuals of 1433 litters in the dominant lethal assay plotted against jittered exposure group. The fitted Altham model has one p and one θ parameter for every exposure level. The circle corresponds to the large outlier seen in Fig. 9.1, labelled as c in Tables 9.1 and 9.4. The four *ed observations are identified in Table 9.1 and by dark bubbles in Fig. 9.1.

High, and a group of unexposed Controls. The original data is given in Paul (1982) with subsequent analyses performed by George and Kodell (1996), among others.

The full data is given in Table 9.5. Paul (1982) points out that every fertilized egg can results in a reabsorption, an early or late fetal death, or delivery of a live fetus. The frequencies of Table 9.5 list skeletal and visceral deformities among the live fetuses. A total of 122 animals with such deformities were observed among 600 rabbit pups born into the 84 litters.

Table 9.6 provides a number of simple summary statistics for this example. There is a general trend towards smaller litters at higher doses although this trend is not strictly monotone. Higher exposure levels are associated with smaller litter

Table 9.5 The frequencies of rabbit litters of size n having i animals with birth defects in the Shell Toxicology Laboratory experiment. Each of the pregnant mothers was exposed to a chemical agent at one of four different levels described as Low; Medium; High; and unexposed, Control. Source: Paul (1982).

	Birth defects	Number of rabbits in litter, n												
Level	i	1	2	3	4	5	6	7	8	9	10	11	12	13
C	0				1		2	4	3	1	3			
	1		1					1	1			1	1	
	2							1	1	1		1		
	3												1	
	4						1*	1*						
	5								1*					
L	0	1			1	1	3	2	1	1				
	1					1	2	1				1		
	2												1	
	3									2				
	5									1*				
M	0			1	1		2	1	1					
	1							1	1					
	2				1					2				
	3				1			1			1			
	4						1			1		1		
	5								1					
	6						2*							1
H	0				1	1	1				1			
	1			2	1	1	1	1	1	1				
	2					1	1							
	3								1					
	4				1*				1					

Notes: The seven litters with *s are identified as outliers in Fig. 9.3 and in Table 9.8.

sizes, suggesting that toxicity effects manifest in different teratologic outcomes simultaneously such as birth defects as well as early *in utero* mortality and reabsorption. Fitted parameters and goodness of fit statistics for several models to this data are given in Table 9.7.

Estimates of the risk of malformation per live fetus and the number of malformations per litter peak in the Middle exposure level group. This may be due to the relatively large average litter size of 7.19 in the Middle exposure, which is larger than the average litter size of the Low exposure level.

Table 9.6 Simple summary statistics for the Shell Toxicology Experiment.

	Exposure level				
	C	L	M	H	Overall
# of live fetuses	215	133	151	101	600
# of litters	27	19	21	17	84
# deformities, m	29	18	52	23	122
Average litter size	7.96	7.00	7.19	5.94	7.14
Malformation rate per fetus	.135	.135	.344	.228	.203
Malformation rate per litter	1.07	.95	2.48	1.35	1.45

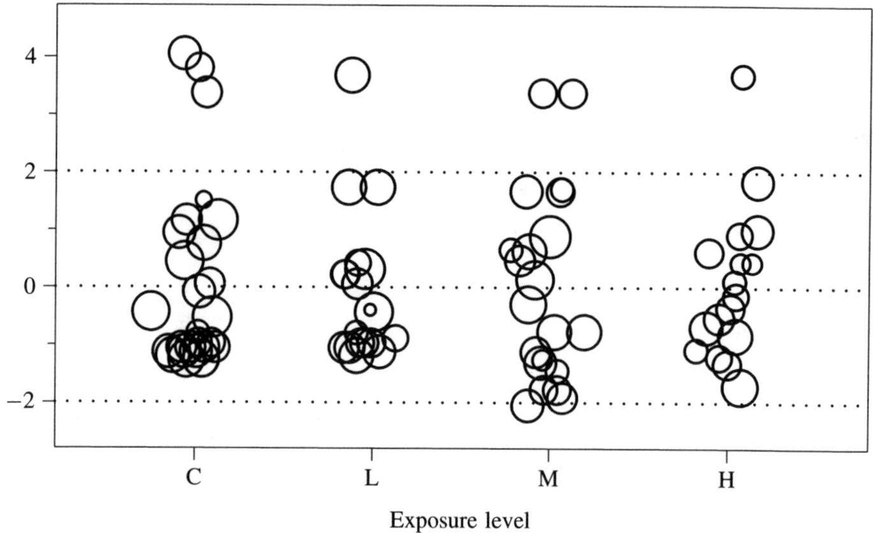

Figure 9.3 Bubble plot of response residuals for the Shell Toxicology Experiment with a separate binomial model fitted to each exposure level. Bubble areas are proportional to litter size. The seven outliers at the top are indicated by *s in Table 9.5.

Our examination of this data differs from previous analyses that concentrated on the incidence of birth defects. We also examined how uniformly the risks are spread across litters within the same level of exposure. The examination of this data shows that increasing exposure not only increases the incidence of defects but also increases their concentration in relatively fewer litters.

Table 9.7 Fitted parameters of models stratified by exposure level for the Shell Toxicology Experiment.

Exposure level	Fitted model	Estimated parameters Value	S.E.	2Λ 1 df	χ^2	Dev.
Control	Hypergeometric				279.19	49.72
$N = 215$	Binomial	$\widehat{p}$ =.135	.02		232.30	48.39
$m = 29$	Altham	$\widehat{p}$ =.322	.02	10.46	51.82	37.94
		$\widehat{\theta}$ =.226	.02			
	FH	$\widehat{p}$ =.078	.01	12.28	51.76	36.21
		$\widehat{p'}$ =.330	.06			
	IR	$\widehat{\alpha} = -2.38$	.16	12.18	50.67	36.33
		$\widehat{\beta} = .928$	.34			
Low	Hypergeometric				134.43	29.90
$N = 133$	Binomial	$\widehat{p}$ =.135	.03		97.39	28.96
$m = 18$	Altham	$\widehat{p}$ =.144	.08	.01	90.08	28.93
		$\widehat{\theta}$ =.014	.03			
	FH	$\widehat{p}$ =.093	.02	3.63	35.10	25.33
		$\widehat{p'}$ =.246	.06			
	IR	$\widehat{\alpha} = -2.23$	.19	4.47	33.01	24.48
		$\widehat{\beta}$ =.626	.19			
Medium	Hypergeometric				636.15	66.64
$N = 151$	Binomial	$\widehat{p}$ =.344	.04		528.66	65.25
$m = 52$	Altham	$\widehat{p}$ =.428	.02	9.45	103.31	55.80
		$\widehat{\theta}$ =.174	.03			
	FH	$\widehat{p}$ =.164	.03	15.73	98.80	49.52
		$\widehat{p'}$ =.619	.08			
	IR	$\widehat{\alpha} = -1.54$	.15	14.29	84.19	50.97
		$\widehat{\beta} = 1.08$	.26			
High	Hypergeometric				180.66	29.70
$N = 101$	Binomial	$\widehat{p}$ =.228	.04		148.68	29.03
$m = 23$	Altham	$\widehat{p}$ =.342	.03	4.20	31.80	24.82
		$\widehat{\theta}$ =.202	.04			
	FH	$\widehat{p}$ =.206	.04	.27	110.90	28.75
		$\widehat{p'}$ =.263	.06			
	IR	$\widehat{\alpha} = -1.45$	.17	1.44	67.26	27.58
		$\widehat{\beta}$ =.393	.19			

The bubble plot in Fig. 9.3 displays the response residuals of all 84 litters. The model is a set of four separate binomial distributions with estimated p parameters as given in Table 9.6. The residuals of these four separate binomial models are centered about their means. The area of each bubble in Fig. 9.3 is proportional to the size of the litter. The exposure level is jittered slightly to improve our perception of the data.

Although most litters fall within ± 2 standard deviations in their number of observed malformations, every exposure level includes between one and three litters with an unusually large number of malformations. The seven extreme outliers are listed in Table 9.8. These outliers are an indication of within-litter correlations that are present even in the unexposed control group. These outliers also motivate the use of bimodal distributions with a small second local mode about 3 to 4 standard deviations above the mean.

All of the models described in Chapter 8 are fitted to these data and are summarized in Table 9.9. The Altham model with a p parameter for each exposure level and one θ parameter common to all levels provides a huge improvement over the four separate binomial models. The Altham model with four p's and four θ's is also a significant improvement over this binomial model but represents only a negligible advance over the simpler Altham model with only one θ parameter for all exposure levels. Both of these Altham models have the smallest χ^2 values of all models summarized in Table 9.9. A plot of the response residuals of these Altham models (not given here) looks almost the same as those for the binomial model plotted in Fig. 9.3. The same outliers identified by this plot are also outliers under either of the Altham models. These seven outliers are listed in Table 9.8 and are, on average, about 0.9 standard deviations smaller than those of the binomials model but remain as outliers in the Altham model.

The summary of this example is that a large variation in litter size due to fetal death or reabsorption may mask trends in the outcome of interest, in this case, fetal malformations. This suggests that multivariate outcomes should be modeled in data of this type. That is, smaller litters and greater rates of malformations, in this example. Outliers are to be expected even in carefully conducted teratology experiments.

9.4 Toxicology of 2,4,5 T

This is another large study of birth defects in litters of laboratory animals. The data presented in Table 9.13 is given by Bowman and George (1995) summarizing a portion of an experiment conducted by the U.S. National Center for Toxicological Research. Different strains of pregnant mice were exposed to daily doses of the herbicide 2,4,5 trichlorophenoxyacetic acid (2,4,5 T) between days 6 and 14 of gestation. The data summarized in this table is limited to the CD-1 outbred mouse strain. The number of implant sites was recorded for every litter within each dam. A number of fetal endpoints were recoded for each implant site including death,

Table 9.8 Seven extreme frequency and response residuals under binomial and Altham models. The first line has a frequency of $x_{6,6} = 2$ for the M exposure level. All of the binomial response residuals are plotted in Fig. 9.3. Outliers identified by one residual method are also detected by the other.

Exposure level	n	i	Response residual: Binomial	Response residual: Altham	Binomial frequency residual
M	6	6	3.38	2.44	21.8
C	7	4	3.38	2.40	4.13
H	4	4	3.68	2.83	11.0
L	9	5	3.69	3.49	8.73
C	6	4	3.81	2.57	9.37
C	8	5	4.06	3.15	10.0

Table 9.9 Summary statistics of models from Chapters 6 and 8 fitted to the Shell Toxicology Experiment. The likelihood ratio statistic Λ is the difference of deviances and its p-value compares models to the binomial.

Model	df	χ^2	Dev.	Λ	df(Λ)	p-value
Hypergeometric	251	1230.43	175.96			
Binomial	251	1007.04	171.63			
Altham (one θ)	250	249.56	150.51	21.12	1	$<10^{-5}$
Altham (four θ's)	247	276.44	147.49	24.14	4	$<10^{-4}$
Trunc. Neg. Poisson	251	460.52	149.23			
Quadratic (4 η's, 4 β's)	247	601.60	153.51	18.12	4	.001
Family History Log-linear Model	247	494.27	144.77	26.86	4	10^{-4}
FH+Quadratic	243	447.47	141.07	30.56	8	10^{-4}

resorption and cleft palate malformations. There were six levels of exposure: 0, 30, 45, 60, 75 and 90 mg/kg. Additional details and analysis of other outcome measures are included in Holson *et al.* (1981) and Chen and Taylor (1992).

Table 9.10 contains a list of simple summary statistics. Litter sizes do not vary much across the six different exposure doses. The rate of combined malformation endpoints per fetus is monotone with dose, increasing from 7.6% in the unexposed control group up to over 95% at the highest 90 mg/kg exposure level. Similarly, the rate of malformations per litter displays a monotonic increase from less than one, on average, in the control group, to ten per litter in the mouse litter with the highest exposure level.

Table 9.10 Summary statistics for the 2,4,5 T data.

	Exposure level in mg/kg						
	0	30	45	60	75	90	Total
Implants	802	952	1126	806	482	254	4422
Litters	73	87	98	76	44	25	403
Malformations	59	124	338	390	372	242	1525
Average litter size	10.99	10.94	11.49	10.61	10.95	10.16	10.97
Rate per fetus	.074	.130	.300	.484	.772	.953	.345
Rate per litter	.81	1.43	3.45	5.13	8.45	9.68	3.78

Fig. 9.4 plots response residuals against a jittered exposure group. A separate binomial model is fitted to each dose level d. The estimated binomial $\widehat{p}_d$ parameters are given in Table 9.10 and also listed at the bottom of Fig. 9.4. These estimated values are very different from each other. The residuals in this figure are centered about their means and standardized to have comparable variances.

Overall, the binomial model is a poor fit for this data. There is a large amount of overdispersion no matter which sets of residuals we examine. Among the chi-squared residuals for the frequencies x_{ni}, there were 31 residuals greater than 10 in absolute magnitude. Out of the 403 litters, 48 response residuals were greater than 3.0 in absolute value.

At the unexposed and two lowest exposure levels, most of these residuals appear skewed with long upper tails. In these three groups, most of the litters showed few of the combined malformations. At the two highest exposure levels, the opposite pattern appears. Specifically, at the two highest exposure doses the residuals are skewed downward reflecting the high percentage of individuals exhibiting one of the combined outcomes.

The variability in this figure is generally increasing from low to high exposure levels. At the highest exposure level of 90 mg/kg there was an 0.953 rate of combined endpoints, so most litters at this level exhibited malformations in all of their members. This leaves no room for extreme positive residuals and many are bunched up at the top of their range at this exposure level.

This is the pattern we would expect to see in the binomial distribution, plotted in Fig. 1.1. When the binomial p parameter is less than 1/2, there will be a longer upper tail. Similarly, when p is close to one, there should be a longer lower tail.

Fig. 9.4 demonstrates a large amount of extra-binomial variability. A large number of residuals appear outside of ± 4 standard deviations in this figure. In the 60 mg/kg-exposure group, there appears to be evidence of a bimodal distribution.

We can also fit Altham models to these data. Table 9.11 summarizes the deviance and fit of the binomial model with one p per dose and two Altham

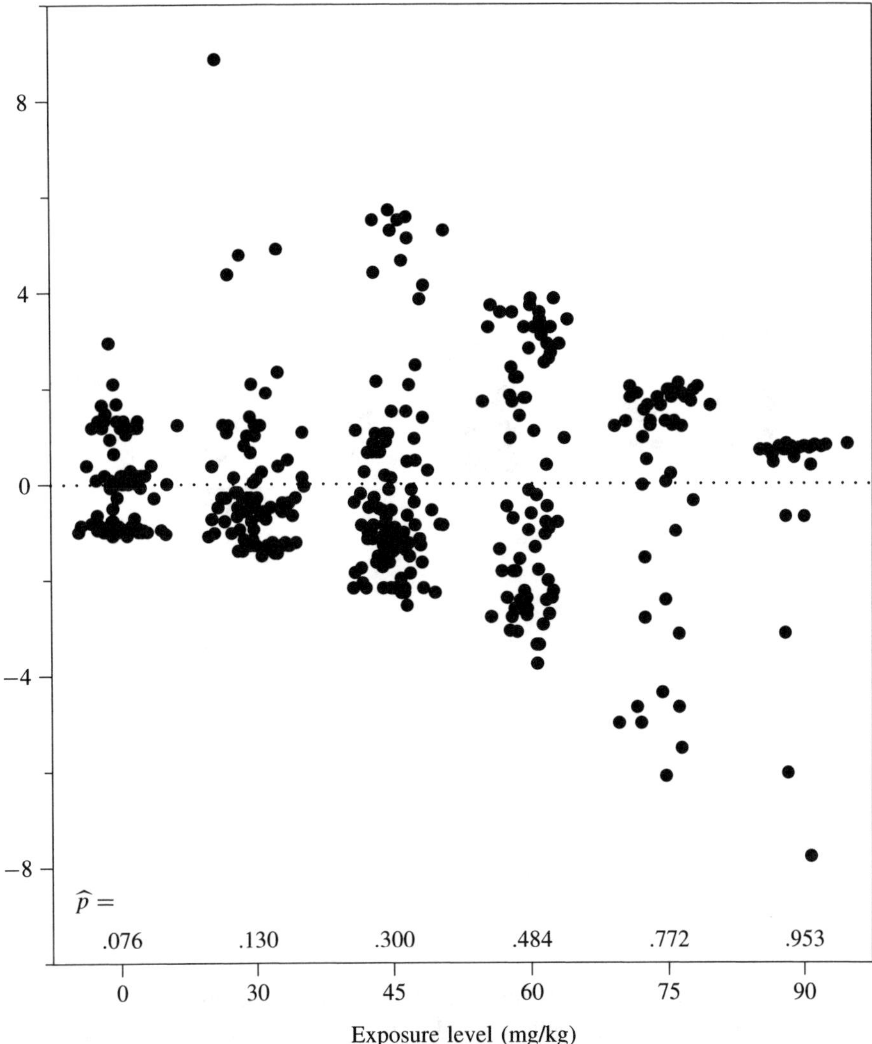

Figure 9.4 Response residuals for 2,4,5 T data plotted against jittered exposure level category. One binomial model is fitted to each exposure level. The estimates of p are given along the bottom.

models. Both of these Altham models have one p parameter for each exposure level. The first of these has one θ for all doses and the second has a separate θ for every dose. The response residuals for this second Altham model are plotted in Fig. 9.5. These two Altham models have much fewer outliers than the separate binomial model. These two models show that the addition of a small number of parameters can result in a large reduction in the deviance. Specifically, even the

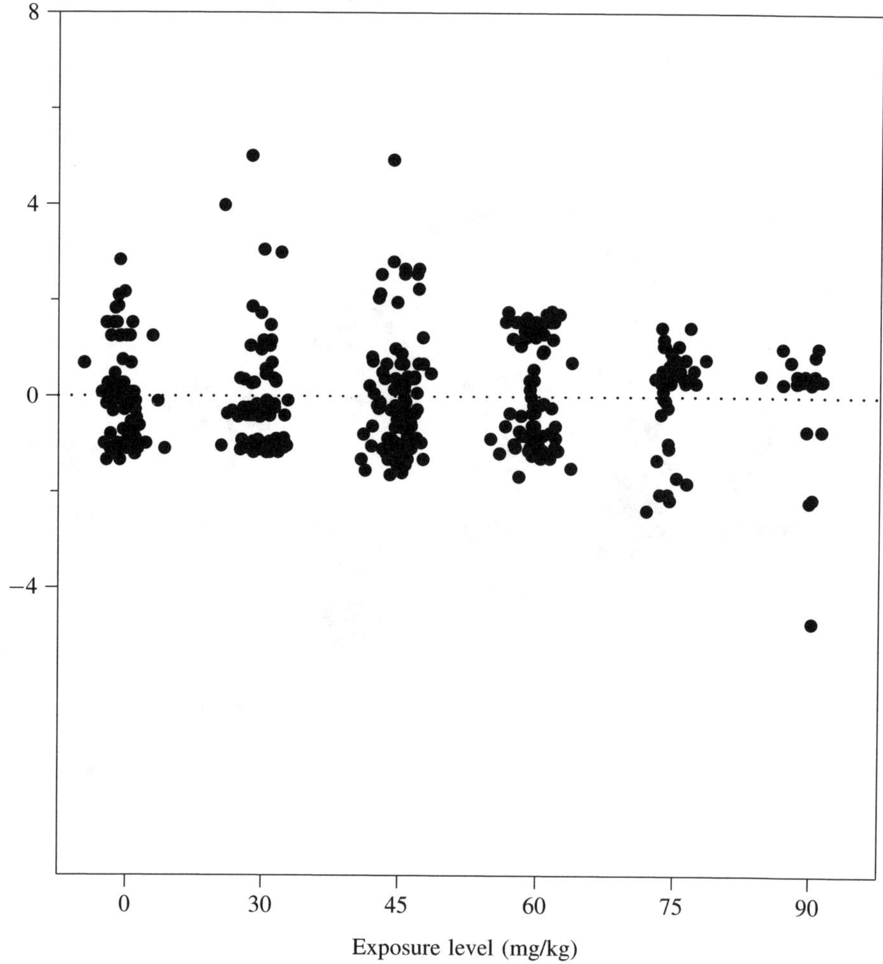

Figure 9.5 Response residuals for 2,4,5 T data plotted against jittered exposure level category. A separate Altham model is fitted to each exposure level. The estimates of p and θ are given in Table 9.12. One huge outlier with value 13.9 in the 30 mg/kg dose is omitted from this figure.

addition of a single parameter in Table 9.11 more than reduced the deviance by half. There is also a marked decrease from the binomial model, in the number of extreme outliers observed following the fit of these models. None of the other weighted models described in Chapter 8 proved useful for this dataset.

The response residuals for the six separate Altham models are plotted in Fig. 9.5. This figure is plotted on the same scale as Fig. 9.4 and shows that the Altham model greatly improves the overdispersion seen in the binomial model. One extreme outlier is omitted from Fig. 9.5. This extreme observation is the litter

Table 9.11 Deviance of models for 2,4,5 T data. The outliers count the number of response residuals greater than 3.0 in absolute magnitude and the number of chi-squared frequency residuals greater than 10.0 in absolute magnitude.

			Outliers	
Model	df	Deviance	Response	Frequency
Hypergeometric	729	1349.2		
Binomial	729	1339.2	48	31
Altham (one θ)	728	622.5	11	3
Altham (separate θ's)	723	556.8	6	6

Table 9.12 Estimated parameters and their standard errors for separate Altham models fitted to each level of exposure in the 2,4,5 T data.

Dose d in mg/kg	0	30	45	60	75	90
$\widehat{p}_d$	.0251	.311	.455	.498	.543	.637
SE's	.02	.04	.009	.007	.01	.07
$\widehat{\theta}_d$	−.126	.150	.181	.230	.265	.326
SE's	.08	.02	.01	.01	.02	.05

Table 9.13 Combined outcomes following exposure to 2,4,5 T (Bowman and George (1995)).

	Unexposed controls				
Litter	Number in litter with birth defects				
size	0	1	2	3	4
1	1				
3	1				
5	1	1			
6	1				
7	2				
8	1				
9	5	2	1		
10	4	1	1		
11	6	7	5		
12	7	6	3		
13	2	5		1	
14	2	2	1	1	
16				1	
17		1	1		

Table 9.13 continued.

Exposure = 30 mg/kg										
Litter	Number in litter with birth defects									
size	0	1	2	3	4	5	6	7	8	15
2	1									
3	1									
4	2									
6	2									
7	2	1	2							
8	1	1	2							
9	2	2					1			
10	4	8	1							
11	8	4	1	1						
12	2	5	2	3	1					
13	3	5	1	2	1			1		
14	2	2	2						1	
15	1	2	1	1		1				
18										1*

The * observation is extreme.

Exposure = 45 mg/kg																
	Number in litter with birth defects															
Litter size	0	1	2	3	4	5	6	7	8	9	10	11	12	13	14	18
1	1															
3	1	1														
4	1															
5		1	1													
6			1													
7	1	1														
8	1	1														
9		3	1		1				1							
10	1	2				1	1			1						
11	8	4	5	1		1					1					
12	3	3	4	2	1	1	2	1				1	2			
13		1	3	3		3			1					2		
14		1	2	1	2	1	3							1	1	
15	1	1	1	1	1	1	1									
16				1			1									
21																1

Table 9.13 continued.

Exposure = 60 mg/kg															
	Number in litter with birth defects														
Litter size	0	1	2	3	4	5	6	7	8	9	10	11	12	13	14
1	1														
3				2											
4		1													
5					1										
6						2	1								
7			1					1							
8	1		1	1					2						
9		2	1		1		1		1	1					
10	1	2	1								5				
11		4			2					2	1	2			
12	3	2				2				1			3		
13		1	4	3		1		1	2			1		2	
14		1		1											2
15	1		1					1							
16						1									

Exposure = 75 mg/kg																
	Number in litter with birth defects															
Litter size	0	1	2	3	4	5	6	7	8	9	10	11	12	13	14	15
5						2										
8		1				1			1							
9	1			1		1		1		3						
10					1				1	1	1					
11	1		2						1			4				
12			2								1	2	3			
13											1		4	3		
14								1							2	
15																1

Table 9.13 continued.

	Exposure = 90 mg/kg												
	Number in litter with birth defects												
Litter size	0	1	2	3	4	5	6	7	10	11	12	13	14
3	1			1									
4					1								
6							1						
7								1					
8					1								
10									4				
11									2	2			
12											6		
13									1			2	
14													2

of size $n = 18$ with $i = 15$ malformations in the 30 mg/kg-exposure group. This litter has a response residual of 13.2, making it large even when judged in light of the overdispersion.

The estimated parameters for the six separate Altham models are given in Table 9.12 along with their standard errors. Not surprising is the monotone increase in the values of the estimated p parameters, as is the case with the binomial model. There is also a monotone increase in the values of the estimated $\widehat{\theta}$'s. The estimated $\widehat{\theta}$ for the unexposed control group is negative, indicating a slight negative correlation of birth defects among animals in the same litter. The estimated correlation in outcome status is positive and increasing in all exposed groups of litters. In other words, we see that the malformation rate increases with dose along with its within-litter correlation. That is, the number of malformations increased and these appear concentrated in fewer litters.

This pattern of dependence is opposite that seen in the dominant lethal assay example of Section 9.2. The parameter estimates of the Altham '†' model in Table 9.3 show a greater death rate at higher levels, but are also more independent of their litter mates.

Contrast the conclusion of the present example with the analysis of the Brazilian children in Section 8.3 using the Altham model. In that dataset, we witness a decrease in correlation to independence and a corresponding increase in incidence as the size of the family increases.

Complements

This is a short list of open-ended problems that the reader may wish to work on.

1. Describe properties of the beta-maximum negative binomial distribution corresponding to the marginal distribution of Y in Section 2.4.3. Motivate this distribution with an example.

2. Describe properties of the minimum negative hypergeometric distribution given in (3.5) including modes, moments and estimation of the m parameter. Motivate this distribution with a practical example.

3. Suppose all individuals in a population can be classified as belonging to one of k strata with known frequencies $\pi_1, \ldots, \pi_k$. In stratified or quota sampling, describe the distribution of the number of randomly sampled individuals necessary in order to observe at least $n_1, \ldots, n_k$ individuals in these strata.

4. In Section 5.6.2, propose additional methods for modeling the dependence of the sequence of dependent Bernoulli indicators.

5. Find an algorithm to facilitate the determination of exact significance levels of family frequency data in Section 6.2.1.

6. In Section 7.2, find other useful models for the conditional probability $C_n(i)$ that have intuitive or computational appeal.

7. In Section 7.2.4, we see that the beta-binomial distribution is both a conditional model and also the sum of exchangeable Bernoulli random variables. Is this the only distribution with this property?

8. In Section 8.1, propose distributions with weights $w(i)$ that have a useful interpretation.

Discrete Distributions Daniel Zelterman
 ISBN: 0-470-86888-0 (PPC)

References

Abramowitz M and Stegun IA 1972 *Handbook of Mathematical Functions*. New York, Dover Publications.

Altham PME 1978 Two generalizations of the binomial distribution. *Applied Statistics* **27**, 162–7.

Andel J 2001 *Mathematics of Chance*. New York, John Wiley.

Anderson JE, Louis TA, Holm NV and Harvald B 1992 Time-dependent association measures for bivariate survival distributions. *Journal of the American Statistical Association* **87**, 641–50.

Bahadur RR 1960 Some approximations to the binomial distribution function. *Annals of Mathematical Statistics* **31**, 43–54.

Balakrishnan N and Koutras MV 2002 *Runs and Scans with Applications*. New York, John Wiley & Sons.

Balasubramanian K, Viveros R and Balakrishnan N 1993 Sooner and later waiting time problems for Markovian Bernoulli trials. *Statistics & Probability Letters* **18**, 153–61.

Bedrick EJ and Hill JR 1996 Assessing the fit of the logistic regression model to individual matched sets of case-control data. *Biometrics* **52**, 1–9.

Berry DA, Parmigiani G, Sanchez J, Schildkraut J and Winer E 1997 Probability of carrying a mutation of breast-ovarian cancer gene BRCA1 based on family history. *Journal of the National Cancer Institute* **89**, 227–38.

Betensky RA and Whittemore AS 1996 An analysis of correlated binary data: application to familial cancers of the ovary and breast. *Applied Statistics* **45**, 411–29.

Birch MW 1963 Maximum likelihood in three-way contingency tables. *Journal of the Royal Statistical Society, Series B* **25**, 220–33.

Bonney GE 1987 Logistic regression for dependent binary observations. *Biometrics* **43**, 951–73.

Bowman D and George EO 1995 A saturated model for analyzing exchangeable binary data: applications to clinical and developmental toxicity studies. *Journal of the American Statistical Association* **90**, 871–9.

Britton T 1997 Tests to detect clustering of infected individuals within families. *Biometrics* **53**, 98–109.

Chen JJ and Gaylor DW 1992 Correlations of developmental end points observed after 2,4,5trichlorophenoxyacetic acid exposure in mice. *Teratology* **45**, 241–6.

Chow YS and Teicher H 1988 *Probability Theory*, 2nd edition. New York, Springer-Verlag.

Discrete Distributions Daniel Zelterman

ISBN: 0-470-86888-0 (PPC)

Claus EB 1995 The genetic epidemiology of cancer. In *Genetics and Cancer: A Second Look*, (eds. Ponder BAL, Cavenee WK and Solomon E), pp. 13–26. Cold Spring Harbor, Cold Spring Harbor Press.

Commenges D and Abel L 1996 Improving the robustness of weighted pairwise correlation test for linkage analysis. *Genetic Epidemiology* **13**, 559–73.

Commenges D, Jacqmin H, Letenneur L and Van Dujin CM 1995 Score test for familial aggregation in probands studies: application to Alzheimer's disease. *Biometrics* **51**, 542–51.

Curtsinger JW, Fukui HH, Townsend DR and Vaupel JW 1992 Demography of genotypes: failure of the limited life-span paradigm in Drosophila melanogaster. *Science* **258**, 461–3.

Dempster AP, Laird N and Rubin DB 1977 Maximum likelihood from incomplete data via the EM algorithm. *Journal of the Royal Statistical Society, Series B* **39**, 1–38.

Ebneshahrashoob M and Sobel M 1990 Sooner and later waiting time problems for Bernoulli trials: frequency and run quotas. *Statistics & Probability Letters* **9**, 5–11.

Ekholm A, Smith PWF and McDonald JW 1995 Marginal regression analysis of a multivariate binary response. *Biometrika* **82**, 847–54.

Elandt-Johnson R 1971 *Probability Models and Statistical Methods in Genetics*. New York, John Wiley.

Elston RC and Sobel E 1979 Sampling considerations in the gathering and analysis of pedigree data. *American Journal of Human Genetics* **31**, 62–9.

Etz Hayim. Torah and Commentary 2001 New York, The Rabbinical Assembly.

FitzGerald PEB and Knuiman MW 1998 Interpretation of regressive logistic regression coefficients in analysis of familial data. *Biometrics* **54**, 909–20.

Fries JF 1980 Aging, natural death, and the compression of morbidity. *New England Journal of Medicine* **303**, 130–5.

Gail MH, Lubin JH and Rubinstein LV 1981 Likelihood calculations for matched case-control studies and survival studies with tied death times. *Biometrika* **68**, 703–7.

George EO and Bowman D 1995 A full likelihood procedure for analysing exchangeable binary data. *Biometrics* **51**, 512–23.

George EO and Kodell RL 1996 Tests of independence, treatment heterogeneity, and dose-related trend with exchangeable binary data. *Journal of the American Statistical Association* **91**, 1602–10.

Goldgar DE, Cannon-Albright LA, Oliphant A, Ward JH, Linker G, Swensen J, Tran TD, Fields P, Uharriet P and Skolnick MH 1993 Chromosome-*17q* linkage studies of 18 Utah breast-cancer kindreds. *American Journal of Human Genetics* **52**, 743–8.

Grimson RC 1993 Disease clusters, exact distributions of maxima, and p-values. *Statistics in Medicine* **12**, 1773–94.

Grimson RC and Oden N 1996 Disease clusters in structured environments. *Statistics in Medicine* **15**, 851–71.

Haberman SJ 1974 *The Analysis of Frequency Data*. Chicago, University of Chicago Press.

Haberman SJ 1977 Log-linear models and frequency tables with small expected cell counts. *Annals of Statistics* **5**, 1148–69.

Haseman JK and Soares ER 1976 The distribution of fetal death in control and its implications on statistical tests for dominant lethal effects. *Mutation Research* **41**, 277–88.

Haseman JK, Zeiger E, Shelby MD, Margolin BH and Tennant RW 1990 Predicting rodent carcinogenicity from four *in vitro* genetic toxicity assays: an evaluation of 114 chemicals studied by the national toxicology program. *Journal of the American Statistical Association* **85**, 964–71.

Hauge M, Harvald B, Fischer M, Gotlieb JK, Joel-Nielson N, Raebild J, Shapiro R and Videbech T 1968 The Danish twin register. *Acta Geneticæ et Gemellologiæ* **17**, 315–32.

Holson JF, Gaines TB, Nelson CJ, LaBorde JB, Gaylor DW, Sheehan DM and Young JF 1981 Developmental toxicity of 2,4,5trichlorophenoxyacetic acid I: Dose-response studies in four inbred strains and one outbred strain stock of mice. *Fundamentals of Applied Toxicology* **19**, 286–97.

Hougaard P, Harvald B and Holm NV 1992 Assessment of dependence in the life times of twins (with discussion). In *Survival Analysis: State of the Art*, (eds. Klein JP and Goel PK), pp. 77–97. Dordrecht, Kluwer Publishers.

Innes JRM, Ulland BM, Valerio MG, Petrucelli L, Fishbein L, Hart ER, Pallotta AJ, Bates RR, Falk HL, Gart JJ, Klein M, Mitchell I and Peters J (1969) Bioassay of pesticides and industrial chemicals for tumorigenicity in mice: a preliminary note. *Journal of the National Cancer Institute* **42**, 1101–14.

Johnson NL and Kotz S 1977 *Urn Models and Their Application: An Approach to Modern Discrete Probability Theory*. New York, John Wiley.

Johnson NL, Kotz S and Balakrishnan N 1997 *Discrete Multivariate Distributions*. New York, John Wiley & Sons.

Johnson NL, Kotz S and Kemp AW 1992 *Univariate Discrete Distributions*, 2nd edition. New York, John Wiley.

Kaigh WD and Lachenbruch PA 1982 A generalized quantile estimator. *Communications in Statistics - Theory and Methods* **11**, 2217–38.

Kemp AW 1968 A wide class of discrete distributions and the associated differential equations. *Sankhyā, Series A* **30**, 401–10.

Klaren HM, van't Veer LJ, van Leeuwen FE and Rookus MA 2003 Potential for bias in studies on efficacy of prophylactic surgery for BRCA1 and BRCA2 mutation. *Journal of the National Cancer Institute* **95**, 941–7.

Knuth D 1981 *The Art of Computer Programming*, Vol. 2: *Seminumerical Algorithms*, 2nd edition. Reading, Addison-Wesley.

Kocherlakota S and Kocherlakota K 1990 Tests of hypothesis for the weighted binomial distribution. *Biometrics* **46**, 645–56.

Kolchin VF, Sevast'yanov BA and Chistyakov VP 1978 *Random Allocations*. Washington, VH Winston & Sons/Wiley. (Translation from original *Случайные размещения* by Balakrishnan AV).

Kupper LL and Haseman JK 1978 The use of a correlated binomial model for the analysis of certain toxicological experiments. *Biometrics* **34**, 69–76.

Lange K 1997 *Mathematical and Statistical Methods for Genetic Analysis*. New York, Springer-Verlag.

Lehmann EL 1983 *Theory of Point Estimation*. New York, John Wiley.

Li FP, Fraumeni JF Jr, Mulvihill JJ, Blattner WA, Dreyfus MG, Tucker MA and Miller RW 1988 A cancer family syndrome in twenty-four kindreds. *Cancer Research* **48**, 5358–62.

Li H, Yang P and Schwartz AG 1998 Analysis of age of onset data from case-control family studies. *Biometrics* **54**, 1030–9.

Liang KY and Zeger SL 1986 Longitudinal data analysis using generalized linear models. *Biometrika* **73**, 13–22.

Liang KY, Zeger SL and Qaqish B 1992 Multivariate regression analyses for categorical data (with discussion). *Journal of the Royal Statistical Society, Series B* **54**, 3–40.

Lingappiah GS 1987 Some variants of the binomial distribution. *Bulletin of the Malaysian Mathematical Society* **10**, 82–94.

Lipsitz SR, Laird NM and Harrington DP 1991 Generalized estimating equations for correlated binary data: using the odds ratio as a measure of association. *Biometrika* **78**, 153–60.

Louis TA 1982 Finding observed information using the EM algorithm. *Journal of the Royal Statistical Society Series B* **44**, 98–130.

McGue M, Vaupel JW, Holm N and Harvald B 1993 Longevity is moderately heritable in a sample of Danish twins born 1870–1880. *Journal of Gerontology: Biological Sciences* **48**, B237–B44.

Miller AB 1993 Cancer screening. In *Cancer Principles & Practice of Oncology*, Vol. I, 4th edition. (eds. DeVita VT Jr, Hellman S and Rosenberg SA). Ch. 21, Section 6, pp. 564–73. Philadelphia, Lippincott

Moore DF, Park, CK and Smith W 2001 Exploring extra-binomial variation in teratology data using continuous mixtures. *Biometrics* **57**, 490–4.

Morris CN 1963 A note on direct and inverse sampling. *Biometrika* **50**, 544–5.

NSABP 1999 Study of tamoxifen and raloxifene (STAR) for the prevention of breast cancer. National Surgical Adjuvant Breast and Bowel Project. P-2: Clinical protocol and amendments, June 24, 1999.

O'Hara Hines RJ 1998 Comparison of two covariance structures in the analysis of clustered polytomous data using generalized estimating equations. *Biometrics* **54**, 312–6.

Ord JK 1967 On a system of discrete distributions. *Biometrika* **54**, 649–56.

Patil GP and Rao CR 1978 Weighted distributions and size biased sampling with applications to wildlife and human families. *Biometrics* **34**, 179–89.

Paul SR 1982 Analysis of proportions of affected foetuses in teratological experiments. *Biometrics* **38**, 361–70.

Pesarin F 2001 *Multivariate Permutation Tests With Applications in Biostatistics*. New York, John Wiley.

Piegorsch WW and Casella G 1996 Empirical Bayes estimation for logistic regression and extended parametric regression models. *Journal of Agricultural, Biological, and Environmental Statistics* **1**, 231–47.

Pregibon D 1984 Data analytic methods for matched case-control studies. *Biometrics* **40**, 639–51.

R 2002 ©The R Development Core Team, Version 1.6.1 Available at `http://www.r-project.org/`

Rai K and Van Ryzin J 1985 A dose-response model for teratological experiments involving quantal responses. *Biometrics* **41**, 1–9.

Sastry N 1997 A nested frailty model for survival data, with an application to the study of child survival in northeast Brazil. *Journal of the American Statistical Association* **92**, 426–34.

Schneider EL and Brody JA 1983 Aging, natural death, and the compression of morbidity: another review. *New England Journal of Medicine* **309**, 854–6.

Shattuck-Eidens D, Oliphant A, McClure M, McBride C, Gupte J, Rubano TME, Pruss D, Tavtigian SV, Teng DH.F, Adey N, Staebell M, Gumpper K, Lundstrom R, Hulick M, Kelly M, Holmen J, Lingenfelter B, Manley S, Fujimura F, Luce M, Ward B, Cannon-Albright L, Steele L, Offit K, Gilewski T, Norton L, Brown K, Schulz C, Hampel H, Schluger A, Giulotto E, Zoli W, Ravaioli A, Nevanlinna H, Pyrhonen S, Rowley P, Loader S, Osborne MP, Daly M, Tepler I, Weinstein PL, Scalia, Jennifer L, Michaelson R, Scott RJ, Radice P, Pierotti MA, Garber JE, Isaacs C, Peshkin B, Lippman ME, Dosik MH, Caligo MA, Greenstein RM, Pilarski R, Weber B, Burgemeister R, Frank TS, Skolnick MH, Thomas A 1997 *BRCA*1 sequence analysis in women at high risk for susceptibility mutations. *Journal of the American Medical Association* **278**, 1242–50.

Smith PG and Pike MC 1976 Generalization of two tests for the detection of household aggregation of disease. *Biometrics* **32**, 817–28.

Stirzaker D 2003 *Elementary Probability*, 2nd edition. Cambridge, Cambridge University Press.

Stuart A and Ord JK 1987 *Kendall's Advanced Theory of Statistics*, Vol 1, *Distribution Theory*, 5th edition. Oxford, Oxford University Press.

Student 1907 On the error of counting with a haemacytometer. *Biometri ka* **5**, 351–60.

Ten Have TR, Kunselman AR, Pulkstenis EP and Landis JR 1998 Mixed effects logistic regression models for longitudinal binary response data with informative drop-out. *Biometrics* **54**, 367–83.

Uppuluri VRR and Blot WJ 1970 A probability distribution arising in a riff-shuffle. In *Random Counts in Scientific Work, 1: Random Counts in Models and Structures*, (ed. Patil GP), pp. 23–46. College Park, Pennsylvania State University Press.

Waller LA and Zelterman D 1997 Log-linear modeling with the negative multinomial distribution. *Biometrics* **53**, 971–82.

Wingo PA, Lee NC, Ory HW, Beral V, Peterson HB and Rhodes P 1993 Age-specific differences in the relationship between oral-contraceptive use and breast-cancer. *Cancer* Supplement S **71**, 1506–17.

Wong GY and Mason WM 1985 The hierarchical logistic regression model for multilevel analysis. *Journal of the American Statistical Association* **80**, 513–24.

Yu C, Waller LA and Zelterman D 1998 Discrete distributions for use in twin studies. *Biometrics* **54**, 546–57.

Yu C and Zelterman D 2001 Exact inference for family disease clusters. *Communications in Statistics: Theory and Methods* **30**, 2293–305.

Yu C and Zelterman D 2002 Statistical inference for familial disease clusters. *Biometrics* **58**, 481–91.

Yu C and Zelterman D 2002 Sums of dependent Bernoulli random variables and disease clustering. *Statistics & Probability Letters* **57**, 363–73.

Zhang Z, Burtness BA and Zelterman D 2000 The maximum negative binomial distribution. *Journal of Statistical Planning and Inference* **87**, 1–19.

Zelterman D 1987 Goodness-of-fit tests for large sparse multinomial distributions. *Journal of the American Statistical Association* **82**, 624–9.

Zelterman D 1992 A statistical distribution with an unbounded hazard function and its application to a theory from demography. *Biometrics* **48**, 807–18.

Zelterman D 1999 *Models for Discrete Data.* Oxford, Oxford University Press.

Zelterman D and Curtsinger JW 1995 Survival curves subjected to occasional insults. *Biometrics* **51**, 1140–6.

Zelterman D, Grambsch PM, Le CT, Ma JZ and Curtsinger JW 1994 Piecewise exponential survival curves with smooth transitions. *Mathematical Biosciences* **120**, 233–50.

Index

Discrete Distributions Daniel Zelterman
 ISBN: 0-470-86888-0 (PPC)

WILEY SERIES IN PROBABILITY AND STATISTICS

ESTABLISHED BY WALTER A. SHEWHART AND SAMUEL S. WILKS

The ***Wiley Series in Probability and Statistics*** is well established and authoritative. It covers many topics of current research interest in both pure and applied statistics and probability theory. Written by leading statisticians and institutions, the titles span both state-of-the-art developments in the field and classical methods.

Reflecting the wide range of current research in statistics, the series encompasses applied, methodological and theoretical statistics, ranging from applications and new techniques made possible by advances in computerized practice to rigorous treatment of theoretical approaches.

This series provides essential and invaluable reading for all statisticians, whether in academia, industry, government, or research.

ABRAHAM and LEDOLTER · Statistical Methods for Forecasting
AGRESTI · Analysis of Ordinal Categorical Data
AGRESTI · An Introduction to Categorical Data Analysis
AGRESTI · Categorical Data Analysis, *Second Edition*
ALTMAN, GILL, and McDONALD · Numerical Issues in Statistical Computing for the Social Scientist
AMARATUNGA and CABRERA · Exploration and Analysis of DNA Microarray and Protein Array Data
ANDĚL · Mathematics of Chance
ANDERSON · An Introduction to Multivariate Statistical Analysis, *Third Edition*
*ANDERSON · The Statistical Analysis of Time Series
ANDERSON, AUQUIER, HAUCK, OAKES, VANDAELE, and WEISBERG · Statistical Methods for Comparative Studies
ANDERSON and LOYNES · The Teaching of Practical Statistics
ARMITAGE and DAVID (editors) · Advances in Biometry
ARNOLD, BALAKRISHNAN, and NAGARAJA · Records
*ARTHANARI and DODGE · Mathematical Programming in Statistics
*BAILEY · The Elements of Stochastic Processes with Applications to the Natural Sciences
BALAKRISHNAN and KOUTRAS · Runs and Scans with Applications
BARNETT · Comparative Statistical Inference, *Third Edition*
BARNETT · Environmental Statistics: Methods & Applications
BARNETT and LEWIS · Outliers in Statistical Data, *Third Edition*
BARTOSZYNSKI and NIEWIADOMSKA-BUGAJ · Probability and Statistical Inference
BASILEVSKY · Statistical Factor Analysis and Related Methods: Theory and Applications
BASU and RIGDON · Statistical Methods for the Reliability of Repairable Systems
BATES and WATTS · Nonlinear Regression Analysis and Its Applications
BECHHOFER, SANTNER, and GOLDSMAN · Design and Analysis of Experiments for Statistical Selection, Screening, and Multiple Comparisons
BELSLEY · Conditioning Diagnostics: Collinearity and Weak Data in Regression
BELSLEY, KUH, and WELSCH · Regression Diagnostics: Identifying Influential Data and Sources of Collinearity

*Now available in a lower priced paperback edition in the Wiley Classics Library.

BENDAT and PIERSOL · Random Data: Analysis and Measurement Procedures, *Third Edition*
BERNARDO and SMITH · Bayesian Theory
BERRY, CHALONER, and GEWEKE · Bayesian Analysis in Statistics and Econometrics: Essays in Honor of Arnold Zellner
BHAT and MILLER · Elements of Applied Stochastic Processes, *Third Edition*
BHATTACHARYA and JOHNSON · Statistical Concepts and Methods
BHATTACHARYA and WAYMIRE · Stochastic Processes with Applications
BILLINGSLEY · Convergence of Probability Measures, *Second Edition*
BILLINGSLEY · Probability and Measure, *Third Edition*
BIRKES and DODGE · Alternative Methods of Regression
BLISCHKE AND MURTHY (editors) · Case Studies in Reliability and Maintenance
BLISCHKE AND MURTHY · Reliability: Modeling, Prediction, and Optimization
BLOOMFIELD · Fourier Analysis of Time Series: An Introduction, *Second Edition*
BOLLEN · Structural Equations with Latent Variables
BOROVKOV · Ergodicity and Stability of Stochastic Processes
BOULEAU · Numerical Methods for Stochastic Processes
BOX · Bayesian Inference in Statistical Analysis
BOX · R. A. Fisher, the Life of a Scientist
BOX and DRAPER · Empirical Model-Building and Response Surfaces
*BOX and DRAPER · Evolutionary Operation: A Statistical Method for Process Improvement
BOX, HUNTER, and HUNTER · Statistics for Experimenters: An Introduction to Design, Data Analysis, and Model Building
BOX and LUCEÑO · Statistical Control by Monitoring and Feedback Adjustment
BRANDIMARTE · Numerical Methods in Finance: A MATLAB-Based Introduction
BROWN and HOLLANDER · Statistics: A Biomedical Introduction
BRUNNER, DOMHOF, and LANGER · Nonparametric Analysis of Longitudinal Data in Factorial Experiments
BUCKLEW · Large Deviation Techniques in Decision, Simulation, and Estimation
CAIROLI and DALANG · Sequential Stochastic Optimization
CHAN · Time Series: Applications to Finance
CHATTERJEE and HADI · Sensitivity Analysis in Linear Regression
CHATTERJEE and PRICE · Regression Analysis by Example, *Third Edition*
CHERNICK · Bootstrap Methods: A Practitioner's Guide
CHERNICK and FRIIS · Introductory Biostatistics for the Health Sciences
CHILÈS and DELFINER · Geostatistics: Modeling Spatial Uncertainty
CHOW and LIU · Design and Analysis of Clinical Trials: Concepts and Methodologies, *Second Edition*
CLARKE and DISNEY · Probability and Random Processes: A First Course with Applications, *Second Edition*
*COCHRAN and COX · Experimental Designs, *Second Edition*
CONGDON · Applied Bayesian Modelling
CONGDON · Bayesian Statistical Modelling
CONOVER · Practical Nonparametric Statistics, *Second Edition*
COOK · Regression Graphics
COOK and WEISBERG · Applied Regression Including Computing and Graphics
COOK and WEISBERG · An Introduction to Regression Graphics
CORNELL · Experiments with Mixtures, Designs, Models, and the Analysis of Mixture Data, *Third Edition*
COVER and THOMAS · Elements of Information Theory
COX · A Handbook of Introductory Statistical Methods
*COX · Planning of Experiments
CRESSIE · Statistics for Spatial Data, *Revised Edition*
CSÖRGÖ and HORVÁTH · Limit Theorems in Change Point Analysis
DANIEL · Applications of Statistics to Industrial Experimentation
DANIEL · Biostatistics: A Foundation for Analysis in the Health Sciences, *Sixth Edition*

*Now available in a lower priced paperback edition in the Wiley Classics Library.

*DANIEL · Fitting Equations to Data: Computer Analysis of Multifactor Data, *Second Edition*
DASU and JOHNSON · Exploratory Data Mining and Data Cleaning
DAVID and NAGARAJA · Order Statistics, *Third Edition*
*DEGROOT, FIENBERG, and KADANE · Statistics and the Law
DEL CASTILLO · Statistical Process Adjustment for Quality Control
DENISON, HOLMES, MALLICK and SMITH · Bayesian Methods for Nonlinear Classification and Regression
DETTE and STUDDEN · The Theory of Canonical Moments with Applications in Statistics, Probability, and Analysis
DEY and MUKERJEE · Fractional Factorial Plans
DILLON and GOLDSTEIN · Multivariate Analysis: Methods and Applications
DODGE · Alternative Methods of Regression
*DODGE and ROMIG · Sampling Inspection Tables, *Second Edition*
*DOOB · Stochastic Processes
DOWDY and WEARDEN, and CHILKO · Statistics for Research, *Third Edition*
DRAPER and SMITH · Applied Regression Analysis, *Third Edition*
DRYDEN and MARDIA · Statistical Shape Analysis
DUDEWICZ and MISHRA · Modern Mathematical Statistics
DUNN and CLARK · Applied Statistics: Analysis of Variance and Regression, *Second Edition*
DUNN and CLARK · Basic Statistics: A Primer for the Biomedical Sciences, *Third Edition*
DUPUIS and ELLIS · A Weak Convergence Approach to the Theory of Large Deviations
*ELANDT-JOHNSON and JOHNSON · Survival Models and Data Analysis
ENDERS · Applied Econometric Time Series
ETHIER and KURTZ · Markov Processes: Characterization and Convergence
EVANS, HASTINGS, and PEACOCK · Statistical Distributions, *Third Edition*
FELLER · An Introduction to Probability Theory and Its Applications, Volume I, *Third Edition*, Revised; Volume II, *Second Edition*
FISHER and VAN BELLE · Biostatistics: A Methodology for the Health Sciences
*FLEISS · The Design and Analysis of Clinical Experiments
FLEISS · Statistical Methods for Rates and Proportions, *Second Edition*
FLEMING and HARRINGTON · Counting Processes and Survival Analysis
FULLER · Introduction to Statistical Time Series, *Second Edition*
FULLER · Measurement Error Models
GALLANT · Nonlinear Statistical Models
GHOSH, MUKHOPADHYAY, and SEN · Sequential Estimation
GIESBRECHT and GUMPERTZ · Planning, Construction, and Statistical Analysis of Comparative Experiments
GIFI · Nonlinear Multivariate Analysis
GLASSERMAN and YAO · Monotone Structure in Discrete-Event Systems
GNANADESIKAN · Methods for Statistical Data Analysis of Multivariate Observations, *Second Edition*
GOLDSTEIN and LEWIS · Assessment: Problems, Development, and Statistical Issues
GREENWOOD and NIKULIN · A Guide to Chi-Squared Testing
GROSS and HARRIS · Fundamentals of Queueing Theory, *Third Edition*
*HAHN and SHAPIRO · Statistical Models in Engineering
HAHN and MEEKER · Statistical Intervals: A Guide for Practitioners
HALD · A History of Probability and Statistics and their Applications Before 1750
HALD · A History of Mathematical Statistics from 1750 to 1930
HAMPEL · Robust Statistics: The Approach Based on Influence Functions
HANNAN and DEISTLER · The Statistical Theory of Linear Systems
HEIBERGER · Computation for the Analysis of Designed Experiments
HEDAYAT and SINHA · Design and Inference in Finite Population Sampling
HELLER · MACSYMA for Statisticians

*Now available in a lower priced paperback edition in the Wiley Classics Library.

HINKELMAN and KEMPTHORNE: · Design and Analysis of Experiments, Volume 1: Introduction to Experimental Design
HOAGLIN, MOSTELLER, and TUKEY · Exploratory Approach to Analysis of Variance
HOAGLIN, MOSTELLER, and TUKEY · Exploring Data Tables, Trends and Shapes
*HOAGLIN, MOSTELLER, and TUKEY · Understanding Robust and Exploratory Data Analysis
HOCHBERG and TAMHANE · Multiple Comparison Procedures
HOCKING · Methods and Applications of Linear Models: Regression and the Analysis of Variance, *Second Edition*
HOEL · Introduction to Mathematical Statistics, *Fifth Edition*
HOGG and KLUGMAN · Loss Distributions
HOLLANDER and WOLFE · Nonparametric Statistical Methods, *Second Edition*
HOSMER and LEMESHOW · Applied Logistic Regression, *Second Edition*
HOSMER and LEMESHOW · Applied Survival Analysis: Regression Modeling of Time to Event Data
HØYLAND and RAUSAND · System Reliability Theory: Models and Statistical Methods
HUBER · Robust Statistics
HUBERTY · Applied Discriminant Analysis
HUNT and KENNEDY · Financial Derivatives in Theory and Practice, *Revised Edition*
HUSKOVA, BERAN, and DUPAC · Collected Works of Jaroslav Hajek—with Commentary
IMAN and CONOVER · A Modern Approach to Statistics
JACKSON · A User's Guide to Principle Components
JOHN · Statistical Methods in Engineering and Quality Assurance
JOHNSON · Multivariate Statistical Simulation
JOHNSON and BALAKRISHNAN · Advances in the Theory and Practice of Statistics: A Volume in Honor of Samuel Kotz
JUDGE, GRIFFITHS, HILL, LÜTKEPOHL, and LEE · The Theory and Practice of Econometrics, *Second Edition*
JOHNSON and KOTZ · Distributions in Statistics
JOHNSON and KOTZ (editors) · Leading Personalities in Statistical Sciences: From the Seventeenth Century to the Present
JOHNSON, KOTZ, and BALAKRISHNAN · Continuous Univariate Distributions, Volume 1, *Second Edition*
JOHNSON, KOTZ, and BALAKRISHNAN · Continuous Univariate Distributions, Volume 2, *Second Edition*
JOHNSON, KOTZ, and BALAKRISHNAN · Discrete Multivariate Distributions
JOHNSON, KOTZ, and KEMP · Univariate Discrete Distributions, *Second Edition*
JUREČKOVÁ and SEN · Robust Statistical Procedures: Asymptotics and Interrelations
JUREK and MASON · Operator-Limit Distributions in Probability Theory
KADANE · Bayesian Methods and Ethics in a Clinical Trial Design
KADANE AND SCHUM · A Probabilistic Analysis of the Sacco and Vanzetti Evidence
KALBFLEISCH and PRENTICE · The Statistical Analysis of Failure Time Data *Second Edition*
KARIYA and KURATA · Generalized Least Squares
KASS and VOS · Geometrical Foundations of Asymptotic Inference
KAUFMAN and ROUSSEEUW · Finding Groups in Data: An Introduction to Cluster Analysis
KEDEM and FOKIANOS · Regression Models for Time Series Analysis
KENDALL, BARDEN, CARNE, and LE · Shape and Shape Theory
KHURI · Advanced Calculus with Applications in Statistics, *Second Edition*
KHURI, MATHEW, and SINHA · Statistical Tests for Mixed Linear Models
KLEIBER and KOTZ · Statistical Size Distributions in Economics and Actuarial Sciences
KLUGMAN, PANJER, and WILLMOT · Loss Models: From Data to Decisions
KLUGMAN, PANJER, and WILLMOT · Solutions Manual to Accompany Loss Models: From Data to Decisions

*Now available in a lower priced paperback edition in the Wiley Classics Library.

KOTZ, BALAKRISHNAN, and JOHNSON · Continuous Multivariate Distributions, Volume 1, *Second Edition*
KOTZ and JOHNSON (editors) · Encyclopedia of Statistical Sciences: Volumes 1 to 9 with Index
KOTZ and JOHNSON (editors) · Encyclopedia of Statistical Sciences: Supplement Volume
KOTZ, READ, and BANKS (editors) · Encyclopedia of Statistical Sciences: Update Volume 1
KOTZ, READ, and BANKS (editors) · Encyclopedia of Statistical Sciences: Update Volume 2
KOVALENKO, KUZNETZOV, and PEGG · Mathematical Theory of Reliability of Time-Dependent Systems with Practical Applications
LACHIN · Biostatistical Methods: The Assessment of Relative Risks
LAD · Operational Subjective Statistical Methods: A Mathematical, Philosophical, and Historical Introduction
LAMPERTI · Probability: A Survey of the Mathematical Theory, *Second Edition*
LANGE, RYAN, BILLARD, BRILLINGER, CONQUEST, and GREENHOUSE · Case Studies in Biometry
LARSON · Introduction to Probability Theory and Statistical Inference, *Third Edition*
LAWLESS · Statistical Models and Methods for Lifetime Data, *Second Edition*
LAWSON · Statistical Methods in Spatial Epidemiology
LE · Applied Categorical Data Analysis
LE · Applied Survival Analysis
LEE and WANG · Statistical Methods for Survival Data Analysis, *Third Edition*
LePAGE and BILLARD · Exploring the Limits of Bootstrap
LEYLAND and GOLDSTEIN (editors) · Multilevel Modelling of Health Statistics
LIAO · Statistical Group Comparison
LINDVALL · Lectures on the Coupling Method
LINHART and ZUCCHINI · Model Selection
LITTLE and RUBIN · Statistical Analysis with Missing Data, *Second Edition*
LLOYD · The Statistical Analysis of Categorical Data
MAGNUS and NEUDECKER · Matrix Differential Calculus with Applications in Statistics and Econometrics, *Revised Edition*
MALLER and ZHOU · Survival Analysis with Long Term Survivors
MALLOWS · Design, Data, and Analysis by Some Friends of Cuthbert Daniel
MANN, SCHAFER, and SINGPURWALLA · Methods for Statistical Analysis of Reliability and Life Data
MANTON, WOODBURY, and TOLLEY · Statistical Applications Using Fuzzy Sets
MARDIA and JUPP · Directional Statistics
MASON, GUNST, and HESS · Statistical Design and Analysis of Experiments with Applications to Engineering and Science, *Second Edition*
McCULLOCH and SEARLE · Generalized, Linear, and Mixed Models
McFADDEN · Management of Data in Clinical Trials
McLACHLAN · Discriminant Analysis and Statistical Pattern Recognition
McLACHLAN and KRISHNAN · The EM Algorithm and Extensions
McLACHLAN and PEEL · Finite Mixture Models
McNEIL · Epidemiological Research Methods
MEEKER and ESCOBAR · Statistical Methods for Reliability Data
MEERSCHAERT and SCHEFFLER · Limit Distributions for Sums of Independent Random Vectors: Heavy Tails in Theory and Practice
*MILLER · Survival Analysis, *Second Edition*
MONTGOMERY, PECK, and VINING · Introduction to Linear Regression Analysis, *Third Edition*
MORGENTHALER and TUKEY · Configural Polysampling: A Route to Practical Robustness
MUIRHEAD · Aspects of Multivariate Statistical Theory

*Now available in a lower priced paperback edition in the Wiley Classics Library.

MURRAY · X-STAT 2.0 Statistical Experimentation, Design Data Analysis, and Nonlinear Optimization
MURTHY, XIE, and JIANG · Weibull Models
MYERS and MONTGOMERY · Response Surface Methodology: Process and Product Optimization Using Designed Experiments, *Second Edition*
MYERS, MONTGOMERY, and VINING · Generalized Linear Models. With Applications in Engineering and the Sciences
NELSON · Accelerated Testing, Statistical Models, Test Plans, and Data Analyses
NELSON · Applied Life Data Analysis
NEWMAN · Biostatistical Methods in Epidemiology
OCHI · Applied Probability and Stochastic Processes in Engineering and Physical Sciences
OKABE, BOOTS, SUGIHARA, and CHIU · Spatial Tesselations: Concepts and Applications of Voronoi Diagrams, *Second Edition*
OLIVER and SMITH · Influence Diagrams, Belief Nets and Decision Analysis
PALTA · Quantitative Methods in Population Health: Extensions of Ordinary Regressions
PANKRATZ · Forecasting with Dynamic Regression Models
PANKRATZ · Forecasting with Univariate Box-Jenkins Models: Concepts and Cases
*PARZEN · Modern Probability Theory and It's Applications
PEÑA, TIAO, and TSAY · A Course in Time Series Analysis
PIANTADOSI · Clinical Trials: A Methodologic Perspective
PORT · Theoretical Probability for Applications
POURAHMADI · Foundations of Time Series Analysis and Prediction Theory
PRESS · Bayesian Statistics: Principles, Models, and Applications
PRESS · Subjective and Objective Bayesian Statistics, *Second Edition*
PRESS and TANUR · The Subjectivity of Scientists and the Bayesian Approach
PUKELSHEIM · Optimal Experimental Design
PURI, VILAPLANA, and WERTZ · New Perspectives in Theoretical and Applied Statistics
PUTERMAN · Markov Decision Processes: Discrete Stochastic Dynamic Programming
*RAO · Linear Statistical Inference and Its Applications, *Second Edition*
RENCHER · Linear Models in Statistics
RENCHER · Methods of Multivariate Analysis, *Second Edition*
RENCHER · Multivariate Statistical Inference with Applications
RIPLEY · Spatial Statistics
RIPLEY · Stochastic Simulation
ROBINSON · Practical Strategies for Experimenting
ROHATGI and SALEH · An Introduction to Probability and Statistics, *Second Edition*
ROLSKI, SCHMIDLI, SCHMIDT, and TEUGELS · Stochastic Processes for Insurance and Finance
ROSENBERGER and LACHIN · Randomization in Clinical Trials: Theory and Practice
ROSS · Introduction to Probability and Statistics for Engineers and Scientists
ROUSSEEUW and LEROY · Robust Regression and Outlier Detection
RUBIN · Multiple Imputation for Nonresponse in Surveys
RUBINSTEIN · Simulation and the Monte Carlo Method
RUBINSTEIN and MELAMED · Modern Simulation and Modeling
RYAN · Modern Regression Methods
RYAN · Statistical Methods for Quality Improvement, *Second Edition*
SALTELLI, CHAN, and SCOTT (editors) · Sensitivity Analysis
*SCHEFFE · The Analysis of Variance
SCHIMEK · Smoothing and Regression: Approaches, Computation, and Application
SCHOTT · Matrix Analysis for Statistics
SCHOUTENS · Levy Processes in Finance: Pricing Financial Derivatives
SCHUSS · Theory and Applications of Stochastic Differential Equations

*Now available in a lower priced paperback edition in the Wiley Classics Library.

SCOTT · Multivariate Density Estimation: Theory, Practice, and Visualization
*SEARLE · Linear Models
SEARLE · Linear Models for Unbalanced Data
SEARLE · Matrix Algebra Useful for Statistics
SEARLE, CASELLA, and McCULLOCH · Variance Components
SEARLE and WILLETT · Matrix Algebra for Applied Economics
SEBER · Multivariate Observations
SEBER and LEE · Linear Regression Analysis, *Second Edition*
SEBER and WILD · Nonlinear Regression
SENNOTT · Stochastic Dynamic Programming and the Control of Queueing Systems
*SERFLING · Approximation Theorems of Mathematical Statistics
SHAFER and VOVK · Probability and Finance: Its Only a Game!
SMALL and McLEISH · Hilbert Space Methods in Probability and Statistical Inference
SRIVASTAVA · Methods of Multivariate Statistics
STAPLETON · Linear Statistical Models
STAUDTE and SHEATHER · Robust Estimation and Testing
STOYAN, KENDALL, and MECKE · Stochastic Geometry and Its Applications, *Second Edition*
STOYAN and STOYAN · Fractals, Random Shapes and Point Fields: Methods of Geometrical Statistics
STYAN · The Collected Papers of T. W. Anderson: 1943–1985
SUTTON, ABRAMS, JONES, SHELDON, and SONG · Methods for Meta-Analysis in Medical Research
TANAKA · Time Series Analysis: Nonstationary and Noninvertible Distribution Theory
THOMPSON · Empirical Model Building
THOMPSON · Sampling, *Second Edition*
THOMPSON · Simulation: A Modeler's Approach
THOMPSON and SEBER · Adaptive Sampling
THOMPSON, WILLIAMS, and FINDLAY · Models for Investors in Real World Markets
TIAO, BISGAARD, HILL, PEÑA, and STIGLER (editors) · Box on Quality and Discovery: with Design, Control, and Robustness
TIERNEY · LISP-STAT: An Object-Oriented Environment for Statistical Computing and Dynamic Graphics
TSAY · Analysis of Financial Time Series
UPTON and FINGLETON · Spatial Data Analysis by Example, Volume II: Categorical and Directional Data
VAN BELLE · Statistical Rules of Thumb
VESTRUP · The Theory of Measures and Integration
VIDAKOVIC · Statistical Modeling by Wavelets
WEISBERG · Applied Linear Regression, *Second Edition*
WELSH · Aspects of Statistical Inference
WESTFALL and YOUNG · Resampling-Based Multiple Testing: Examples and Methods for p-Value Adjustment
WHITTAKER · Graphical Models in Applied Multivariate Statistics
WINKER · Optimization Heuristics in Economics: Applications of Threshold Accepting
WONNACOTT and WONNACOTT · Econometrics, *Second Edition*
WOODING · Planning Pharmaceutical Clinical Trials: Basic Statistical Principles
WOOLSON and CLARKE · Statistical Methods for the Analysis of Biomedical Data, *Second Edition*
WU and HAMADA · Experiments: Planning, Analysis, and Parameter Design Optimization
YANG · The Construction Theory of Denumerable Markov Processes

*Now available in a lower priced paperback edition in the Wiley Classics Library.

*ZELLNER · An Introduction to Bayesian Inference in Econometrics
ZELTERMAN · Discrete Distributions: Applications in the Health Sciences
ZHOU, OBUCHOWSKI, and McCLISH · Statistical Methods in Diagnostic Medicine

*Now available in a lower priced paperback edition in the Wiley Classics Library.